MW00607932

IMAGERY-ENHANCED CBT FOR SOCIAL ANXIETY DISORDER

Also Available

Fight or Flight: Overcoming Panic and Agoraphobia [video]
Featuring Ronald M. Rapee

I Think They Think . . . : Overcoming Social Phobia [video]
Featuring Ronald M. Rapee

Imagery-Enhanced CBT for
Social Anxiety Disorder

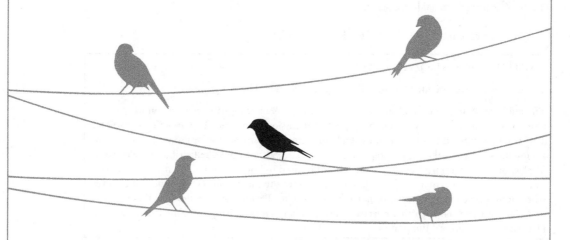

Peter M. McEvoy
Lisa M. Saulsman
Ronald M. Rapee

THE GUILFORD PRESS
New York   London

Copyright © 2018 The Guilford Press
A Division of Guilford Publications, Inc.
370 Seventh Avenue, Suite 1200, New York, NY 10001
www.guilford.com

All rights reserved

Except as indicated, no part of this book may be reproduced, translated, stored in a retrieval
system, or transmitted, in any form or by any means, electronic, mechanical, photocopying,
microfilming, recording, or otherwise, without written permission from the publisher.

Printed in the United States of America

This book is printed on acid-free paper.

Last digit is print number: 9   8   7   6   5   4   3   2   1

LIMITED DUPLICATION LICENSE

These materials are intended for use only by qualified mental health professionals.

The publisher grants to individual purchasers of this book nonassignable permission to
reproduce all materials for which photocopying permission is specifically granted in a footnote.
This license is limited to you, the individual purchaser, for personal use or use with clients. This
license does not grant the right to reproduce these materials for resale, redistribution, electronic
display, or any other purposes (including but not limited to books, pamphlets, articles, video- or
audiotapes, blogs, file-sharing sites, Internet or intranet sites, and handouts or slides for lectures,
workshops, or webinars, whether or not a fee is charged). Permission to reproduce these
materials for these and any other purposes must be obtained in writing from the Permissions
Department of Guilford Publications.

The authors have checked with sources believed to be reliable in their efforts to provide
information that is complete and generally in accord with the standards of practice that are
accepted at the time of publication. However, in view of the possibility of human error or
changes in behavioral, mental health, or medical sciences, neither the authors, nor the editors and
publisher, nor any other party who has been involved in the preparation or publication of this
work warrants that the information contained herein is in every respect accurate or complete, and
they are not responsible for any errors or omissions or the results obtained from the use of such
information. Readers are encouraged to confirm the information contained in this book with
other sources.

Library of Congress Cataloging-in-Publication Data

Names: McEvoy, Peter M., author.
Title: Imagery-enhanced CBT for social anxiety disorder / Peter M. McEvoy,
   Lisa M. Saulsman, Ronald M. Rapee.
Description: New York : The Guilford Press, [2018] | Includes bibliographical
   references and index.
Identifiers: LCCN 2017023840 | ISBN 9781462533053 (paperback : alk. paper) |
   ISBN 9781462535491 (hardcover : alk. paper)
Subjects: LCSH: Social phobia—Treatment. | Cognitive therapy. | BISAC:
   PSYCHOLOGY / Psychopathology / Anxieties & Phobias. | MEDICAL / Psychiatry
   / General. | SOCIAL SCIENCE / Social Work.
Classification: LCC RC552.S62 M39 2018 | DDC 616.85/225—dc23
LC record available at *https://lccn.loc.gov/2017023840*

About the Authors

Peter M. McEvoy, PhD, is Professor in the School of Psychology and Speech Pathology at Curtin University in Perth, Australia. He is also Clinical Research Director at the Centre for Clinical Interventions of the Western Australia Department of Health. An associate editor of the *Journal of Anxiety Disorders* and the *Journal of Experimental Psychopathology*, Dr. McEvoy has published articles on the treatment of anxiety and depression, transdiagnostic approaches to mental disorders, and mechanisms of change.

Lisa M. Saulsman, PhD, has spent the majority of her career as a senior clinical psychologist at the Centre for Clinical Interventions of the Western Australia Department of Health. She is experienced in providing individual and group interventions for adults with anxiety and depression and training mental health professionals in evidence-supported treatments for emotional disorders. Dr. Saulsman has published articles on the use of imagery to enhance CBT and the role of personality in psychopathology. She is now Director of Cognitive Behaviour Therapy Services, Western Australia, offering CBT-based training and workshops to professionals, businesses, and the general public.

Ronald M. Rapee, PhD, is Distinguished Professor of Psychology at Macquarie University, in Sydney, Australia, and former Director of the University's Centre for Emotional Health. He is best known for his theoretical models of the development of anxiety disorders and his creation of empirically validated intervention programs that are widely used internationally. Dr. Rapee is a recipient of the Distinguished Career Award from the Australian Association for Cognitive and Behaviour Therapy and the Distinguished Contribution to Science Award from the Australian Psychological Society. He is an Australian Research Council Laureate Fellow and has been appointed as a Member of the Order of Australia for his contributions to clinical psychology.

Preface

Human beings are social creatures living in a world built around relationships, so almost any life circumstance can be seen as threatening to socially anxious persons. From direct group or individual social interactions of any kind, to the possibility of being observed when stepping out of the front door of their home, to the inadequacy of their "performance" on virtually any task—social threat can be perceived everywhere. Social anxiety disorder (SAD) is a common and distressing condition that, without being treated, can be disabling and lifelong.

SAD can be challenging for therapists, but it is also tremendously rewarding to treat. People with SAD want to relate well to people—they desire close, genuine, and fulfilling relationships. They are *people* people, although they may not believe this about themselves when they first seek help. People with SAD care about others, have a high degree of empathy, and are keen to please—personal qualities that are highly valued by others. The problem is they care too much. The probability and cost of not pleasing others are perceived to be extremely high. Social situations are seen as threatening, which triggers a cascade of anxiety symptoms, negative beliefs, and avoidant behaviors. In severe SAD, "life" is threatening and virtually nowhere is safe. We hope the treatment in this book helps to ease the suffering of people with SAD by helping them to abandon the psychological factors that maintain their constant expectation of social catastrophe, while allowing them to retain the wonderful personal qualities they have that facilitate genuine and fulfilling relationships.

Cognitive-behavioral therapy (CBT) has been shown to be very helpful for SAD over many research trials with clients who have severe and complex cases of the disorder. CBT has been successfully delivered on a one-to-one basis and in groups, and in both research units and "real-world" clinics. As our understanding of the mechanisms behind SAD has improved, specific treatment enhancements have been designed to target these mechanisms to attain even better outcomes. The core components of the program in this book have been extensively evaluated and shown to work, and they are more effective than traditional cognitive–behavioral approaches. The novel contribution of this book is the detailed description of an innovation from our own clinic—imagery-enhanced CBT for SAD—that has been shown to improve our clients' engagement and outcomes. Since including the imagery enhancements in our protocol, treatment completion rates have increased from 65% to 90%, and the impact on social anxiety symptoms has also greatly improved.

Imagery-based CBT "enhances" traditional approaches by emphasizing the benefits of facilitating cognitive and emotional change via the imagery mode. Multisensory imagery is highly emotionally evocative, and more so than verbal activity. If our primary aim in therapy is to enable our clients to change their extreme emotional reactions, it follows that therapy will be more potent within the imagery mode. Clients are encouraged to incorporate vivid, multisensory imagery into every aspect of the treatment described in this book.

We are bringing this book to you in the hope that your clients can benefit from the very latest therapeutic developments. We hope these innovations help you to enjoy working with clients suffering from SAD as much as we do and, most important, to ease their suffering.

A brief note about pronouns: With the exception of specific examples, we alternate between masculine and feminine pronouns throughout the book to avoid awkward sentences.

Acknowledgments

We owe a considerable debt of gratitude to the clinicians and clinical researchers (and their clients) whose contributions this book builds on. Arnoud Arntz, David Barlow, Aaron Beck, Judith Beck, James Bennett-Levy, Chris Brewin, David M. Clark, Albert Ellis, Melanie Fennell, Jessica Grisham, Ann Hackmann, Richard Heimberg, Emily Holmes, Michael Liebowitz, Michelle Moulds, David Moscovitch, Christine Padesky, and Jennifer Wild are just a few of the giants on whose achievements our work relies. Colleagues in our own services have also been tremendously influential, including Paula Nathan, Jonathan Gaston, Maree Abbott, Bruce Campbell, and Mark Summers. We are grateful to the National Health and Medical Research Council of Australia for its support of our work through Project Grant APP1104007. We would also like to express our appreciation to our families for their love and support. Finally, we acknowledge the courageous socially anxious clients who have participated in this treatment within our programs. Your experiences have helped shape this treatment and taught us so much.

Contents

PART II. TREATMENT MODULES

Purchasers of this book can download and print copies of the handouts and worksheets
at *www.guilford.com/mcevoy-forms* for personal use or use with clients
(see copyright page for details).

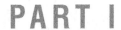

PART I

Overview of Social Anxiety and Its Treatment

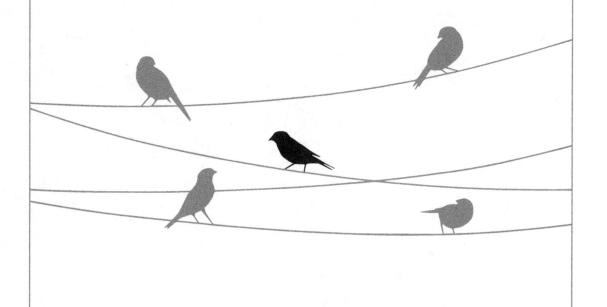

CHAPTER 1

What Is Social Anxiety Disorder?

Jacquie, a single 22-year-old woman, described herself as having been a quiet and "bookish" child who enjoyed her own company. Her parents were both loving and supportive, and they had high expectations for her academic and social performance. Her mother always encouraged her to "put her best foot forward" and seemed disappointed with her shyness in social situations. Jacquie's father was more sympathetic and also seemed to prefer to stay at home with the family rather than socialize with others. When she was old enough, he would often allow Jacquie to stay home if the family was going to visit family or friends.

Jacquie attended a small local primary school before moving to a large high school when she was 13 years old, which she remembered as being a particularly difficult experience. She found it hard to make friends, and she remembered having to give formal presentations in front of the class for the first time, which she found terrifying. Jacquie tried to avoid these presentations by pretending to be sick, but her parents were both teachers and would always send her to school anyway.

Jacquie remembered one particularly traumatic presentation when she was 15 years old. She had dreaded speaking in front of the class for weeks beforehand as she had vivid images of herself stammering and then being paralyzed by fear. She knew that she blushed when she was embarrassed, so she imagined all her classmates laughing at her bright red cheeks. In her mind's eye, her peers could clearly see how awkward and incompetent she was, and she feared that the few friends she had managed to make would ridicule and reject her. On the day of the presentation Jacquie awoke feeling unwell and anxious. She recalled having a headache and feeling too nauseous to eat breakfast. Just before her presentation her heart and thoughts were racing, her palms were sweaty, and she had a strong urge to escape.

Jacquie doesn't recall much about the actual speech itself other than the overwhelming sense of shame she felt about her performance. She had written her speech word for word so that she didn't forget anything, and so she could look down at the paper rather than see the weird looks she thought her classmates must have been giving her. She remembered stumbling over her words, having her mind go blank, and being on the brink of tears. She was sure that her voice was trembling and quiet. She sat down without making eye contact with anyone and felt humiliated.

Unfortunately for Jacquie the trauma didn't end when the presentation was over. She continued to ruminate about her poor performance in the hours, days, and weeks afterwards. She repeatedly criticized herself, asking herself why she was so stupid. In the years that followed, negative thoughts and images of how she must have looked during the presentation came to mind every time Jacquie thought she was the focus of attention (e.g., when eating or drinking in public, or even walking down the street). Jacquie believed this image warned her of imminent humiliation and occasionally caused her anxiety to escalate to the point where she would have a panic attack.

Jacquie decided that she would start to protect herself from criticism and rejection by rarely speaking in social situations, and in fact she became an expert in avoiding social situations altogether by making excuses that she was unwell or had other plans. Jacquie's social anxiety became so severe at times that she was unable to walk down the street in case she saw someone she knew, or a stranger attempted to speak to her. When she did go out in public she would walk down the most isolated streets, avoid any eye contact with other people, and would cross the road to avoid passing another person. When Jacquie could not avoid social situations, she learned to ask questions so people talked about themselves and she did not need to disclose anything about herself.

After high school Jacquie studied to become a librarian because she loved books and it meant that she would not be expected to interact with people very often. Unfortunately, as Jacquie isolated herself more and more, even brief interactions she had with other staff and patrons began causing her significant anxiety. Jacquie knows she is introverted and does not necessarily want to change this, but she recognizes that her anxiety is more severe and debilitating than it need be. Jacquie presented for treatment because she would like a family one day, but she feels depressed because she does not believe this is possible for her.

Max's Story

Max is a 27-year-old actor who needs to attend auditions regularly. He has been experiencing panic attacks with increasing frequency, particularly when he is anticipating auditions or having to interact with colleagues. Max presented as a sociable and bright individual who is eager to please but nonetheless reported having been shy for his whole life. When he was young he remembers hiding behind his parents when other people were around. Max reports having had some friends at school, but he would often listen from the periphery of the group rather than actively contribute to the discussions. He figured that if he was quiet he would avoid saying something stupid or boring, and people would tolerate him. As a consequence he usually felt disconnected from others, and he had few close friends. Max believes his love of acting came from his curiosity about people, but he also enjoys the fact that he has a clear script to work from. Max reported that he thrives onstage where he can play a character and his lines are written for him. However, whenever he has to interact as himself he "falls to pieces." Max's social anxiety increased when he left school and he had to meet new people in college, and again when he left college to become a professional actor. He noticed that over time he started to feel apprehensive in more and more social situations, to the point where he even felt anxious with his family. He began drinking alcohol to "settle his nerves" in the evenings and on weekends, and he recently started to carry around a hip flask of whiskey so that he could have a sip before having to meet other actors or directors.

As time has gone on Max has become more and more self-conscious about his anxiety. He scrutinizes the warmth in his cheeks and the sweatiness of his palms before interacting with others. He also closely studies his colleagues' facial expressions for any sign that they can see just how anxious he is. Although no one ever says anything to him directly, he believes he can read their minds from the expressions on their faces. Max notices that his thoughts are dominated by expectations of failure and negative evaluation from others before, during, and after social situations. In his mind's eye, he repeatedly sees an image of his colleagues looking at him strangely, which just confirms that he has failed and no longer enjoys their respect. He even interprets positive feedback as a sign of "pity," and he has started to find auditions intolerable. Max has also recently started avoiding seeing his friends and family by making excuses that he is too busy to see them. Max presented for treatment because alcohol is no longer working, and his increasing panic attacks mean that he can no longer concentrate on his acting career. It took Max a while to realize that he has significant social anxiety because he has always been able to bluff his way through social events with the use of alcohol. Max had also thought it was impossible for him to have social anxiety, given that he could comfortably perform onstage in front of a large audience. However, Max now recognizes his anxiety is excessive and wants to do something about it.

Jacquie and Max present just two of the many faces of social anxiety disorder (SAD). This book is designed to equip clinicians with new ways of integrating imagery- and verbally based strategies when working with clients like Jacquie and Max who suffer from SAD. The first part of the book provides clinicians with key information on SAD, including the unique aspects and advantages of imagery-enhanced cognitive-behavioral therapy (CBT) and the model that guides the treatment.

The second part of the book describes the components of imagery-enhanced CBT in sufficient detail so that they can be easily applied clinically. We provide sample scripts that can be used with clients, detailed step-by-step descriptions of each treatment strategy, suggested questions to optimize clients' learning, and sample dialogues. We also provide some clinical anecdotes that we hope will help therapists appreciate how the various strategies have been used with our clients. Throughout the book we describe potential difficulties that have arisen in our clinical work and suggest how these can be managed. At the end of the book we provide client-friendly handouts that describe the rationale for each treatment component, as well as worksheets that can be used as a framework to guide the application of specific treatment strategies and record clients' examples.

We have used this treatment in both group and individual formats with success. In Chapter 3 we provide a suggested structure for group treatment, which we have used in our treatment evaluation trials (McEvoy, Erceg-Hurn, Saulsman, & Thibodeau, 2015; McEvoy & Saulsman, 2014). To maximize the flexibility with which the treatment can be used in individual therapy, we have not written the book in a session-by-session structure. Instead, in Part II, we have devoted one chapter to each key maintaining factor in the model that guides the treatment: (1) negative thoughts and images, (2) avoidance and safety behaviors, (3) negative self-image, (4) attention biases, and (5) core beliefs. Some clients might require more or fewer sessions targeting each of these maintaining factors, and clinicians should be guided by their case formulation and experience when determining the appropriate "dose" of each component. In the final chapter of the book we discuss relapse prevention. Although this book is designed to enable clinicians to "hit the ground running," where possible it is highly recommended that relatively inexperienced clinicians receive supervision by therapists who are accredited and experienced in cognitive-behavioral approaches.

In the rest of this chapter we provide clinicians with a working knowledge of SAD, including its symptoms, common comorbidities, and how to distinguish it from other disorders. It is also helpful to have an understanding of the epidemiology and causes of SAD because clients are often surprised (and very reassured) by just how common the disorder is, and they are interested in the factors that may have contributed to their problem.

What Is SAD?

The core characteristic of people with SAD is excessive worry about or fear of other people thinking badly of them in some way. The particular fears or worries vary slightly from person to person—some people worry that others will think they are odd or weird, that they are "uncool," incompetent, unlikable, weak, rude, and so on. But in all cases, there is a basic concern that others will evaluate them negatively. As a result, people with SAD find any situation where there is a possibility for scrutiny by another person to be highly anxiety provoking. They avoid a wide range of situations where they might be observed or might have to interact with others. Again, the specific situations will vary from person to person, but some of the common ones include meeting new people, being the center of attention, work meetings, social functions, using public toilets, or eating, drinking, or writing in front of others.

When working with socially anxious people, it is probably not critically important whether they meet the full diagnostic criteria for SAD. However, there are times when a formal diagnosis is needed, and most research on treatments for SAD has been conducted on people who meet formal diagnostic criteria. Therefore having an appreciation of SAD diagnostic criteria (e.g., the fifth edition of the *Diagnostic and Statistical Manual of Mental Disorders* [DSM-5; American Psychiatric Association, 2013]) and using diagnostic information to assist treatment planning is advisable.

Jacquie and Max report long-standing and severe shyness, inhibition, and social avoidance across a variety of social situations because they anticipate being judged and rejected for failing to meet others' standards. When these social situations cannot be avoided they report suffering from extreme anxiety symptoms and panic attacks, which Max has tried to self-medicate with alcohol. As is the case for other emotional disorders, a diagnosis of SAD can only be given after other psychological or physiological causes or medical conditions have been ruled out as better explanations. For instance, if a client reports that he only loses his confidence and worries about negative evaluation when he is in the middle of a depressive episode, then a diagnosis of major depressive disorder rather than SAD should be considered. For both Jacquie and Max their social anxiety is chronic, persistent, pervasive, and not due to another condition. It is also important to consider sociocultural context when deciding whether anxiety is out of proportion to the actual threat because there are cross-cultural variations in the prevalence, nature, and meaning of social anxiety (Furmark, 2002). As with any mental disorder, the key issue is life impairment. Many people report being shy or quiet in some situations, but a diagnosis is only appropriate when that shyness impacts significantly on one's life. Max and Jacquie both acknowledge that their social fears are excessive, and their social and occupational functioning has clearly been chronically and severely affected by their social anxiety.

Epidemiology and Impact of SAD

SAD is one of the most common anxiety disorders. Lifetime rates of SAD vary depending on the assessment method, but it appears to be most common in Western countries such as the United States (18.2%), Australia (8.4%), and the nations of Europe (5.8–12%), and less common in Africa (e.g., 3.3% in Nigeria) and Asia (2.4–5.3%; Demyttenaere et al., 2004; McEvoy, Grove, & Slade, 2011). SAD typically begins in early adolescence (around 10 to 13 years of age), which is several years earlier than other anxiety and affective disorders except specific phobias (Kessler et al., 2005; McEvoy et al., 2011). New cases of SAD are uncommon after age 25, and people who report experiencing SAD from an earlier age tend to be more severely affected (Grant et al., 2005).

A range of factors increases the chances of having SAD. There are mixed findings on gender differences in children or adolescents, with some studies finding no difference in rates between boys and girls (Beidel, Turner, & Morris, 1999; Wittchen, Stein, & Kessler, 1999) and others finding higher rates in girls (Kessler et al., 2012). A consistent finding is that more women than men in the general population have SAD (Asher, Asnaani, & Aderka, 2017; Kessler, Petukhova, Sampson, Zaslavsky, & Wittchen, 2012; Wittchen et al., 1999), so we might expect more women than men to seek treatment. Interestingly, however, this is not the case. Within clinical samples the ratio of women to men is relatively even (Rapee, 1995). Cultural expectations for men to be more dominant and assertive may result in greater impairments in social and occupational functioning for men than women with SAD, and therefore higher rates of treatment seeking (Asher et al., 2017).

Some important cross-cultural differences in the expression of SAD have been documented (Furmark, 2002; Rapee & Spence, 2004). *Taijin kyofusho* ("interpersonal fear disorder" in Japanese) is a culturally specific expression of social anxiety where the fear is of acting in ways that are inadequate or offensive *to* others, rather than fear of negative evaluation *by* others in SAD. DSM-5 (American Psychiatric Association, 2013) lists a range of specific fears of offending others due to emitting an offensive body odor (olfactory reference syndrome), facial blushing (erythrophobia), too much or too little eye gaze, awkward body movements or expression (e.g., stiffening), or body deformity. Eastern collectivist cultures value introversion and humility, and prioritize "the other" over "the self," which may, at least in part, explain the higher prevalence of SAD in Western countries, which value individualism and extraversion (Cain, 2012). The higher value placed on individual achievement and performance in Western countries may then create the perception of a more evaluative environment, and thus higher rates of SAD, for more introverted individuals. In collectivist cultures, where the communal rather than individual good is prioritized, the documented prevalence of SAD is lowest. This literature highlights the need to understand mental disorders within an individual's sociocultural context.

SAD tends to be chronic without treatment. One study found that only 35% of a clinical sample with SAD experienced full remission over an 8-year period, with a rapidly diminishing rate of remission after the first 2 years (Yonkers, Dyck, & Keller, 2001). SAD has the lowest remission rate of all anxiety disorders, with a median length of illness of 25 years (deWit, Ogborne, Offord, & MacDonald, 1999). A recent review found that full remission rates in prospective studies of SAD varied between 36 and 66%, whereas partial remission rates (i.e., not fulfilling all of the diagnostic criteria but continuing to have some social fears) varied between 54 and 93% (Vriends, Bolt, & Kunz, 2014). These findings might suggest that a reasonably high proportion of individuals spontaneously remit over time, or alternatively that SAD follows a waxing and waning course (Vriends et al., 2014). A range of factors was associated with an increased likelihood of remission, including having a nongeneralized subtype of social anxiety, no panic attacks, less avoidance, higher age of onset, less severe impairment, no comorbid mental disorders, no alcohol use, being older than 65, being employed, being in a relationship, higher socioeconomic status, fewer critical life events, and no parental history of SAD or depression.

Due to its high prevalence SAD has been found to account for a similar degree of disability in the population as schizophrenia and bipolar affective disorder (Mathers, Vos, & Stevenson, 1999). Individuals with SAD are more likely to have poorer academic functioning, to be unemployed, and to be single (Davidson, Hughes, George, & Blazer, 1993; Kessler, Stein, & Berglund, 1998). SAD is therefore an early-onset, common, chronic, and debilitating anxiety disorder that does not tend to remit without treatment. Unfortunately some studies have suggested that as few as 5% of individuals seek treatment for social anxiety (Keller, 2003) and, for those that do, the mean age of presentation for treatment is around 30 years (Rapee, 1995). People with SAD tend to wait longer to seek treatment than other anxiety disorders, which leads to an extended period of disability. Given the interpersonal nature of the disorder, the fact that most activities humans do in life involve interpersonal interactions, and the substantial delay in treatment seeking, SAD can have a pervasive impact on people's lives.

What Causes SAD?

As a truism, the causes of SAD almost certainly include a combination of nature and nurture. Although individual studies show some variability in results, overall, evidence from twins points to a consistent inherited component for social anxiety (Scaini, Belotti, & Ogliari, 2014). It is interesting that the heritable component seems to be almost twice as strong for symptoms of social anxiousness than for the actual clinical diagnosis of SAD. This might suggest that whereas social anxiousness reflects more of a fundamental personality trait, whether a highly shy person develops the clinical syndrome (SAD) might depend more on environmental factors (Spence & Rapee, 2016). There is some evidence that SAD "breeds true" so that individuals with SAD are more likely to have offspring with SAD compared to individuals without mental disorders (Fyer, Mannuzza, Chapman, Martin, & Klein, 1995) and compared to individuals with a different disorder (Lieb et al., 2000). However, most of the genetic influence seems to increase vulnerability to emotional disorders in general rather than SAD in particular. In other words, what is inherited seems to mostly be a general tendency to be "emotional"—often referred to as neuroticism. Neuroticism refers to a general tendency to experience negative emotional states and sensitivity to stress (Watson, Gamez, & Simms, 2005) and is a common temperamental vulnerability factor for a range of emotional disorders.

Personality and temperamental factors can increase the risk of developing SAD. Children who display a general tendency to be submissive, anxious, socially avoidant, and behaviorally inhibited are more likely to develop SAD (Clauss & Blackford, 2012; Rapee, 2014). Other personality dimensions have also been associated with SAD, particularly the combination of high neuroticism and low extraversion, and the personality style of low effortful control. Thus SAD is likely to result from a complex interplay between temperamental factors.

A range of environmental factors has been associated with SAD, but most of the evidence is based on retrospective self-report and correlational designs. It is therefore unclear if the relationships are causal, unidirectional, or reciprocal. Environmental risk factors also appear to be similar across mental disorders rather than specific to SAD (Kendler et al., 2011). Examples of social traumas that have been associated with anxiety disorders in general and SAD in particular include bullying by peers, abuse, and a dysfunctional family of origin (Spence & Rapee, 2016).

Insecure attachment styles have also been associated with an increased risk of SAD (Shamir-Essakow, Ungerer, & Rapee, 2005). Trust in caregivers promotes exploration of the social world, development of social skills, and self-efficacy, whereas an absence of a secure, trusting, and responsive caregiver may adversely impact social skills and confidence. Parents of sociable and socially competent children tend to be warm and supportive and set clear expectations. In contrast, parents of shy and socially withdrawn children tend to be more overcontrolling, overprotective, distant, insensitive, rejecting, less sociable, stress the importance of others' opinions, and use shame for discipline (McLeod, Wood, & Weisz, 2007; Wong & Rapee, 2016).

It is important to emphasize again that these associations have been weak and mostly based on correlations and retrospective recall. It is plausible that parents adopt these styles *in response to* their children's inhibition. For instance, a parent may take more control as a way of trying to encourage a shy child to engage more fully with her peers with the laudable aim of enhancing her social skills and confidence. Alternatively, sensitive to their shy child's discomfort, other parents might allow him to predominantly engage in solitary activities. "Overcontrolling" and '"overprotective" parenting may thus be a response to the child's fearfulness and distress in social situations. In turn, reciprocal relationships between a child's temperament and parenting styles may serve to reinforce threat expectations and avoidant coping strategies (Spence & Rapee, 2016; Wong & Rapee, 2016).

In summary, the development of SAD probably involves a complex and reciprocal interaction among a range of genetic, temperamental, and environmental factors. Genetic and temperamental factors can elicit responses from the environment that reinforce or strengthen tendencies toward behavioral inhibition, and environmental factors may act upon preexisting temperamental characteristics to reduce or increase the risk for SAD. Each individual may be influenced by these factors to differing degrees, and a wide range of idiosyncratic experiences are also likely to complicate the picture. On an individual basis, when you meet a client with SAD, it is impossible to know exactly what factors led to his presenting problems. For this reason, treatment is not aimed at the "causes" of the disorder but rather at the current processes that maintain the problem. We discuss these processes in a later section.

Comorbidity

SAD rarely occurs in isolation. In fact SAD frequently co-occurs with other mental disorders, especially depression, other anxiety disorders, substance use disorders, and personality disorders (Grant et al., 2005). At least half the people presenting for treatment with SAD will have a comorbid disorder (McEvoy et al., 2015), so it is important for assessing clinicians to be "on the lookout" for additional problems. Mood disorders are the most common co-occurring disorders, followed by other anxiety disorders (Grant et al., 2005). SAD is one of the earliest-onset mental disorders, so most clients' comorbid disorders will have started after their SAD.

Concurrent conditions can interfere with treatment progress (Lincoln et al., 2003, 2005; McEvoy, 2007), so treating clinicians need to carefully consider how they might need to feature in their case formulations and treatment plans. For instance, if major depression is the most debilitating problem when the client presents for treatment, this might need to be prioritized even if the depression started after the SAD. If left untreated, depression symptoms such as lethargy, avolition, and profound hopelessness may interfere with treatment engagement. Substance dependence may also interfere with progress by causing anxiety symptoms (especially during short-term withdrawal), which can reduce the effectiveness of the treatment strategies and ultimately reduce clients' confidence in the SAD treatment. However, it may be difficult for the client to reduce her substance use if the social anxiety is not addressed. In these cases an integrative approach to treating social anxiety and substance abuse is indicated, where both problems are treated simultaneously by the same or complementary services (Stapinski et al., 2015).

It can sometimes be difficult to determine which problem should be treated first, and this will typically be a decision that is made collaboratively with the client. We will often have an open discussion with clients about the treatment options and the pros and cons of each approach. In our experience, clients are usually well equipped to decide whether, for instance, their depressed mood is likely to interfere with their ability to regularly attend treatment sessions and apply treatment strategies for their SAD. If the client is suffering from severe depression and agrees that this needs to be addressed first, we will prescribe psychological and/or pharmacological treatments for depression before targeting his SAD. Once a collaborative decision has been made on the preferred treatment focus, the clinician can monitor comorbid problems and shift focus if it becomes clear that they are interfering with treatment. Group treatment is less flexible in this regard, so at times it might be necessary to remove a client from a SAD group if it becomes clear that comorbid problems are inhibiting treatment progress. After the comorbid issue is addressed she can then recommence treatment for SAD.

Differential Diagnoses

Some psychological disorders can present in similar ways to SAD, but the differences can have important treatment implications. Recurrent panic attacks can occur in SAD but are not diagnosed as panic disorder unless uncued (unexpected) panic attacks that are unrelated to social triggers are present (American Psychiatric Association, 2013). The core negative cognitions differ between SAD and panic disorder, with the former revolving around themes of evaluation and the latter around themes of catastrophic consequences of somatic symptoms (e.g., heart attack). Individuals with panic disorder may fear some social consequences of having a panic attack, but their panic attacks are not invariably triggered by social cues, and the primary fear is of having a panic attack or the consequences of a panic attack rather than of negative evaluation. Agoraphobic avoidance may also resemble avoidance in SAD, but the function of avoidance in agoraphobia is to prevent fear and panic attacks, whereas the function of avoidance in SAD is to prevent social evaluation.

Body dysmorphic disorder (BDD) is another mental disorder that shares features with SAD. People with BDD believe they have an abhorrent and unacceptable physical flaw in their appearance (American Psychiatric Association, 2013). Individuals with BDD and SAD can present with some similar affective, physiological, interpersonal, and behavioral symptoms. Individuals with both disorders may report feeling anxiety, shame, and humiliation, and they might appear behaviorally inhibited, avoid social contact, and fear attention from others. Both disorders may also be associated with fear of negative evaluation based on appearance, which may result in mirror gazing, camouflaging, and excessive grooming behaviors. However, with BDD the cognitions tend to be more focused on rejection as a consequence of a specific perceived or exaggerated physical flaw (e.g., skin defects, nose size), and sufferers may have low insight into the discrepancy between their perception and reality. Individuals with SAD tend to have more general fears of rejection as a consequence of their social performance not meeting others' standards, which may extend to and include aspects of physical appearance. It is important to do a careful assessment for the presence of comorbid BDD because elements of treatment for SAD can be particularly grueling for these individuals (e.g., video feedback, see Chapter 7). When BDD is associated with very poor insight and is of almost delusional intensity, differential diagnosis is critical and relatively straightforward. However, in milder cases there is substantial overlap, and the concerns about aspects of physical appearance can be missed without careful assessment.

Avoidant personality disorder (PD) is characterized by a pervasive pattern of social inhibition, feelings of inadequacy, and hypersensitivity to negative evaluation (American Psychiatric Association, 2013) and reflects a more severe variant of SAD. Individuals with an avoidant personality will present as being more chronic, comorbid (e.g., depression, substance abuse), and debilitated by their social anxiety. Negative core beliefs about the self being inadequate, unlikable, and inferior, and of others being hostile, judgmental, and superior, are likely to be "stickier" than for those without avoidant PD. Avoidance behaviors will also be more pervasive, long-standing, and rigid. These individuals can be effectively treated using similar interventions as for SAD but may require a larger dose of therapy to achieve comparable outcomes to clients without avoidant PD. Research has found similar rates of improvement between those with and without comorbid avoidant personality, but fewer individuals with avoidant PD achieve full remission (Cox, Turnbull, Robinson, Grant, & Stein, 2011).

Occasionally individuals with schizoid PD are referred for treatment of SAD. Schizoid PD is characterized by a lack of interest in close interpersonal relationships and, like avoidant PD and SAD, is associated with high neuroticism and low extraversion

(Saulsman & Page, 2004). One 19-year-old man referred to our clinic was accompanied by his very concerned father, who reported that his son had always been uninterested in engaging with his peers and family unless it was necessary. A detailed assessment revealed that the son simply did not find social interactions rewarding, and so he preferred solitary activities. He described apathy rather than anxiety in social situations, and he did not meet criteria for major depression or dysthymia. Clearly this client was not a good candidate for treatment of SAD, as he did not experience the primary feature of this disorder, fear of negative evaluation.

SAD and depression often co-occur and have overlapping features. Like SAD, depression is often associated with social withdrawal, inactivity, low self-esteem, negative beliefs and perceptions about the self and others, and negative ruminations about social interactions. Given its earlier average age of onset, it is more common for SAD to precede rather than follow depression, suggesting that social anxiety and associated withdrawal can lead to depression. Many clients will report this pattern when asked what they recall first, feeling anxious in social situations or feeling depressed. For other clients it will be more difficult to tease these symptoms apart. If clients deny feeling socially anxious in between depressive episodes, this suggests that the primary disorder is depression, and if this is successfully treated the social anxiety should resolve. If the client reports that depression typically follows a period of social anxiety, then depression may be masking an underlying SAD. In these cases, it may still be important to treat the depression before the social anxiety, but we will often make this decision based on client preference and whether the depression is so severe that it is likely to interfere with engagement in SAD treatment.

A final issue we discuss here is a recognition that some clients referred for SAD may genuinely elicit frequent rejection or interpersonal disputes. Individuals with SAD fear negative evaluation, but almost invariably this is *perceived* evaluation. Friends or family members might express some frustration at their inhibited behavior, or the individual might avoid establishing social contact with others, but it is rare that someone with SAD *is* overtly rejected by others. Clients who present with clear evidence of negative evaluation and rejection may require a different form of treatment from what we describe in this book, such as social skills training, anger management, interpersonal psychotherapy, or dialectical behavior therapy. It is noteworthy that while there is evidence that children with SAD demonstrate social skills deficits, most adults with SAD have perfectly adequate social skills (Rapee & Spence, 2004). The problem is that they don't *think* they have adequate social skills. One of the most important goals of treatment is for clients to learn that there is a large discrepancy between their *perceived* and *actual* social skills. Avoidant behaviors (e.g., not making eye contact, staying quiet) may masquerade as social skills deficits, but as these fall away during treatment one of the great pleasures of treating clients with SAD is observing their natural social skills flourish. Many SAD clients feel relatively comfortable with clinicians, so some of these skills are often apparent in the initial assessment. Individuals with SAD desire relationships with others, they are sensitive to others' opinions and needs, and they are caring (albeit too much).

Social Anxiety: Dimension versus Subtypes

Normal shyness is typically considered to be a relatively mild social awkwardness that does not significantly interfere with functioning. Up to 40% of nonclinical samples report having felt shy at some point in their lives (Rapee, 1995), suggesting that it is a common and normal experience. We have all probably had the experience of feeling awkward within social situations. Perhaps you can recall an experience when everyone else appeared to be engaged in conversations while you were standing alone in the corner of the room with an hors d'oeuvre in your hand? Suddenly, the food or an item of furniture became extremely fascinating as you attempted to appear preoccupied by choice (rather than just appearing to be awkward and a loner). Perhaps you pretended to look busy with your cell phone as you considered excuses for making a hasty exit (perhaps you were Googling "how to make a hasty but subtle exit from a party")? We have all also had the experience of engaging in a pretty dull conversation or putting our "foot in our mouth." These are normal experiences that are very specific to particular situations (e.g., when we don't know anyone) and mercifully quite rare, and the awkwardness generally passes quickly. Even if these fleeting experiences occur relatively frequently and we identify as being a shy person, we might not let them overly affect our life. On the other hand, if we start to notice that these experiences are occurring frequently, are associated with significant anxiety in anticipation of social situations, start to promote avoidant behavior, and are having a negative impact on our life, then we have moved beyond "normal" shyness into SAD territory.

Previous editions of the DSM (American Psychiatric Association, 1987, 1994, 2000) distinguished between circumscribed (specific) and generalized social phobia. Specific social phobia was diagnosed when clinically significant social anxiety was triggered by one or two situations, whereas generalized social phobia was diagnosed when the client experienced social anxiety in most social situations. The validity of this subtyping was controversial, with researchers questioning whether the distinctions were more quantitative (different severities) than qualitative (different forms of the disorder) (see Skocic, Jackson, & Hulbert, 2015). Compared to specific social phobia, generalized social phobia tends to be associated with an earlier onset, greater chronicity, more severe anxiety, more avoidance and impairment, and more suicidal behavior (Furmark, Tillfors, Stattin, Ekselius, & Fredrikson, 2000; Hook & Valentiner, 2001; Stein, Torgrud, & Walker, 2000). Avoidant PD is even more severe on each of these variables.

DSM-5 (American Psychiatric Association, 2013) removed the specific and generalized specifiers and instead introduced a "performance only" subtype. The performance subtype is given when a client's fear of being observed or scrutinized is limited to situations such as presentations, job interviews, and when eating or drinking in public, but they do not fear interacting with people (Hofmann, Newman, Ehlers, & Roth, 1995; Stein & Deutsch, 2003). Epidemiological research suggests that the performance subtype of SAD is quite rare (Burstein et al., 2011). Apart from the specific subtype, and public speaking fears in particular, SAD may best be considered along a continuum based on the number of feared situations and the associated degree of distress and disability (Skocic et al., 2015). Avoidant PD remained as a separate disorder in DSM-5 despite evidence that it is a more severe variant of SAD.

Summary

Jacquie and Max, our clinical cases at the start of this chapter, are typical examples of what the diagnostic criteria and research tell us about SAD. They report long-standing shyness and behavioral inhibition, and in Jacquie's case there is some suggestion that her father was introverted and her mother had high expectations of social performance. Although they are young adults, they have already suffered for a number of years with their social anxiety, and they have presented for treatment at a time when they are highly debilitated by their symptoms. Throughout this book we provide case examples of individuals we have worked with who have undertaken the challenging but ultimately rewarding journey through treatment. The aim of treatment is for our clients to feel that they can make genuine choices in their lives without their social anxiety dictating what they can and cannot do. Both Jacquie and Max have aspirations for a relationship, career, and family. The ultimate marker of treatment success is when clients believe that they can pursue their aspirations and lead fulfilling lives. Unfortunately, many individuals like Jacquie and Max suffer through every facet of life in silence, either indefinitely or for many years before seeking help.

In the next chapter we review cognitive-behavioral models that describe factors that maintain SAD and therefore inform the treatment described in Part II of this book. It is important for clinicians to have a working understanding of these models because they provide an understanding of why SAD persists and underpin the treatment rationale.

CHAPTER 2

Cognitive-Behavioral Models and Treatments for SAD

SAD has been treated using a diverse range of psychological models, although CBT has the strongest evidence from both stringent randomized controlled trials in research settings and effectiveness studies within real-world clinics. A range of CBT-based treatments has been evaluated, including those that emphasize behavioral exposure, cognitive change, social skills training, and a combination of these components. This chapter begins with a brief review of two of the most influential cognitive-behavioral models of SAD and then review the key mechanisms from these models that will be targeted by the treatment in Part II of this book. We then briefly review evidence that cognitive-behavioral approaches are effective for many people with SAD, but also that a substantial minority of clients are not sufficiently helped by existing treatments. Finally, we describe the rationale for enhancing CBT for SAD using imagery-based techniques.

Cognitive-Behavioral Models of SAD

The classification of SAD as an anxiety disorder in the third edition of the *Diagnostic and Statistical Manual of Mental Disorders* (DSM-III; American Psychiatric Association, 1980) prompted a rapid escalation of research in the area. As our understanding of SAD improved, further refinements to diagnostic criteria and theoretical models followed. Two influential cognitive-behavioral models of the maintenance of SAD were initially published by David Clark and Adrian Wells (1995) and Ron Rapee and Richard Heimberg (1997). Rapee and Heimberg's model has since been updated and elaborated (Heimberg, Brozovich, & Rapee, 2010, 2014). Interested readers are referred to Wong,

Gordon, and Heimberg (2014) for a description of additional models that have also increased our understanding of SAD.

Clark and Wells (1995)

Clark and Wells's (1995) cognitive model of SAD describes factors that serve to maintain and exacerbate social anxiety despite repeated exposure to social situations. The model also describes processes that occur before and after social situations that reinforce negative beliefs and, in turn, increase vulnerability to future social anxiety. Clark and Wells (1995; Clark, 2001) argue that individuals with SAD develop assumptions about themselves and their social world based on early life experiences. These assumptions are divided into three categories: excessively high standards for social performance (e.g., "I must never show signs of anxiety and weakness"), conditional beliefs concerning the consequences of performing in a certain way (e.g., "If I express my opinion, I'll be rejected"), and unconditional negative beliefs about the self (e.g., "I am unlikable"). These assumptions cause the individual to anticipate social threat due to an expected failure to meet social standards, and to misinterpret ambiguous social cues as being consistent with their negative assumptions (e.g., smiles from other people are interpreted as sympathy for anxiety or poor performance rather than genuine approval).

The model suggests that a range of processes prevent disconfirmation of these negative beliefs. One of these processes is self-focused attention. The model suggests that individuals with SAD closely scrutinize themselves within social contexts, including their performance, anxiety levels, and physiological symptoms (Clark & Wells, 1995). Information gathered from this self-focused attention is then used to guide a self-image of how the individual believes he is seen by others, that is, from the observer perspective. Unfortunately, the individual's preexisting negative assumptions in conjunction with his anxiety symptoms conspire to negatively bias this self-image. The anxiety symptoms are believed to be obvious to others and are therefore seen as evidence of failure to meet social standards. Negative evaluation is expected to follow. In this way, emotional reasoning, where the individual believes that because he feels anxious his symptoms must be obvious to others, along with a "felt sense" of performing poorly, reinforce the negative self-image and associated negative assumptions.

Another process in the model builds on earlier work by Paul Salkovskis (1991, 1996) and suggests that individuals with SAD engage in a range of safety behaviors. Safety behaviors are subtle avoidance behaviors that are used in an attempt to prevent fears from coming true. However, although on some occasions safety behaviors may provide a temporary sense of control over the perceived threat and thus a reduction in acute anxiety, Clark and Wells (1995) suggest that they actually serve to maintain perceived social threat and SAD in the longer term. One way safety behaviors maintain the perception of social threat is by individuals attributing the nonoccurrence of social catastrophe to the use of the safety behavior, rather than as evidence that the perceived probability or cost of the threat needs to be modified. For example, if an individual with SAD does not disclose any personal information during a conversation and there is no evidence of rejection, she may attribute the absence of rejection to the fact that the other person had no information that would have invariably led to rejection. Negative core beliefs such as "I am unlikable" and "others are judgmental" are therefore maintained, when in fact if the person took the risk of self-disclosing she might learn that she is far more likable and others far more accepting than expected.

Another way safety behaviors can maintain SAD is by "contaminating" the social situation, which then becomes a self-fulfilling prophecy. Extending the previous social interaction example, if the individual with SAD remains quiet and fails to reciprocate during the discussion, her conversational partner might conclude that she is aloof or disinterested and abruptly terminate the conversation. By using the safety behavior for the purpose of preventing negative evaluation, the individual with SAD has unknowingly elicited negative evaluation. Another example is if someone uses alcohol as a social lubricant, which leads to obnoxious or otherwise inappropriate behavior and, in turn, negative evaluation.

Safety "behaviors" can include cognitive attempts to prevent social failure, such as rehearsing conversations or hesitating to speak one's mind for so long that the topic has moved on and the point is no longer relevant. These processes maintain a preoccupation with potential social failure and threat and distract people from the task at hand (e.g., the actual topic of the conversation or noticing cues from the conversational partner that can be used to naturally formulate responses). As a consequence of being "stuck in one's head," the individual with SAD may appear uninterested or even arrogant. In these ways, safety behaviors may be interpreted by others as a lack of social skills, when in fact the anxiety and associated attempts to prevent feared outcomes *inhibit* the individual's natural social skills—social skills that come to the fore when the person is not anticipating negative evaluation (e.g., when in the psychologist's office or with a trusted loved one).

Excessive self-focused attention means that people with SAD are unable to notice when they receive positive or neutral feedback from others. On occasions when they are able to "look outside of themselves" feedback from others is often filtered through their negative core beliefs, and they scan for any confirmation of social inadequacy. Feedback that can be interpreted as evidence of social failure is more likely to be noticed, to the exclusion of feedback that disconfirms this belief. An absence of positive feedback will also be seen as confirmation of negative evaluation. In fact, it's not uncommon for people with SAD to interpret unambiguously *positive* feedback as evidence of social failure. For example, encouragement from a boss might be interpreted as evidence of a need to improve work quality rather than as a reward for meeting standards. Recent theory and research suggest that positive feedback can elicit a fear of evaluation for people with SAD. Either way, these are striking examples of the power of underlying assumptions to negatively influence the processing of ambiguous (and even unambiguous) social cues.

Clients with SAD will tell you that the suffering does not start and end with the social situation itself. Social events may be anticipated hours, days, weeks, months or even years ahead of time. One client dreaded giving a speech at his daughter's wedding well before she even had a partner, let alone a proposal! As clients with SAD envision an upcoming social situation, they imagine their social fears playing out (i.e., negative evaluation and rejection). This primes them to perceive a threat, and to become physically aroused and self-focused, even before the event has occurred. Clark and Wells (1995; Clark, 2001) argue that this anticipatory process kick-starts the in-situation processing biases described earlier. This anticipatory processing and anxiety can even result in wholesale avoidance, which of course denies people any opportunity to disconfirm their fears.

Biased anticipatory and in-situation processing can also drive biased postevent processing, whereby the individual scrutinizes his social performance in a negative way after the social event (Clark & Wells, 1995). Because people with SAD preferentially attend to any possible sign of negative social feedback within social situations, they are naturally going to have a negative impression of the event afterwards. Attention is the "microscope of the mind" and dictates what will be encoded in memory. In the case of SAD, benign and positive feedback falls out of the microscope's range, so it is ignored and lost forever. The individual therefore leaves the social situation believing his social fears have been confirmed, which further reinforces his negative core beliefs and assumptions. Each "social failure" is recalled within the context of a long history of perceived failures, which then influences what is expected in future social situations, and so the cycle continues.

In summary, Clark and Wells's (1995) model emphasizes the importance of negative assumptions and core beliefs, negative automatic thoughts, attentional biases (self-focus), negative self-images from the "observer-perspective," avoidance, safety behaviors, and anticipatory and postevent processing. Interventions targeting these processes have proven to be highly effective in treating social anxiety (Clark et al., 2003, 2006).

Rapee and Heimberg (1997)

Rapee and Heimberg (1997) suggest that individuals with SAD hold assumptions that (1) others are generally critical and are likely to judge them negatively, and (2) there is a high perceived cost to negative evaluation from others. Similar to Clark and Wells's (1995; Clark, 2001) model, Rapee and Heimberg also acknowledge that perceived social threat can trigger anxiety regardless of whether the social situation is anticipated (anticipatory processing), actually encountered in the present moment (in-situation processing), or retrospectively reflected on (postevent processing).

Central to Rapee and Heimberg's (1997) model is that people with SAD form a mental representation of the self, creating a vivid impression of how others see them (i.e., the observer perspective). Critically, this mental representation is not based on objective feedback, but rather is internally constructed based on a combination of long-term memory (e.g., photos of the self, previous experiences within social situations), internal cues (e.g., physical symptoms such as blushing, self-images), and observable feedback from others. The model suggests that the person's attention is focused primarily on negative aspects of this mental representation (e.g., signs of anxiety perceived to be obvious to others, such as blushing or shaking) and on monitoring for external threat from others.

For people with SAD, monitoring of potential external threat involves scanning the social environment for any sign of evaluation, such as frowns, yawns, or essentially any ambiguous feedback that could possibly be consistent with negative evaluation (e.g., a couple laughing in the opposite corner of the room). Dividing attention across sources of internal and external threat, along with the task at hand, is cognitively demanding and can interfere with social performance.

Rapee and Heimberg's (1997) model proposes that the mental representation of the self is compared to the audience's perceived social standards, and people with SAD believe they fall woefully short of the mark. The magnitude of this discrepancy will determine the perceived likelihood of negative evaluation from others. The perceived likelihood and "cost" (i.e., consequences) of negative evaluation together determine the perceived severity of the social threat, which, in turn, maintains physiological, cognitive, and behavioral symptoms. For instance, the more likely or costly an individual believes rejection to be, blushing will intensify and, in turn, the individual assumes her anxiety is even more obvious to others. The self-image therefore becomes even more distorted, and the use of subtle avoidance behaviors to prevent evaluation (e.g., not contributing to the conversation, averting eye gaze to the ground) reinforces beliefs of social incompetence. The discrepancy between the mental representation of the self and perceived social standards widens, maintaining the cycle.

Heimberg and colleagues (2010, 2014) updated and extended Rapee and Heimberg's (1997) model in several ways, but most relevant here was a renewed focus on imagery as a treatment target and mode of intervention. We return to this point in detail later in this chapter. Wong, Moulds, and Rapee (2014) describe subtle differences between existing models of SAD, but there are also substantial commonalities in the key maintaining factors across the models.

Key Cognitive-Behavioral Maintaining Factors

Three key maintaining factors across these cognitive-behavioral models relate to negative cognitive content (i.e., negative automatic thoughts, negative self-images, and negative core beliefs), behavioral avoidance and safety behaviors, and attentional problems (self- and environment-focused attention). We summarize these processes briefly to highlight the importance of targeting them in treatment. Each of these processes is shown in the client-friendly model used to guide the treatment in Part II of this book (see Chapter 3, Figure 3.1).

Negative Cognitive Content: Thoughts, Images, and Core Beliefs

Negative cognitive content is considered to be of central importance to SAD, including negative automatic thoughts and images. *Negative thoughts and images* in SAD relate to the probability and cost of past, present, or future social threats. Perceptions of threat stem from beliefs that one will fail to meet expected social standards due to some combination of (1) personal inadequacy, (2) high external social standards, and (3) judgmental others. Moscovitch (2009) suggested that perceptions of personal inadequacy could be due to individuals believing that they have poor social skills and behaviors, visible signs of anxiety, problems in physical appearance, and/or a flawed character (i.e., personality). Extensions to Rapee and Heimberg's (1997) model, based on evolutionary models (Gilbert, 2001), also suggest that positive evaluation can be socially threatening for individuals with SAD (Heimberg et al., 2014). Exposure of perceived self-deficiencies and potential negative evaluation, or of upward threats to the social hierarchy in the case of positive evaluation (i.e., standing out for good reasons, possibly resulting in peer jealousy), are expected to be both highly probable and highly costly (e.g., lead to rejection).

Distorted mental self-images regarding social performance are guided by perceived past failures and are reinforced by vigilance toward symptoms of physiological arousal, which the individual assumes are obvious to others. In anticipation of social situations, negative thoughts and images can serve to prime self-focused attention and anxiety. After the social event, negative beliefs and images about the self and others are heavily reinforced during the cognitive "postmortem" because in-situation self-processing was so negatively biased. Negative automatic thoughts and images derive from *negative core beliefs* about the self (e.g., "I'm socially inept and unlikable") and others (e.g., "others are judgmental and hostile"). Clearly it is critical for treatment to target negative thoughts and images, self-images, and core beliefs.

Behavioral Avoidance and Safety Behaviors

Behavioral avoidance is a critical maintaining factor of negative thoughts and imagery in all models. Negative cognitions cannot be optimally activated, challenged, and modified without exposure to the perceived threat. Early negative social experiences will continue to be highly influential in driving perceptions of social threat if new, more realistic, competing memories are not created. *Safety behaviors* are subtle forms of avoidance that (1) prevent negative cognitions from being genuinely and comprehensively tested and modified, (2) conceal perceived self-deficiencies, which deprives the individual of opportunities to learn that the probability or consequences of exposing these aspects of the self are far less likely and/or catastrophic than expected, (3) lead individuals to attribute the nonoccurrence of the perceived catastrophe to the use of the safety behavior, thus undermining the perceived need to recalibrate probability and cost estimates, (4) attract negative evaluation themselves, thus becoming self-fulfilling prophecies, and (5) reinforce self-focused attention and self-consciousness. People with SAD are usually acutely aware that they are using safety behaviors, which thereby increases self-focused rather than task-focused attention. If threat perceptions are to be therapeutically modified, it is therefore important that social fears are not avoided, but instead genuinely confronted in the absence of safety behaviors.

Attentional Problems: Self- and Environment Focus

Anxiety is designed to narrow attention on threats and away from extraneous (nonthreatening) stimuli, which is critical for survival in genuinely threatening situations. In the case of SAD an important perceived threat is self-deficiency. Inflexible *self-focused* attention increases hypervigilance to signs of physiological arousal, which, in combination with negative thoughts and images, escalates the perception of social threat. For example, an individual with social anxiety who becomes aware of warmth in her cheeks may become more focused on these sensations. As a consequence, in her mind's eye she might envision herself blushing bright neon red, which increases the perceived likelihood of humiliation and rejection. With any remaining attentional capacity she will strategically scan the *environment* for (often ambiguous) sources of external social threat (e.g., two people laughing in the corner of the room), which may be personalized (e.g., "They are laughing at me").

Self- and environment-focused attention (rather than task-focused attention) can directly result in a failure to meet social standards. For instance, by not focusing on the topic of a conversation, individuals with SAD may miss important social cues for them to contribute. Social awkwardness may ensue, which, in turn, leads to the appearance of a social skills deficit. Training clients to redeploy their attention onto functional aspects of social situations is important to break down many of the vicious cycles maintaining acute social anxiety and SAD.

Now that we have an understanding of the key factors that maintain SAD, below we summarize outcomes from treatments that target these factors.

What Treatments Work?

CBT Is the Treatment of Choice for SAD

Meta-analyses offer the highest level of evidence for the effectiveness of a particular treatment because they combine outcomes from multiple trials. Several recent meta-analyses have compared active treatments to wait-list controls or alternative treatments. Acarturk, Cuijpers, van Straten, and de Graaf (2009) conducted a meta-analysis of psychological interventions (mainly forms of CBT) for SAD based on 29 randomized controlled trials (RCTs) (N participants = 1,628) and found large effect sizes on measures of social-evaluative cognitions, depression, and general anxiety (Cohen's d's = 0.70–0.80). Treatment outcomes did not differ based on age group (university students vs. older adults), type of SAD (specific vs. generalized), intervention format (individual vs. group), recruitment source (community volunteers vs. clinical population), or type of psychological interventions (with vs. without cognitive restructuring; with vs. without exposure; with vs. without social skills training). Overall, the findings of this meta-analysis revealed that CBT is more effective than wait-list and placebo control groups, and that few client or treatment factors moderate these outcomes. These findings are consistent with earlier meta-analyses that also failed to find significant differences between exposure-based, cognitive-therapy based, and combined exposure plus cognitive-therapy treatments, or treatment format (group vs. individual therapy; Powers, Sigmarsson, & Emmelkamp, 2008; although see Aderka, 2009). Two RCTs that directly compared individual to group treatment found an advantage of individual treatment (Mörtberg, Clark, Sundin, & Åberg Wistedt, 2007; Stangier, Heidenreich, Peitz, Lauterbach, & Clark, 2003), but the group effect sizes in these trials were substantially smaller than is commonly found for group CBT (Heimberg et al., 1990; McEvoy, 2007; McEvoy, Nathan, Rapee, & Campbell, 2012; McEvoy et al., 2015; Rapee, Gaston, & Abbott, 2009).

Canton, Scott, and Glue (2012) recently conducted a systematic literature review of pharmacotherapies and psychotherapies for SAD. CBT was identified as the psychological treatment of choice, with interpersonal psychotherapy or mindfulness-based therapies being potential alternatives for those who do not respond. Selective serotonin reuptake inhibitors (SSRIs) and dual serotonin–norepinephrine reuptake inhibitors (SNRIs) were recommended as first-line pharmacotherapies based on their efficacy and tolerability. The authors suggested that nonselective monoamine oxidase inhibitors (MAOIs) may be more potent, but they should be restricted to those who fail to benefit from SSRIs or SNRIs due to their side-effect profile, including interactions with a range of foods.

Canton and colleagues (2012) reported that SSRIs and psychological treatments appear to be equally effective, although there is some evidence that cognitive therapy may be superior (Clark et al., 2003). Several studies have also demonstrated that cognitive therapy is superior to medication in terms of long-term maintenance of gains (Haug et al., 2003; Liebowitz et al., 1999). Studies comparing medication alone to combined medication plus CBT have found nonsignificant trends favoring the combined treatment, although one study of benzodiazepines found a significant advantage of the combined treatment (Canton et al., 2012). Studies of psychological treatment compared to combined medication plus psychological treatment have also reported nonsignificant trends favoring the combined treatment, although some studies have found clear evidence of superiority for combination treatments (see Blanco et al., 2010). Canton and colleagues note that many studies used relatively small sample sizes and so may have been underpowered to detect differences.

Mayo-Wilson and colleagues (2014) conducted the largest and most recent network meta-analysis of psychological and pharmacological interventions for SAD in adults. This study included 101 trials (N participants $= 13{,}164$) of 41 interventions or control conditions. Psychological treatments found to be superior to wait-list control (in order of effect size) were individual CBT, group CBT, exposure and social skills training, self-help with support, self-help without support, and psychodynamic psychotherapy. Exercise promotion and other psychological therapy (interpersonal psychotherapy, mindfulness training, and supportive therapy) were not superior to wait-list controls. Combined psychological and medication interventions were also superior to wait-list controls. Of the psychological treatments, only CBT based on Clark and Wells's (1995) model, individual CBT, and enhanced CBT (Rapee et al., 2009) had greater effects than psychological placebo. Pharmacological treatments found to be superior to pill placebos include MAOIs, SSRIs (except citalopram), and SNRIs. Mayo-Wilson and colleagues reported that there was no consistent evidence of differential efficacy within pharmacotherapies. The authors concluded that due to lower risk of side effects, comparable efficacy, and superior longer-term outcomes, psychological interventions should be the first line treatment for SAD.

The consistent indication across systematic reviews, meta-analyses, and the most recent National Institute for Health and Care Excellence (NICE; 2013) guidelines is that CBT is the most effective psychological treatment for SAD. Individual CBT consistently outperforms a range of other treatments, and group CBT is also highly effective. A large body of evidence also suggests that CBT is effective and cost-effective when delivered over the Internet (Andersson, Cuijpers, Carlbring, Riper, & Hedman, 2014; Andrews, Cuijpers, Craske, McEvoy, & Titov, 2010; Arnberg, Linton, Hultcrantz, Heintz, & Jonsson, 2014; Boettcher, Carlbring, Renneberg, & Berger, 2013), although there is some evidence that Internet-based treatments may be less effective at improving broader measures of quality of life (Hofmann, Wu, & Boettcher, 2014). SSRIs and SNRIs are the pharmacological treatments of choice due to their combined effectiveness and side-effect profiles, with MAOIs being effective but more poorly tolerated.

The National Institute for Health and Care Excellence (NICE; 2013) guidelines suggest that other psychological treatments should not be routinely offered as a first-line treatment, and should only be offered if clients refuse or do not respond to CBT that is designed for SAD. Although there is early evidence that acceptance and mindfulness-based approaches, interpersonal psychotherapy, and psychodynamic psychotherapies may be helpful for SAD, meta-analyses and treatment comparison studies consistently show that CBT is either superior or that the alternative treatments are at best equally effective (e.g., Goldin et al., 2016). Research evaluating these alternative therapies also tends to be limited by a range of methodological problems and potential biases, including publication bias, uneven "doses" across comparison treatments, unclear descriptions of treatments and clinician training, a lack of power analyses, the use of superiority rather than noninferiority designs with appropriate equivalence analyses, and a lack of data on adherence to and competence of treatment delivery, interrater reliability of diagnosis, or credibility ratings (Norton, Abbott, Norberg, & Hunt, 2015; Öst, 2014; although see Goldin et al., 2016, for a recent exception). Consistent with recommendations from a number of professional bodies, CBT should be the first treatment offered to people with SAD. If clients have a strong preference against CBT and their concerns cannot be addressed, or they do not respond, they could be offered pharmacotherapy or an alternative psychological treatment including exposure and social skills, self-help, or short-term psychodynamic psychotherapy specifically designed for SAD (Mayo-Wilson et al., 2014; National Institute for Health and Care Excellence, 2013).

Enhanced CBT Is Superior to Traditional CBT

Rapee and colleagues (2009) conducted an RCT comparing three group treatments: traditional CBT, enhanced CBT, and stress management. Traditional CBT involved cognitive restructuring (e.g., thought challenging) and graded *in vivo* exposure based on a habituation model (i.e., repeated exposure will reduce anxious responding). Cognitive restructuring targeted negative automatic thoughts but not core beliefs. Enhanced CBT targeted more of the key maintaining factors reviewed earlier in this chapter (i.e., negative cognitive content–negative automatic thoughts, negative self-images, and negative core beliefs; avoidance and safety behaviors; and self-focused attention). Cognitive restructuring and in vivo exposure were important components of the enhanced treatment, but exposure was conducted as behavioral experiments with a cognitive rationale (hypothesis testing and evidence gathering) rather than a habituation rationale. Enhanced CBT also included challenging of negative underlying core beliefs, *in vivo* exercises aimed at eliminating safety behaviors, attention retraining, and video feedback. The stress management treatment included general psychoeducation about the fight-or-flight response that was not specific to social threat, relaxation skills, problem solving, time management, and healthy lifestyle habits.

Rapee and colleagues (2009) found that the enhanced and traditional treatments were both more effective than stress management in terms of the proportion of clients meeting diagnostic criteria for SAD at posttreatment. Clinically significant change indicates that an individual's symptom severity falls within the normative (nonclinical) range after treatment. On symptom measures, a significantly higher proportion of clients in the enhanced group (31–42%) achieved clinically significant change compared to the traditional group (18–22%). The enhanced group also had superior outcomes on a measure of clinician-rated severity. Therefore, overall enhanced CBT was superior to more traditional CBT, and the findings suggest that broadly targeting the key cognitive-behavioral maintaining factors improves outcomes.

Other studies evaluating individual CBT that incorporated imagery-based strategies have found that this treatment is also highly effective. Clark and colleagues' (2003; see also Clark et al., 2006) treatment included strategies to reduce reliance on safety behaviors and self-focused attention, and to shift attention onto the social situation. Video feedback, behavioral experiments, strategies for reducing anticipatory and postevent processing, and restructuring of dysfunctional assumptions were also core components of the intervention. Clark and colleagues (2003, 2006) found that their approach was associated with very large effect sizes that are among the largest in the literature. The manual on which these treatments are based remains unpublished, although the procedures have been described (Clark, 2001; Wells, 1997, pp. 167–199).

But Enhanced CBT Is Still Not Good Enough

CBT currently has the strongest evidence for its efficacy, but many people continue to suffer with symptoms after completing gold-standard treatment (Mayo-Wilson et al., 2014; McEvoy et al., 2012). Although effect sizes are large, with symptoms reducing by around one standard deviation or more on average, most effectiveness studies have found that only a minority of clients' symptoms fall within the normative range after treatment (McEvoy et al., 2012; Rapee et al., 2009). Moreover, attrition rates of 25–35% are not unusual (Hofmann & Suvak, 2006; Lincoln et al., 2005; McEvoy et al., 2012). We decided to revisit theory and recent research on emotion and treatment innovations in an attempt to improve treatment engagement and outcomes, which led us to inject a more comprehensive dose of imagery-based strategies throughout Rapee and colleagues' (2009) enhanced CBT protocol. Before describing the imagery-based enhancements in Chapter 3, we first present the evidence that led us to believe that this could be a fruitful avenue to pursue.

Imagery as an Important Treatment Target for SAD

A distorted mental representation of the self that is highly discrepant with perceived external standards is central to Rapee and Heimberg's (1997) conceptualization of SAD, and thus is a key treatment target. More recently Heimberg and colleagues (2010, 2014) extended Rapee and Heimberg's model by considering the potent role that imagery plays in maintaining negative affect more broadly. Heimberg and colleagues (2010) also elaborated the contribution of negative self-imagery to SAD in particular by reviewing evidence that negative self-imagery is common in SAD, reflects recollections of past social situations from the observer perspective, and adversely affects performance in social situations.

Negative Self-Imagery Is Common in SAD

Accumulating evidence strongly suggests that individuals with SAD experience more negative images of past social situations than nonanxious or low-social-anxiety controls, before, during, and after social situations (Hackmann, Clark, & McManus, 2000; Hackmann, Surawy, & Clark, 1998; Hinrichsen & Clark, 2003). Compared to controls, these images are also more distorted in people with SAD, reflecting negative self-referential themes and feared predictions of negative evaluation. Consistent with the cognitive models reviewed earlier in this chapter, the images also tend to be from the observer perspective (through the audience's eyes) rather than the field perspective (looking outward from one's own eyes) for those with SAD (Hackmann et al., 1998; Wells, Clark, & Ahmad, 1998), particularly for highly anxiety provoking situations (Coles, Turk, Heimberg, & Fresco, 2001). Hackmann and colleagues (2000) found that 100% of a SAD sample ($N = 22$) reported negative, multisensory social imagery within social situations, and the negative imagery tended to be associated with social traumas occurring around the onset of the disorder ("ghosts from the past"; see Hackmann, Bennett-Levy, & Holmes, 2011, p. 133). Hackmann and colleagues further speculated that the imagery may have therefore contributed to the development of the disorder, or at least to the exacerbation of symptoms. This finding is consistent with Clark and Wells's (1995) and Rapee and Heimberg's (1997) models, which suggest that current negative cognitions are informed by past social experiences.

Subsequent research has found that most individuals high in social anxiety report negative social imagery (Chiupka, Moscovitch, & Bielak, 2012). Importantly, Moscovitch, Gavric, Merrifield, Bielak, and Moscovitch (2011) found that although low socially anxious individuals also reported negative imagery, high socially anxious individuals retrieve a higher ratio of negative-to-positive images and less detailed positive images. Moreover, high socially anxious individuals experienced stronger negative affect and less positive affect when retrieving negative images, and both Moscovitch and colleagues and Chiupka and colleagues (2012) found that images in high socially anxious individuals contained more negative self-related themes and had a greater adverse influence on beliefs about themselves, others, and the world. Chiupka and colleagues suggested that the negative *meanings* high socially anxious individuals attach to their negative imagery may distinguish high versus low socially anxious individuals, rather than the occurrence of negative imagery per se, which is common across the social anxiety spectrum. Interestingly, while anticipatory processing prior to a social stressor task was associated with more negative social images and associated negative affect, negative images during postevent processing after a social situation resulted in more self-criticism.

Negative Imagery Adversely Impacts Social Performance

Experimental research has demonstrated that negative self-imagery is associated with adverse cognitive, behavioral, and emotional sequelae in both clinical and nonclinical samples. In socially anxious individuals, holding negative self-images in mind (compared to neutral images) is associated with more negative self-evaluations of anxiety intensity and performance, as well as poorer performance as rated by blind assessors (Hirsch, Clark, Mathews, & Williams, 2003; Hirsch, Mathews, Clark, Williams, & Morrison, 2006; Hirsch, Meynen, & Clark, 2004; Makkar & Grisham, 2011). Makkar and Grisham (2011) used a similar methodology by asking high and low socially anxious participants to hold negative or control self-images in mind during a brief speech task, but these researchers investigated an even broader array of consequences. Participants instructed to hold a negative self-image reported higher anxiety, more self-focused attention, more negative self-cognitions, stronger beliefs that their anxiety was visible to others, more negative appraisals of their performance, and more negative postevent processing, even after controlling for depression. In a systematic review, Ng, Abbott, and Hunt (2014) examined the role of self-imagery in social anxiety and found large effects of negative self-imagery on anxiety, and on observer- and self-rated performance appraisals.

Heimberg and colleagues (2010) cautioned that the act of intentionally holding negative images in mind places considerable cognitive demands on participants that may adversely affect performance independent of the content of the images. Additionally, intentionally holding negative images in mind may not reflect the naturally intrusive images experienced by individuals with SAD. Notwithstanding these caveats, these studies do demonstrate that negative images, compared to control or positive images, have a greater impact on a range of factors theoretically implicated in the maintenance of social anxiety.

Updates to the Role of Negative Self-Imagery in SAD

Heimberg and colleagues' (2010, 2014) updated model includes two key additions to the original model that are relevant to imagery, specifically *observation/image of self and audience behavior* and *postevent processing*. Negative self-imagery is fundamental to the former and also features prominently in the latter. The updated model emphasizes the use of this image of the self and the audience's behavior as a comparator for the audience's expected standard. The more negative and distorted this image, the greater the perceived discrepancy with the audience's perceived standard and, in turn, the higher the perceived probability and cost of evaluation from the audience. This recent addition to the model suggests that strategies that can effectively correct distorted self-images are likely to minimize the discrepancy with the expected standard and thus reduce the behavioral, physical, and cognitive symptoms of SAD. Heimberg and colleagues (2014) also reviewed evidence that negative images from past social failures guide self-images before, during, and after current social situations, and that these past images are more likely to be framed from the observer perspective over time (Coles et al., 2001; Vassilopoulos, 2005).

Positive Imagery Deficits in SAD

In addition to excessive negative imagery, socially anxious individuals also have a paucity of positive and neutral self-images (Amir, Najmi, & Morrison, 2012; Moscovitch et al., 2011). Pictet (2014) reviewed evidence that in addition to targeting negative imagery, eliciting and elaborating positive imagery can be beneficial in social anxiety. SAD is associated with both high negative affectivity and low positive affect (Weeks, 2015), and people with SAD are less likely than others to approach or interpret situations positively (Alden & Taylor, 2004; Kashdan, 2007; Weeks & Heimberg, 2012). Imagining positive events occurring in the future has been found to influence the *perception* that the positive events are likely to occur in the future (Carroll, 1978), and to enhance motivation and goal-oriented behavior (Libby, Shaeffer, Eibach, & Slemmer, 2007; Pictet, Coughtrey, Mathews, & Holmes, 2011). These findings have been found to apply to social anxiety in particular, with evidence that positive imagery is associated with less anxiety and superior performance in speech tasks, compared to when negative images are held in mind (e.g., Stopa, Brown, & Hirsch, 2012; Stopa & Jenkins, 2007). In treatment, individuals with SAD may therefore benefit from both (1) challenging negative images and (2) bolstering positive images.

Imagery as a Mode of Intervention in Emotional Disorders

Imagery as an Emotional Amplifier

In addition to negative imagery being critical in the maintenance of SAD in particular, there is strong evidence that imagery is powerfully associated with emotion more generally. The neural pathways and physiological, behavioral, and conceptual responses activated by imagery are similar to those activated by *in vivo* exposure to threatening stimuli

(Kosslyn, 1994; Lang, 1979). Consistent with this idea, Kosslyn, Ganis, and Thompson (2001) suggested that "mental imagery occurs when perceptual information is accessed from memory, giving rise to the experience of 'seeing with the mind's eye,' 'hearing with the mind's ear,' and so on "(p. 635). Experimental studies that have manipulated participants' use of verbal thoughts and imagery have demonstrated that imagery elicits more intense affective responding than verbal-linguistic activity (Holmes & Mathews, 2010). These findings extend to both negative and positive stimuli, such that negative imagery elicits more intense negative affect than negative verbal activity and positive imagery elicits more intense positive affect than positive verbal activity (Holmes, Lang, & Shah, 2009; Holmes & Mathews, 2005).

This phenomenon is easy to demonstrate. If you read the word "zombie" here, you are unlikely to have a strong emotional response. Now just take a minute to bring to mind vivid images of zombies and note any physiological, affective, behavioral, and cognitive responses you have to the images. Likewise, the words "happy child" may be pleasant, but simply reading them is unlikely to elicit a strong affective response. Again, bringing to mind vivid images of smiling, giggling children is likely to elicit a stronger affective response than simply reading the words, at least for people who are fond of children! Images of one's own happy child might elicit stronger positive affect than those of an unfamiliar child. Images of personal faux pas recalled from the past or anticipated in the future might elicit stronger negative affect than those of others. So regardless of the valence (positive or negative), imagery is likely to elicit more intense affect than reading the words. If imagery intensifies emotional responses, and our aim in therapy is to modify affective responses to social cues (i.e., up-regulating positive affect and down-regulating negative affect), then treatment strategies within the imagery mode are more likely to produce larger and more robust affective change.

Potential Mechanisms of Affective Change in Imagery-Based Interventions

Three potentially complementary psychological models could explain how imagery-based interventions are more effective than verbal-linguistic strategies: avoidance theory (Borkovec, Alcaine, & Behar, 2004), emotional processing theory (Foa & Kozak, 1986), and retrieval competition theory (Brewin, 2006). The avoidance theory of worry (Borkovec et al., 2004) proposes that worry is primarily experienced as verbal-linguistic activity and is negatively reinforced by suppressing more intense physiological responses associated with imagery-based processing. In this way, worry functions as a cognitive avoidance strategy that prevents full emotional processing of fear stimuli and thus serves to maintain emotional disorder. Worry is one form of repetitive negative thinking that shares many features of other forms, such as anticipatory and postevent processing in SAD. Imagery-based approaches encourage clients to directly process arousing negative imagery, thereby circumventing verbal-linguistic suppression of physiological arousal. In contrast, verbally based approaches allow clients to remain in the verbal-linguistic mode, thereby potentially inhibiting full emotional processing of negative imagery and limiting modification of the fear network (Foa, Huppert, & Cahill, 2006).

Foa and Kozak (1986) argue that the entire fear structure, which includes stimulus, response, and meaning propositions, must be accessed for extinction to occur. The emotional processing theory proposes two necessary conditions for extinction: (1) the fear structure must be activated and (2) information that is incompatible with elements of the fear structure must be made available. Foa and Kozak argue that physiological arousal indicates that the fear structure has been activated, and habituation to the feared stimulus indicates emotional processing. Consistent with Borkovec and colleagues (2004), Foa and Kozak's model suggests that higher physiological arousal experienced during imagery-based strategies, compared to verbal strategies, creates the opportunity for more complete emotional processing, which should result in superior outcomes. It has been suggested that imaginal exposure may be even more effective than *in vivo* exposure at activating all aspects of the fear network because it is impossible to create all feared situations, and many feared consequences are rare (Beidel et al., 2014). In contrast, anything is possible within imagery. More recent behavioral accounts argue that the discrepancy between expectancies and actual outcomes (i.e., prediction errors) is most important for new learning (Craske, Treanor, Conway, Zbozinek, & Vervliet, 2014). The capacity for imagery to contain vivid and specific expectancies across a range of contexts that are not limited by practicalities may mean that the opportunities for prediction errors during exposure tasks are maximized.

Brewin's (2006) retrieval competition theory argues that the purpose of therapy is to "alter the relative accessibility of memory representations containing positive and negative information" (p. 773). These memory representations can include knowledge structures, sensory features (e.g., episodic memories, images), somatic and motor responses, and verbal-linguistic activity. Brewin argues that successful therapy helps individuals to create new, more positive representations in memory that effectively compete with original negative representations. Brewin's model therefore predicts that superior interventions will activate positive memories with more potency and valence, which will more effectively compete with and reduce access to older negative memories.

Clearly these theories are highly compatible. Imagery-based interventions circumvent imagery suppression (Borkovec, 1994; Borkovec et al., 2004), which may facilitate more intense arousal and greater activation of the fear network. This facilitates greater potential for habituation (Foa & Kozak, 1986) and inhibitory learning via prediction errors (Craske et al., 2014), which, in turn, allow for more potent and positive memory representations to be newly consolidated (Brewin, 2006). A comprehensive review of these models and the evidence for the proposed mechanisms is beyond the scope of this chapter. Suffice to say that the superiority of imagery compared to verbal-linguistic activity in promoting affective change in psychotherapy is on very safe theoretical and empirical ground.

Summary

Contemporary cognitive-behavioral models suggest that negative thoughts and images (before, during, and after social events), avoidance, safety behaviors, biased self-images, self- and environment-focused attention, and negative core beliefs are critical maintaining factors for SAD. The treatment in Part II of this book is structured around these factors. By targeting these factors, existing treatments have resulted in large effect sizes. Evidence that negative imagery is a common and prominent maintaining factor in SAD, and that imagery is more potent at eliciting affect than verbal-linguistic activity, encouraged us to incorporate imagery-based strategies throughout the treatment outlined in Part II of this book. The use of imagery in psychotherapy is not new (Edwards, 2007), and previous SAD treatments have incorporated some imagery-based strategies (Clark et al., 2003; Rapee et al., 2009). Imagery was always intended to be an important part of CBT (Beck, Rush, Shaw, & Emery, 1979), but until recently it was relatively absent from standard CBT for most emotional disorders, including social anxiety. Typically, verbal-linguistic methods such as "thought" challenging have been emphasized in treatment. While self-imagery has been targeted in CBT for SAD (Clark et al., 2003; Harvey, Clark, Ehlers, & Rapee, 2000), previous treatments have not explicitly and comprehensively incorporated imagery-based strategies into all of their components and thus may not have fully exploited the particularly powerful relationship between imagery and emotion, and its capacity to optimize affective change (McEvoy et al., 2015).

The treatment from which the imagery-enhanced CBT protocol was developed has been extensively evaluated and shown to be effective within research, community clinic, and private practice settings (Gaston, Abbott, Rapee, & Neary, 2006; McEvoy et al., 2012; Rapee et al., 2009). The strategies from this treatment are included in this book, but these have been comprehensively enhanced with additional imagery-based components. The imagery-enhanced protocol described in the book has been evaluated in an initial pilot (McEvoy & Saulsman, 2014) and in a larger open trial (McEvoy et al., 2015). In our open trial the outcomes compared extremely favorably to international benchmarks, exceeding previous group treatments and being comparable to some of the largest effect sizes for individual therapy in the literature.

In Chapter 3 we provide an overview of the imagery enhancements incorporated into Part II of this book, along with some guidance on treatment structure.

Overview of Imagery-Enhanced CBT for SAD

In this chapter we first provide an overview of the model used to guide treatment in Part II of this book, followed by a brief description of the strategies used to target each SAD maintaining factor. We then provide some guidance to therapists about structuring and delivering individual and group-based imagery-enhanced CBT for SAD.

A Model of SAD and Treatment Targets

The theories reviewed in Chapter 2 converge on six key maintaining factors that need to be targeted in treatment for SAD. These factors are prominent in the model we use with clients to formulate their social anxiety and treatment plan (see Figure 3.1). The shaded aspects of the model suggest that particular triggers (social situations) lead to a perception of social threat, which, in turn, leads to the fear response (i.e., fight or flight). The fight-or-flight response includes all the physical symptoms of social anxiety such as sweating, shaking, blushing, hyperventilation, dizziness, urge to escape, and so on. We next review each factor that maintains the perception of social threat, moving clockwise around the model, which reflects the order of treatment. We also discuss the strategies used to target each factor in imagery-enhanced CBT, and ways in which imagery-enhanced CBT may be similar to and different from other approaches.

Negative Social Thoughts and Images

The first focus of SAD treatment is to identify and target *negative social thoughts and images* that elicit and maintain a perception of social threat. It makes intuitive sense that if people hold more neutral or positive thoughts and images regarding social situations, then other maintaining factors within the SAD model will resolve (i.e., avoidance, safety

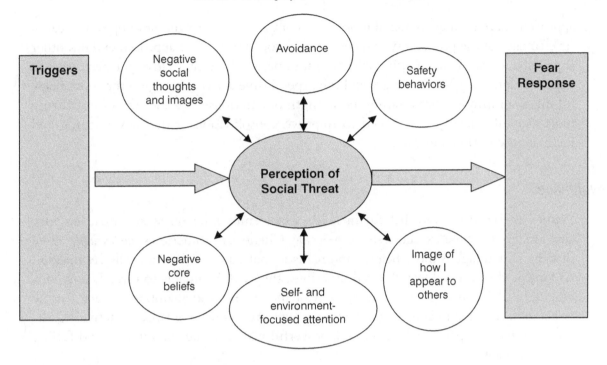

FIGURE 3.1. A client-friendly model of SAD.

behaviors, negative self-image, and self-focused attention). These additional maintaining factors are essentially attempts to prevent negative social thoughts and images from coming true. While the relationship between all these maintaining factors is reciprocal (i.e., modifying avoidance, safety behaviors, negative self-image, and self-focused attention can alter negative social thoughts and images), within these relationships cognition still holds a central and causal role. The therapist first needs to be aware of the specific details of the client's perceived social threat, revealed by the negative social thoughts and images, as this allows the function of the other maintaining factors to be better understood, and hence targeted with maximum effect later in treatment.

The approach to targeting negative thoughts and images shares key features with other treatments that focus predominantly on negative thoughts, including monitoring and then challenging unhelpful cognitions. Our approach diverges from most other treatments in its explicit focus on imagery-based cognitions. Imagery-enhanced CBT describes an extensive rationale to clients for focusing on imagery rather than only negative thoughts (i.e., imagery increases specificity, elicits stronger emotions, and facilitates behavioral experiments). Rather than using thought records to monitor and challenge cognitive products, imagery-enhanced CBT uses imagery records. Negative thoughts about the probability and cost of social fears are still monitored and targeted, but from the first session, clients are socialized to attend to naturally occurring negative images and to transform thoughts into images.

Once clients are able to identify thoughts and imagery, the restructuring process can begin. At this stage clients are prompted to identify negative images and, as in other approaches, are then encouraged to identify contrary evidence and develop more realistic estimates of the probability and cost of their social fears. Our approach extends other approaches by then encouraging clients to summarize these alternative perspectives into a more helpful or realistic image, and then spend time actively bringing the more helpful image to mind before rerating the strength of emotions. The addition of visualizing more helpful imagery is designed to improve consolidation of the new learning and increase its emotional impact.

Avoidance

While entertaining more helpful imagery when embarking on social situations may ease anxiety to some extent, *seeing is believing*. Clients can sometimes *intellectually* agree that the new image is more helpful and realistic, but emotionally they still *feel* anxious. As long as clients avoid feared social situations, they will be unable to directly and convincingly test their negative images, so avoidance is the next maintaining factor to be targeted in treatment via behavioral experiments. Reversing avoidance by actively gathering evidence experientially is often a powerful way to bring the intellect and feeling into alignment.

Behavioral experiments offer a structured way of directly testing negative social images in the real world to maximize learning, and they are the most important component of SAD treatment. Behavioral experiments resemble *in vivo* exposure in most respects, with both techniques challenging expectancies, and in practice it is virtually impossible to isolate behavioral from cognitive change. Although behavioral experiments are initially labor intensive, as clients fully embrace and internalize this process they become less formal. The empiricism promoted by behavioral experiments becomes the new philosophy by which clients approach social situations they are apprehensive about—being curious about their anticipatory imagery, participating fully in the situation rather than avoiding, and then reflecting on the difference between imagination and reality.

Behavioral experiments will initially need to be meticulously planned and conducted and comprehensively debriefed within the session. Imagery challenging can initially be used to prepare clients to engage in behavioral experiments that they find particularly anxiety-provoking, but as clients have more success imagery challenging may not be required. Most aspects of behavioral experiments used in this treatment are similar to other CBT interventions, with two key differences. First, clients are asked to describe their predictions using imagery, again so that predictions are as rich in detail, breadth, and specificity as possible. Second, clients are encouraged to consolidate their learning and increase its emotional impact after the behavioral experiment by eliciting a vivid new image of the scenario that incorporates the new evidence observed.

Imagery-enhanced CBT includes coping imagery as an additional treatment strategy to assist with engagement with behavioral experiments. The use of coping imagery can be conceptualized as an imagery-based form of anxiety surfing. Clients are encouraged to create a metaphorical image that represents their anxiety for them (e.g., drowning at sea) and then create a resolution to the problem within the imagery (e.g., envisaging oneself as a powerful Olympic swimmer who is able to overcome the swell and swim to shore with a renewed sense of strength and self-efficacy). Clients are encouraged to attend to the emotional valence (e.g., excited, determined), meanings (e.g., strength, power, confidence, capacity to cope, hope), physical aspects (e.g., body language), and somatic associations that accompany this new image and creatively elaborate the new image to enhance consolidation (e.g., paintings, paired with music or within additional imagery). This new image can then be used in the service of approaching (not avoiding) social situations during behavioral experiments and in social contexts in general.

Safety Behaviors

Avoidance of social situations altogether is only one way clients try to prevent social fears coming true. Not all social situations can be avoided, so clients develop an arsenal of more subtle and creative avoidance behaviors that can be deployed in an attempt to prevent feared outcomes. These are known as safety behaviors and can take many forms (e.g., using alcohol before attending a social function, averting one's gaze from others to reduce social engagement, using heavy makeup to cover blushing). Regardless of their form, safety behaviors share a common purpose—an attempt to prevent social catastrophe. Unfortunately, these strategies actually maintain and exacerbate social anxiety, so they need to be addressed.

The approach used in imagery-enhanced CBT to challenge the helpfulness of safety behaviors, thereby providing a rationale for abandoning them, is similar to that used in other approaches. After you discuss the function and impacts of safety behaviors, clients complete a behavioral experiment that manipulates the use of safety behaviors by contrasting the impact of using versus abandoning them during a social interaction. This experiment ideally assists clients to recognize the unhelpfulness and futility of these strategies. In imagery-enhanced CBT this experiment diverges slightly from other approaches by encouraging clients to elicit in advance vivid images of how they expect the interaction to play out. The aim of this extra step is to maximize prediction errors by creating specific, broad, and vivid predictions that will maximize any discrepancy with the actual outcomes. In addition, imaginal rehearsal of not using safety behaviors can help clients to become more familiar and comfortable with this new way of interacting.

Image of How I Appear to Others

Negative self-images are a key feature of SAD, with sufferers believing that the image in their mind's eye is an accurate representation of what observers are seeing. This self-image is typically highly distorted, often with physical symptoms being far more obvious than they are in reality, which dramatically escalates the perceived likelihood of negative evaluation. As with other negative social images, behavioral experimentation is required to test their accuracy. All contemporary evidence-supported treatments of SAD, including imagery-enhanced CBT, target negative self-images in similar ways. Clients may design experiments where they request feedback from trusted family members, colleagues, teachers, or friends, but the most powerful experiment involves video feedback because it provides an opportunity for clients to directly test negative self-images themselves. When setting up video-feedback experiments in other CBT approaches, clients are usually asked how they *think* they appear to others, and particularly what anxiety symptoms they *think* are most obvious. In imagery-enhanced CBT, clients are asked to elicit a vivid mental *image* of how they appear to others when they are socially anxious. Features of this mental image are then directly compared to a video-recorded image of them completing an anxiety-provoking social task, such as a speech task or social interaction. Imagery-enhanced CBT adds one final step to this process to further consolidate learning, whereby the client is encouraged to elicit the new more objective self-image within a variety of contexts to generalize learning beyond the single behavioral experiment.

Attentional Problems: Self- and Environment Focus

An important source of threat in SAD is the self because people with SAD fear negative evaluation from others if their anxiety symptoms or social incompetence is exposed. As a consequence, people with SAD closely scrutinize their anxiety and behavior to ensure that it is meeting others' perceived standards. In addition to self-focus, people with SAD scrutinize their environment for any sign of negative evaluation from others. For example, while talking to a friend they might be scanning the room for any sign that others are looking in their direction or laughing. The individual with SAD then assumes the laughter is directed toward them, when in reality it is unrelated to their social performance.

One consequence of this self- and environment-focused (i.e., "off-task") attention is that normal behaviors and fluctuations in physical sensations are more likely to be noticed, which then triggers a range of predictions about negative social consequences. Individuals whose attention is off task are also less likely to detect and therefore respond appropriately to social cues, which may then lead to underengagement in conversations and the appearance of aloofness, which, in turn may increase the actual likelihood of negative evaluation. It is therefore critical that people with SAD increase their awareness of when their attention wanders off task (e.g., away from the content of the conversation), and then actively deploy their attention back onto the task at hand. Like other treatments (Clark et al., 2003; Rapee et al., 2009), imagery-enhanced CBT uses behavioral experiments comparing self-focused attention versus task-focused attention during a social interaction to demonstrate the impact of off-task attention on anxiety and social performance. Imagery-enhanced CBT diverges from other approaches by encouraging clients to imagine themselves being task focused prior to completing the interaction. The rationale for this step is to clarify exactly which elements of the social experience they would be attending to if they were more task focused, and prime them to engage in these behaviors during the task so they are less likely to revert to habitual self-focus.

Consistent with other treatments (e.g., Rapee et al., 2009), clients are taught attention-retraining and attention-focusing tasks. These tasks are designed to increase clients' awareness of where they are deploying their attention, first in nonsocial and then in social contexts, and to strengthen their ability to shift their attention onto the task at hand. These strategies are described as approaches for strengthening the "attention muscle," which can then be used when needed in social situations to disengage from unhelpful self-focused attention.

Negative Core Beliefs

Negative core beliefs about the self, others, and the world guide the negative thoughts and images people hold regarding socializing in the here and now. In the social anxiety model used in this treatment, negative core beliefs occupy a bubble that may seem to be on par with the other maintaining factors, but they can be conceptualized as an underlying factor that ultimately gives rise to the other maintaining factors. If someone has a negative core belief about herself (e.g., as defective) and others (e.g., as judgmental), then it makes sense that all the other maintaining factors addressed in the model will emerge as a result of this core belief (i.e., negative social thoughts and images, avoidance, safety behaviors, negative self-image, and self-focused attention). These factors arise as a means of warning and (ostensibly) protecting the client from the threat of negative social consequences once her core "defectiveness" is exposed.

Negative core beliefs drive the various maintaining factors in the model, but the relationship is reciprocal such that the other factors also reinforce core beliefs. For example, if the client has very *negative social thoughts and images* of rejection in an anticipated social situation because of his negative core beliefs, this generates the same felt experience as actual rejection, which serves to fuel his core beliefs. This cycle promotes *avoidance* of the social situation, which deprives the client of the opportunity to have positive or neutral experiences that would contradict his core beliefs. Therefore, core beliefs are not modified and continue to drive the vicious cycle.

If the client does approach the social situation, but only while engaging in *safety behaviors*, then positive or neutral experiences may be attributed to the safety behaviors, again preventing core beliefs from being modified. While in the social situation, if the client is experiencing very *negative self-images*, this will be taken as confirmation of his negative core beliefs regarding the self. Finally, if his *attention is highly self-focused* during the experience, then unpleasant feelings, sensations, and images will be encoded at the expense of more benign aspects of the situation. Heightened anxiety and self-consciousness, which self-focused attention promotes, provides a felt sense that his core belief in his own "defectiveness" is accurate. In addition, when any remaining attentional capacity is focused on perceived threats in the *environment* (e.g., two people sharing a joke and laughing on the other side of a room), this leads to the interpretation of ambiguous social cues in a negative manner ("They are laughing at me!"), providing further confirmation of the accuracy of the client's negative core beliefs regarding others.

Unlike some negative thoughts or images, core beliefs cannot be tested and modified from a single behavioral experiment; instead they only begin to shift following extensive experiential learning. Sufficient experiential learning can only be gained from the accumulation of new positive or neutral social experiences, or by coping with negative social experiences. The cognitive, behavioral, and attentional changes promoted by addressing the previous maintaining factors in the model are likely to be necessary before clients with SAD are in a position to accumulate and process social experiences in an adaptive way. For these reasons, core beliefs are usually explicitly targeted later in treatment.

Consistent with other treatments (e.g., Rapee et al., 2009), imagery-enhanced CBT includes downward-arrowing techniques for identifying core beliefs, and evidence gathering for modifying core beliefs. In addition, imagery-enhanced CBT incorporates two imagery-based strategies for directly modifying core beliefs. The first one is imagery rescripting. Imagery rescripting has been used for a range of disorders and within individual CBT for SAD (e.g., Clark et al., 2003), but we have also successfully used it within our SAD groups. The rescripting approach used in this treatment is informed by Arntz and Weertman's (1999) and Wild and Clark's (2011) imagery rescripting process. In this approach, past traumatic events (i.e., memories) from which negative core beliefs have developed are identified. Within imagery, clients then have the opportunity to reexperience these past events from new perspectives, which can facilitate more functional meanings to the events and hence undermine negative core beliefs.

The second imagery-based strategy targeting negative core beliefs derives from Padesky and Mooney's (2005, cited in Hackmann et al., 2011) "Old System/New System" approach, which recruits positive imagery as a platform for constructing new more helpful and positive core beliefs. These new positive core beliefs can then be strengthened through *in vivo* activities. This process is seen as a more helpful alternative to just breaking down old negative core beliefs because it focuses the client on building a positive view by imagining *how they would like to be* in the world. Imagining this more adaptive way of operating, and then purposely acting in a manner that is consistent with this positive image, can provide a path to building and strengthening new core beliefs over time.

Treatment Structure

Individual Therapy

Individual therapy affords the flexibility of targeting each component of the client's idiosyncratic case formulation. Clinicians are limited only by their creativity in designing behavioral experiments that will provide opportunities to directly test negative thoughts and imagery and maximize the "prediction errors" for each individual. The client and therapist can ensure that time is efficiently and effectively spent working through each component of the treatment, only moving on to each successive component when the client has developed competence and confidence in applying the earlier principles. Individual therapy also offers more flexibility to repeat or complete additional behavioral experiments within the same session or across sessions to consolidate learning.

In individual therapy, the therapist can titrate each component to the client's needs, and the number of sessions will vary depending on client severity, complexity, and engagement. In our clinic we typically plan for 12–15 weekly, 50-minute sessions to work through each of the modules in sufficient depth. Longer sessions can be scheduled (e.g., 90 minutes) if the therapist believes this is required to ensure enough time to fully process and debrief from a strategy (e.g., imagery rescripting) or to complete an extended behavioral experiment session. Although there is some flexibility in treatment length, imagery-enhanced CBT was designed as an efficient and effective time-limited treatment, so we would rarely offer more than 15 sessions plus follow-ups. However, if clients are not engaging well with the treatment, or if they do not seem to be benefiting, obstacles to change need to be addressed as soon as possible before proceeding.

As outlined in the treatment session guide in Table 3.1, we usually spend two to three sessions socializing clients to the model and then introducing thought and imagery monitoring and challenging. The module on avoidance, safety behaviors, and behavioral experiments is the focus for the next three sessions. At least one of the behavioral experiment sessions involves a series of *in vivo* experiments with the therapist out in

TABLE 3.1. Individual Treatment Session Guide

Session	Content	Chapter
Sessions 1–3	Introduction to social anxiety, model, imagery monitoring and challenging	4 and 5
Sessions 4 and 5	Avoidance and behavioral experiments, coping imagery, hierarchies, safety behaviors	6
Session 6	Within-session behavioral experiments, review hierarchies	6
Session 7	Self-imagery: video feedback	7
Session 8	Attention retraining and focusing	8
Session 9	Within-session behavioral experiments (challenging cost using shame attacking)	6
Session 10	Rescripting past imagery	9
Sessions 11 and 12	Positive imagery and action planning: constructing new core beliefs	9
Session 13	Review and relapse prevention	10
Session 14	Follow-up: progress, dealing with setbacks, future imagery	10

Note. Session numbers can vary based on individual client needs.

the "real world." Clients do need to be able to identify the content of their cognitions with minimal prompting but do not need to be highly skilled at imagery challenging before behavioral methods are introduced. Given that behavior change creates the best opportunities for cognitive change, we don't want to delay this by waiting for the client to perfect imagery challenging. Imagery challenging will be a skill they continue to develop over treatment. The skills covered in the first five or six sessions are reviewed at the beginning of each therapy session thereafter, to ensure that the client continues to regularly apply the principles.

One session is then dedicated to challenging negative self-images via video feedback, followed by another session on introducing the concept of self-focused attention and practicing the skills of attention training and focusing. At this point, and before targeting core beliefs, we often schedule another behavioral experiment session with the therapist, but this time with a clear focus on more challenging "shame-attacking" exercises that are designed to evaluate the true cost of drawing attention to ourselves. One or two sessions are dedicated to imagery rescripting, depending on the number of images that require rescripting, followed by another two sessions on developing more positive core beliefs.

It is important not to lose sight of the main aim, which is not to "cure" the client of negative core beliefs. Instead, the aim is to ensure that clients are operating in the world in such a way that they are continually undermining their old negative core beliefs about themselves and others and strengthening their new balanced perspective. It is about placing them on the path to core belief adjustment over time.

A final relapse prevention session involves a review of all the treatment components and of the client's progress, as well as the development of a self-management plan for maintaining and building on progress made during treatment. Two or three monthly follow-up sessions might also be scheduled to check on progress and to ensure the client maintains his momentum.

Therapy is completed when all treatment components have been covered and clients can independently engage in imagery challenging, behavioral experiments without safety behaviors, and task-focused attention in their daily lives. Once they are doing so, their social anxiety should improve in a meaningful way, with some clients experiencing modest improvements and others experiencing large and highly significant shifts. If they have a clear plan for how they can continue to apply the strategies and deal with setbacks, larger gains will be made as they spend more time in the social world.

Group Therapy

Group treatment offers less flexibility than individual treatment but has other advantages. Our clients often nominate meeting other people with SAD as one of the most helpful aspects of the intervention. They find it tremendously destigmatizing and normalizing to meet other people who genuinely understand what it is like to live with SAD. Group treatments offer opportunities for vicarious learning, which can be particularly helpful for clients who would otherwise be reluctant to take risks in therapy. On countless occasions we have observed reticent group members "take the plunge" after observing the success of other group members, which appears to have more impact than only learning about the principles from therapists. Group CBT for SAD has also been found to be highly effective in research trials. Our early outcomes using imagery-enhanced group CBT have been very promising, with effect sizes that are comparable to or exceed those of other individual and group treatments in the literature.

Our group program consists of 12 weekly 2-hour sessions, plus a 1-month follow-up. A group treatment session overview, along with a detailed session outline, are provided in Tables 3.2 and 3.3, respectively. Groups are co-facilitated by two clinicians, usually one clinical psychologist and a trainee therapist. We have facilitated groups with between 6 and 12 clients with success, although we find that around 8–10 clients is ideal for balancing the need for sufficient time and attention for each individual while maintaining a therapeutic group process. One or two clients may discontinue treatment with the group, which can have a disproportionately negative influence on smaller groups. We have also found that larger groups increase the likelihood of having at least a couple of clients who are particularly eager to apply the treatment principles, which appears to have a positive influence on the progress of the group as a whole (including the therapists).

TABLE 3.2. Group Treatment Session Overview

Session	Content	Chapter
Session 1	Introduction to social anxiety, model, imagery monitoring	4 and 5
Session 2	Imagery challenging	5
Session 3	Avoidance and behavioral experiments, coping imagery	6
Session 4	Avoidance and behavioral experiment hierarchies	6
Session 5	Safety behaviors	6
Session 6	Self-imagery: video feedback	7
Session 7	Within-session behavioral experiments, review hierarchies	6
Session 8	Attention retraining and focusing	8
Session 9	Rescripting past imagery	9
Session 10	Within-session behavioral experiments	6
Session 11	Positive imagery and action planning: constructing new core beliefs	9
Session 12	Review and relapse prevention	10
Session 13	Follow-up: progress, dealing with setbacks, future imagery	10

TABLE 3.3. Detailed Group Session Plan

Session	Content	Handouts/worksheets	Chapter
Session 1	Introduction to social anxiety, model, imagery monitoring *Content* • Set agenda • Welcome, housekeeping, program overview, importance of homework, change expectations, group structure and guidelines (20 min) • What is social anxiety disorder and epidemiology? (10 min) • Overview of treatment model (25 min) • Break (5 min) • Role of imagery in SAD (15 min) • Psychoeducation: imagery rationale, SUDS (15 min) • Thought and imagery monitoring (20 min) • Three take-home messages (5 min) • Homework and preview of next session (5 min) *Homework (provide sheet itemizing homework and new list of accumulating skills each week)* • Set agenda • Read handouts • Complete My Model of Social Anxiety • Complete fear and avoidance list • Complete Looking Forward handout • Thought and imagery recording	What Is Social Anxiety Disorder? (H1) Recording Thoughts and Images (H2) My Model of Social Anxiety (W1) Personal Fear and Avoidance List (W2) Looking Forward (W3) Thought and Imagery Record (W5)	4 and 5
Session 2	Imagery challenging *Content* • Set agenda • Homework review (30 min) • Thought/imagery–feeling connection (15 min) • Imagery challenging (15 min) • Break (5 min) • Imagery-challenging practice: personal examples (45 min) • Three take-home messages (5 min) • Homework and preview (5 min) *Homework* • Read handouts • Imagery challenging	Challenging Negative Thoughts and Images (H3) Thought/Image–Feeling Connection (W4) Imagery Challenging Record (W6)	5
Session 3	Avoidance and behavioral experiments; coping (metaphorical) imagery *Content* • Set agenda • Homework review (20 min) • Rationale for tackling avoidance (10 min) • Behavioral experiments (30 min) • Break (5 min) • Coping (metaphorical) imagery (45 minutes)	The Cycle of Avoidance and Anxiety (H4) Behavioral Experiments (H6) Coping (Metaphorical) Imagery (H9) Imagery Challenging Record (W6) Behavioral Experiment Record (W7) Coping Imagery (W10)	6

(continued)

TABLE 3.3. *(continued)*

Session	Content	Handouts/worksheets	Chapter
Session 3 *(continued)*	• Three take-home messages (5 min) • Homework and preview (5 min) *Homework* • Read handouts • Continue imagery challenging • Start generating ideas for behavioral experiments • Elaborate coping image and practice using it daily		
Session 4	Avoidance and behavioral experiment hierarchies *Content* • Set agenda • Homework review (15 min) • Within-session behavioral experiment setup: walking in single file along street (15 min) • Conduct behavioral experiment (20 min) • Break (5 min) • Complete Behavioral Experiment record (5 min) • Debrief behavioral experiment (15 min) • Start developing individualized hierarchies (35 min) • Three take-home messages (5 min) • Homework and preview (5 min) *Homework* • Read handouts provided • Plan two hierarchies • Complete at least four behavioral experiments and records • Continue practicing imagery challenging and coping imagery	Behavioral Experiment Hierarchies (H8) Behavioral Experiment Hierarchy (W9) Behavioral Experiment Record (W7) Imagery Challenging Record (W6)	6
Session 5	Safety behaviors *Content* • Set agenda • Homework review (20 min) • Safety behaviors: psychoeducation (15 min) • Safety behaviors: imagery exercise (25 min) • Break (5 min) • Safety behaviors: experiment (35 min) • Safety behaviors and hierarchies (10 min) • Three take-home messages (5 min) • Homework and preview (5 minutes) *Homework* • Read handouts • Drop safety behaviors within social situations • Complete behavioral experiments on hierarchy • Continue imagery challenging • Use coping imagery to prepare for behavioral experiments	Safety Behaviors (H5) Safety Behaviors Experiment (W8) Behavioral Experiment Record (W7) Imagery Challenging Record (W6)	6

(continued)

TABLE 3.3. *(continued)*

Session	Content	Handouts/worksheets	Chapter
Session 6	Self-imagery: Video feedback *Content* • Set agenda • Homework review (20 min) • Self-imagery: how I appear to others (10 min) • Video speech task (30 min) • Break (5 min) • Watch recordings in session (45 min) • Three take-home messages (5 min) • Homework and preview (5 min) *Homework* • Read handouts • Watch speech another three times, then rerate • Continue dropping safety behaviors and doing behavioral experiments • Continue image challenging and coping imagery	Self-Image: How I *Really* Appear to Others (H10) Speech Form (W11) Speech Rating Form (W12) Behavioral Experiment Record (W7) Imagery Challenging Record (W6)	7
Session 7	Within-session behavioral experiments *Content* • Set agenda • Homework review (20 min) • In-session group behavioral experiments—from menu (45 min) • Break (5 min) • Review individual behavioral experiment hierarchies (40 min) • Three take-home messages (5 min) • Homework and preview (5 min) *Homework* • Read handouts • Complete four planned behavioral experiments • Continue image challenging and coping imagery	Behavioral Experiment Menu (H7) Behavioral Experiment Record (W7) Imagery Challenging Record (W6)	6
Session 8	Attention retraining and focusing *Content* • Set agenda • Homework review (20 min) • Psychoeducation: role of attention (10 min) • Attention retraining (30 min) • Break (5 min) • Attention focusing (30 min) • Behavioral experiment hierarchies (15 min) • Three take-home messages (5 min) • Homework and preview (5 min) *Homework* • Read handouts • Practice attention retraining multiple times daily and monitor • Practice attention focusing during social interactions	Self-, Environment-, and Task-Focused Attention (H11) Attention Retraining and Focusing (H12) Self- versus Task-Focused Attention Experiment (W13) Attention Retraining Record (W14) Task-Focused Attention Exercise (W15) Behavioral Experiment Record (W7) Imagery Challenging Record (W6)	8

(continued)

TABLE 3.3. *(continued)*

Session	Content	Handouts/worksheets	Chapter
Session 8 *(continued)*	• Monitor one conversation during the week using task-focused attention exercise worksheet • Complete four planned behavioral experiments, including attention focus. • Continue previous skills as required.		
Session 9	Rescripting past imagery *Content* • Set agenda • Homework review (15 min) • Imagery rescripting introduction and image identification (20 min) • Identifying the perspective of the "older self" (10 min) • Break (5 min) • Past imagery rescripting (35 min) • Debrief (25 min) • Three take-home messages (5 min) • Homework and preview (5 min) *Homework* • Read handouts provided • Work on behavioral experiment hierarchies • Rescript past images and/or work with image from today's session • Continue previous skills as required	Past Imagery Rescripting (H13) Past Imagery Rescripting (W16) Behavioral Experiment Record (W7) Imagery Challenging Record (W6)	9
Session 10	Within-session behavioral experiments *Content* • Set agenda • Homework review (30 min) • Within-session individual behavioral experiments—from menu (60 min) • Debrief (20 min) • Three take-home messages (5 min) • Homework and preview (5 min) *Homework* • Read session handouts • Continue working on behavioral experiment hierarchies • Continue using previous skills as required • Arrange a meeting with other group members to do between-session behavioral experiments	Behavioral Experiment Menu (H7) Behavioral Experiment Record (W7) Imagery Challenging Record (W6)	6
Session 11	Positive imagery and action planning: constructing new core beliefs *Content* • Set agenda • Homework review (25 min) • Positive imagery rationale (5 min) • New core belief imagery (15 min) • Break (5 min) • Generalize impact of new core beliefs (45 min)	Constructing New Core Beliefs (H14) Constructing New Core Beliefs (W17) New Core Belief Action Plan (W18)	9

(continued)

TABLE 3.3. *(continued)*

Session	Content	Handouts/worksheets	Chapter
Session 11 *(continued)*	• Action plans (15 min) • Three take-home messages (5 min) • Homework and preview (5 min) *Homework* • Identify icon consistent with new system of core beliefs • Start implementing action plans • Continue working on behavioral experiment hierarchies • Continue with previous skills		
Session 12	Review and relapse prevention *Content* • Set agenda • Homework review (30 min) • Review treatment components (15 min) • Relapse prevention and dealing with setbacks (20 min) • Brief imagery exercise: looking forward (10 min) • Take-home messages from the course, questions, follow-up (10 min) • Posttreatment questionnaires (35 min) *Homework* • Continue applying skills	Skills Toolbox (H15) Dealing with Setbacks (W20)	10
Session 13: Follow-up	Progress review, dealing with setbacks, future plans and imagery *Content* • Set agenda • Welcome back (5 min) • Your progress: review (30 min) • Dealing with setbacks: review (20 min) • Brief imagery exercise: looking forward (10 min) • Final questions (10 min) • Follow-up questionnaires (45 min) • Close group	Your Progress (W19)	10

Who Is Qualified to Provide the Treatment?

The treatment protocol outlined in Part II should be delivered by therapists with supervised experience with CBT so that it is applied competently and with fidelity. Our therapists are all registered or trainee clinical psychologists who receive regular and ongoing supervision, but any appropriately trained and supervised mental health professional can deliver the treatment. We would encourage therapists without a period of supervised CBT practice to seek regular supervision from a CBT specialist, at least for the first few times they deliver the intervention. It is also highly recommended that all outcomes be evaluated using validated measures (see the "Measures to Aid Case Formulation and Outcome Evaluation" section in Chapter 4). Clinicians should compare their outcomes to those in the published literature to ensure their clients are benefiting to a similar degree. If not, it is critical that they seek additional professional development.

Therapists who are highly socially anxious themselves and unwilling to challenge social norms may not be well equipped to effectively treat individuals with SAD. It is important that clinicians who themselves are overly fearful of negative evaluation address their own social anxiety using many of the components outlined in this treatment, either independently or with the assistance of a professional. Of course, many of the behavioral experiments can be at least mildly embarrassing, even for the therapist, but the therapist needs to be willing to model to the client that these emotions can be genuinely experienced and tolerated without it being a social or personal catastrophe. It is critical that therapist anxiety does not lead to avoidance of behavioral experiments, particularly if this approach is novel. Sometimes therapists believe their job is to make clients feel good, rather than help them become good at feeling. In fact our job as therapists is to treat the long-term disorder, not the acute anxiety. Comfortable sessions are usually wasted sessions that are ultimately unhelpful for our clients and are more about meeting therapists' needs. We discuss this issue in more detail in Chapter 6 because if this is not addressed it is likely that therapist anxiety will compromise clients' progress.

Who Can Benefit from the Treatment?

Few reliable predictors of treatment outcome have been identified, which may be disappointing to therapists who wish to predict which clients are best suited to this approach. Reviews of the empirical literature fail to identify replicated sociodemographic or clinical predictors of poor treatment outcome. People whose SAD is more severe at the start of treatment tend to remain most severely affected at the end of treatment, but they appear to improve at the same rate as people with less severe cases. Age, chronicity, and gender are poor predictors of outcome.

The good news from there being very few predictors of outcome is that all clients with SAD have more or less the same chance of benefiting from treatment. As long as the clinician closely monitors progress each session and responds to treatment obstacles, then most clients will benefit, at least to some degree. Clients who do not benefit often acknowledge that they are continuing to avoid social situations and are not applying the treatment principles between sessions. If the case formulation and treatment plan is developed collaboratively, many of these compliance problems can be preempted one way or another. Clients who are unwilling to engage in the challenging tasks required in imagery-enhanced CBT will choose to not proceed past the assessment, although this is rare in our clinic.

There is some evidence that comorbid depression can adversely impact outcomes, but again this is inconsistent in the literature. Clients with severe depression would also typically be referred for treatment for their depression first before determining whether they have a separable SAD that warrants treatment. However, if the depression is clearly temporally and functionally secondary to SAD, and the client has a preference for targeting her SAD, she may be treated for SAD first. We routinely exclude clients who have a comorbid substance use disorder that is likely to interfere with engagement and progress. If substance use is clearly secondary to SAD and thus can be easily formulated as a safety behavior, and the client is willing to reduce her use in general and abstain during treatment sessions and behavioral experiments, then she may not be excluded from treatment. However, if her use is daily and involves a probable physical dependence, we would refer her for individual treatment of her substance use first, or for an integrative approach that simultaneously targets social anxiety and substance use.

When deciding which comorbid problem to address first in therapy, it can be useful to assess the functional relationships between the comorbid conditions. A useful question is "If I had a magic wand and could take away your problem (e.g., depression), would you still be anxious in social situations?" This question can then be asked in the opposite way to determine if the client believes the comorbid problem would continue if her social anxiety was removed. If the client believes her social anxiety would disappear if the comorbid problem was addressed, then the comorbid problem should be targeted first. If she believes that her social anxiety would continue if comorbid problems disappeared, then it may be best to start treating her SAD (unless, as previously mentioned, the comorbid disorder is more debilitating at the time of assessment). If the comorbid problem does not resolve as expected after successful treatment for SAD, the remaining issues are likely to need further intervention.

Client selection for group CBT requires careful consideration. Clients with atypical presentations such as comorbid psychosis are routinely excluded from our groups. An important consideration is that a SAD group should be normalizing, destigmatizing, and validating for all participants. If a client's experiences are substantially different from those of other group members, this can have the opposite effect and interfere with group cohesion and process. In a similar way, clients with crisis needs such as suicidal urges or self-harming behaviors can take a disproportionate amount of therapist time in the group and would normally be better placed in individual treatment. If we are in doubt, we would treat the client individually. More studies on the effectiveness of CBT for clients with comorbid substance use, bipolar disorder, and psychosis are required to guide clinical decision making.

Summary

Imagery-enhanced CBT for SAD targets similar maintaining factors to other evidence-based protocols (e.g., Clark et al., 2003; Rapee et al., 2009). The main point of departure is its emphasis on facilitating affective change by using the imagery mode across all strategies. The treatment modules in Part II of this book are structured around socializing clients to the SAD model (Chapter 4) and then focusing practically on how to address the key maintaining factors in the treatment model, which include negative thoughts and imagery (Chapter 5), avoidance and safety behaviors (Chapter 6), negative self-image (Chapter 7), self- and environment-focused attention (Chapter 8), and negative core beliefs (Chapter 9). Finally we look at the process of completing treatment, with a focus on the maintenance of gains and relapse prevention (Chapter 10).

PART II

Treatment Modules

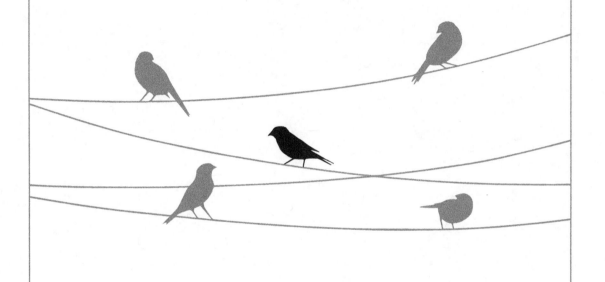

CHAPTER 4

Socializing Clients to the Treatment Model

THERAPIST: Hello, Jacquie, welcome back to the clinic. As we discussed at the end of your assessment last week, the aim of today's session is for us to start putting together a picture of why your social anxiety continues to be a problem. By the end of this session, I am hoping that we will have a shared understanding of what keeps your social anxiety going and, most importantly, what can be done to help you to manage it better and move forward in your life. How does that sound?

CLIENT: Great. But do you really think I can be helped?

THERAPIST: Actually, I am very hopeful that by the end of our sessions together you will have a range of skills and strategies that will help to reduce the impact of social anxiety on your life. This treatment has been shown to be effective for a lot of people just like you.

CLIENT: That's great to hear and I really do want to change, but I think it is going to be very difficult. I've just been this way for so long.

THERAPIST: It certainly sounds like you've really suffered with social anxiety for a long time—it has dictated how you live your life, robbing you of the ability to make genuine choices about what you would like to do. And I'm really sorry to hear that it has been so difficult for you. The good news is that this treatment has been shown to be helpful for people of all ages, regardless of how long they have suffered with social anxiety. You are right to expect that it will be a challenging process. Using some of the strategies might initially be quite anxiety provoking, but I will be here to support you throughout the process and it will get easier with practice. How do you feel about committing to therapy knowing that it is going to be challenging at times?

CLIENT: Well, I can't lie. I am anxious about it, but things have to change. I just can't go on like this.

THERAPIST: It's great to hear that you are ready to make changes, and I'm looking forward to working with you on this. Although it is difficult, it is also tremendously rewarding for people when they start the process of change. And I'll be interested to hear how you're managing at every stage of the process, both when things are going well and when you are struggling. In fact, I can be of most help to you when you're finding it hard. So I hope that you always feel that you can be open with me throughout treatment because to make progress we need to work together as a team. How does that sound?

CLIENT: Scary, but I'll give it a go.

THERAPIST: That's a great answer because it acknowledges that you are committed to the process of change even though you are aware that it will be difficult at times. OK, so let's talk about the factors that are maintaining your social anxiety. Once we understand these factors, it should then be clear why the different strategies you will be learning throughout treatment are going to be helpful to you because the strategies are designed to target each factor. After all, if you're going to be pushing yourself to make changes, it is important that you believe that your efforts will be worthwhile in the longer term.

About This Module: Beginning Treatment

The most important tasks when beginning treatment are to start building rapport and a strong therapeutic alliance, to build cohesion if the program is being delivered in a group format, to instill a strong sense of hope and optimism for change, and to socialize clients to the maintenance model of SAD used to guide treatment. Once the client understands how the model can help to explain what drives his social anxiety, the rationale for the treatment components will become clear. No one would willingly engage in highly distressing tasks in therapy without first being confident that it could be beneficial. Every time we ask our clients to try something new we are asking them to tolerate uncertainty about whether their fears will come true, which is a terrifying prospect for them. This process takes considerable courage and perseverance. Having clients understand the potential payoff, within the context of a supportive therapeutic relationship, is therefore critical to engaging them in the process of change. Time spent collaboratively developing a shared understanding of social anxiety and strategies for better managing the problem is invaluable. This module outlines the process of introducing the treatment approach and model to the client, individualizing the model to the client's presentation, and integrating all sources of available information to develop a case formulation that will guide treatment. At the end of this process the client and therapist should have a shared understanding of what maintains the client's SAD and, most importantly, what changes are needed for treatment to be successful.

Setting the Scene

Building Rapport

It is critical that therapists are able to rapidly build rapport with clients with SAD. The therapist may need to do most of the talking early in the first session until the client's anxiety starts to reduce. Some clients might speak openly from the beginning of the session if they have been in therapy before, or if they believe they are unlikely to be negatively evaluated (i.e., expect unconditional positive regard) by a trained therapist. Other clients will be able to speak more freely as the session progresses, and for others it might take a few sessions before their natural social skills are less inhibited by their anxiety.

If a client appears to find it difficult to interact with the therapist during the first session, there are at least three strategies that could be used. The first option is for the therapist to persevere in asking questions and receiving monosyllabic answers, but this is likely to be inefficient and anxiety provoking for the client. The second option is for the therapist to temporarily change topics and discuss more benign topics, such as the client's hobbies or personal information that is unrelated to social anxiety (e.g., who is in her family, where she was born, travel experiences) until her anxiety subsides somewhat. The therapist will need to be cautious that this does not set a precedent for future sessions, where the client and therapist retreat to "safe" topics to avoid discomfort. The third option is to pay attention to the process in the room by opening up discussion of how the client feels about speaking with the therapist. A sample dialogue might be:

THERAPIST: Tell me more about the sorts of social situations that you find anxiety provoking?

CLIENT: I'm not sure. (*Looks at the floor.*)

THERAPIST: I'm aware that speaking to me about social anxiety can be very difficult. I'm just wondering what's going on for you right now?

CLIENT: Yeah, it's hard. It's all just so stupid. It's embarrassing.

THERAPIST: I'm really sorry that you're feeling uncomfortable right now. It makes sense that it would feel awkward to talk about private experiences that you've been working so hard to hide for so long. I suspect that a lot of the people I see for the first time feel the same way. And they are probably worried that I will judge them if they are open with me about their thoughts and feelings. I'm wondering if this is the case for you?

CLIENT: Yes. I know you're a professional and you're not supposed to judge people, but I still feel embarrassed.

THERAPIST: I think it is very common to feel embarrassed and reluctant to disclose personal information the first time you meet someone. I want you to know that I have seen many people with social anxiety and I understand how difficult this process can be. My hope is that you will never feel judged by me during our time together, but if you do then please let me know so that we can talk about it. You are also welcome to let me know if you would prefer to not answer a question, or if we need to slow down a bit. If it's OK with you, I might just check in now and then about how we are doing together—how you are feeling in the room with me—because it is important to me that you always feel we are working together on the same team. Would that be OK?

CLIENT: Yeah, that's OK. I'm starting to feel a bit more comfortable now.

THERAPIST: That's great to hear. How would you feel about describing some of the social situations that you find most challenging? Feel free to go into as much or little detail as you like . . .

If highly anxious clients continue to find it difficult to describe their social anxiety, at this point the therapist might decide to ask them about topics they are more able to speak freely about, such as work or school, hobbies, pets, or family members. Once the client's anxiety diminishes and rapport has been strengthened, the therapist can venture back to the topic of social anxiety.

Clients with SAD have overcome numerous hurdles just to arrive at the therapist's office. They first needed to identify that they have a significant problem in their lives. This is not an easy task. Many people do not know they are suffering from a diagnosable disorder and that effective treatments are available. Clients may have endured years of anxiety and shame before garnering the courage to admit this to themselves and then disclose the problem.

As a first step toward building rapport, it is important to validate how difficult it is for clients to have made the decision to attend the appointment. Many clients with SAD are not entirely sure that they will attend until the moment they are called from the waiting room, and they may have endured many sleepless nights as the first appointment approaches. Therapists do well by their clients by first acknowledging the important first step toward change they have made simply by attending the appointment. It is often fruitful to ask clients what led to their decision to attend therapy for SAD at this time, as these reasons may need to be revisited at length when treatment becomes particularly challenging.

The Client Is Not Alone

By its very nature SAD is an often lonely disorder that is rarely openly discussed. Our clients generally have never knowingly met another person with SAD so that experiences could be shared, validated, and to some extent normalized. Unsurprisingly, our clients don't go to parties and introduce themselves as someone with SAD, so they have no opportunities to discover just how common it is! An important maintaining factor that needs to be counteracted is self-stigmatization, where people with SAD judge themselves as being weak, different, inadequate, and unacceptable for experiencing social anxiety. These negative self-judgments are often assumed to be shared by others.

It is important that the clinician share how common SAD is in the general community so clients appreciate that they are not alone. Clinicians should also describe some of their experiences of working with social anxiety, so the client is confident that the clinician is genuinely aware of his plight and has expertise in effective treatment approaches. Ensuring clients understand that SAD is one of the most common anxiety disorders and that it affects millions of people can be very helpful. It is useful for therapists to know the approximate rates of SAD in their own country based on relevant population surveys.

There Is Hope

It is also a sad fact that many people suffering from SAD do not seek treatment, and few of those who seek treatment receive an empirically supported intervention. It is important to engender a strong sense of hope by describing outcomes from treatment trials of CBT for SAD and even giving some clients references if they want them. Fortunately the strong evidence that CBT is efficacious in research settings and effective in "real-world" settings gives us reason to be optimistic with our clients about the prospect of a good outcome. It is important that we are generous with this optimism. Part of this discussion may include dispelling any myths about potential obstacles to change, such as age, duration of anxiety, or comorbidities. All clients have the potential to do well if they are willing to take some risks during treatment and regularly apply the treatment strategies.

Expectations of CBT and Change

It may be helpful to discuss clients' expectations of the program. Some clients may have completed treatment before, in which case it is especially important to elicit their expectations from them. Clients may have had good experiences before and want more of the same, or may have had bad experiences and want something different. Identifying what the client sees as the positives and the negatives from her prior therapy experience will be very useful to help adjust current expectations. You can emphasize the similarities of what you are about to do to her prior positive experiences and emphasize how different this will be from her negative experiences. Overall, it is important the client understand that this program is about learning skills for better managing social anxiety. In other words, it is commonsense and practical, and requires active engagement. The program is not about just talking about the problem or focusing only on the past, but rather it is about focusing on what is maintaining the problem in the present, and regularly and repeatedly doing things differently in day-to-day life.

It is often helpful to ask clients how they see the change process playing out—that is, assessing their theory of change. The following questions can be informative:

- "What do you think will help you to improve your social anxiety and achieve your goals?"
- "What do you think needs to change before you are likely to feel less anxious?"

- "Do you expect your anxious feelings to change before you are able to approach social situations, or do you think you will need to change what you do before you can build confidence and manage your anxiety better?"
- "Do you expect improvement to occur smoothly, or do you expect it to be a bit up and down?"
- "If you are finding an aspect of treatment challenging, how do you think we could manage that together so that you continue to move forward?"

CBT is unlikely to be helpful for clients who wish to just talk about their problems without engaging in active behavior change, or for clients who believe they need to feel no anxiety before behavior change can begin. It is critical that therapists collaboratively develop an active theory of change with their clients. The questions listed above are designed to get the client talking about what he believes he needs to do to progress in therapy and manage difficulties. This approach will assist the client rather than the therapist to take ownership of the process of change. We are often candid with our clients, letting them know that we wish we had a "magic wand" that could take their social anxiety away, but realistically the only way we know how to effectively change their social anxiety is by supporting them in making gradual behavioral changes.

The process of change is likely to be rocky, with periods of progress followed by plateaus or even setbacks. Setbacks can be discouraging for clients, so it is useful to challenge any unrealistic expectations. The therapist and client can formulate a plan for managing setbacks so that the client returns to a positive trajectory as soon as possible. This plan can involve recognizing that setbacks are a normal part of the change process, experiencing a setback can help the therapist and client learn more about potential obstacles to change or triggers for lapses, and working through the setback can help to build clients' confidence in their ability to recover from one in the future. Relapse is common in emotional disorders, and it is just as important to learn how to recover from a setback as it is to experience an initial reduction in symptoms. Opportunities to overcome setbacks during therapy should be framed as a positive therapeutic experience that builds resilience. Once clients appreciate that the goal of therapy is not to remove all social anxiety, but instead to learn to manage their anxiety, distress, and uncertainty with more confidence, they may be able to better appreciate that learning to recover from setbacks is an integral part of becoming and staying well.

CBT Is Collaborative

It is critical that clients are on board with the collaborative nature of treatment. Clients are experts in themselves and their lives, and therapists are impotent without mining the riches of this expertise. Therapists bring to the table their knowledge of factors that maintain SAD and treatment strategies that have shown to be effective. Clients need to appreciate that both the client and therapist need to be active participants in treatment to maximize the chances of success. Therapists should normalize that treatment can be challenging and there may be times when the client is unsure whether he wishes to continue. The therapist needs to acknowledge that halting therapy is an option always available to clients, but it is important to emphasize that challenging times are precisely when it is most important to keep the communication channels open. The therapist needs to engender a strong sense of trust that he will be nonjudgmental if the client expresses any concerns, doubts, or reluctance to engage in any aspect of treatment. The client needs to take on the responsibility of discussing any issues with the therapist so that they can be resolved, or treatment deferred if necessary. Maintaining a strong therapeutic alliance needs to be the priority at all times.

The Socratic Method

The Socratic method, which is critical to the collaborative approach of CBT, has been defined as "a method of guided discovery in which the therapist asks a series of carefully sequenced questions to help define problems, assist in the identification of thoughts and beliefs, examine the meaning of events, or assess the ramifications of particular thoughts or behaviors" (Beck & Dozois, 2011, p. 401). The idea is that guiding the client's discovery through reflective questioning will be more productive than simply telling the client what to do and how to do it. If a client is guided by the therapist to articulate a narrative of how his thoughts, emotions, physical sensations, and behaviors interact to maintain his problem, and then to reexamine his assumptions, this will result in more genuine and enduring change than the therapist attempting to provide the client with all the answers. Clients are experts in their own experience, and therapists may not truly understand how the client sees the world if they make assumptions, and therefore treatment may not be optimally targeted to the client's personal experience. The client is also likely to have more "buy-in" to the treatment if she is articulating the principles of change herself, rather than being told by a therapist. An overarching aim of CBT is to develop the client's self-efficacy—confidence in her own ability to manage her problems. The Socratic method helps clients to achieve this by teaching them *how* to think more helpfully, not *what* to think.

Often the most challenging aspect of the Socratic method for new therapists is that it is more time-consuming than more didactic methods. At times therapists may feel that they need to "give the client something" or that they could speed things up and get to the crux of the matter by being more directive. There are certainly times when a more direct approach may be necessary (e.g., when clients are at high risk of harming themselves), but generally speaking therapeutic time is well spent by asking questions that will help clients to consider information that might be outside their awareness so that *they* can reach new perspectives (Beck et al., 1979; Clark & Egan, 2015; Kennerley, 2007). Christine Padesky (1993) suggests that the Socratic method helps clients consider all relevant information and explore alternative explanations in an open, curious, and empathic manner. Synthesizing questions can then be asked to encourage the client to consider whether this new information offers any fresh perspectives compared to their initial beliefs (e.g., "It's interesting that when I asked the last time you were overtly criticized it was hard for you to think of a specific example. What might this tell us about the thought that 'people always think I'm stupid'?"). The Socratic method is invaluable for preventing the therapist and client from reaching an impasse that could derail the therapeutic alliance.

In all of the sample dialogues and questions in this book the therapist adopts the Socratic method. You will notice that the therapist takes a curious, agnostic stance when gently probing clients about their experience. The therapist does not presume that the client's perspective is wrong or misguided, but rather expresses genuine interest in the client's worldview with questions that encourage him to reflect on his own experience in a way that may generate new perspectives.

The Importance of Homework

Homework is not an optional extra in CBT, but is the most important ingredient. It is vital to emphasize this with clients before commencing treatment. Clients have commenced treatment because they want to better manage their anxiety in their lives, not within the four walls of the therapist's office. It is therefore critical that skills practiced in session are applied between sessions. There is a considerable body of evidence that both quantity and quality of homework are associated with better outcomes, and it is important that clients are aware of this before they begin. To clarify any misconceptions about the critical role homework plays in achieving a positive treatment outcome, we will often say to clients something like:

> "Clients often think that coming to these appointments is the 'therapy.' I don't see these appointments as the therapy. These appointments are just preparation for the real therapy, which takes place when you apply the strategies we will be learning in your day-to-day life. Initially these strategies will need to be set as formal homework to maximize their effectiveness. However, at some point the strategies will no longer seem like homework, as they will just become the new way you are living your life."

Session Structure

The clinician should set an agenda at the start of each session so that the client knows what to expect. If the client and therapist collaboratively set homework during the previous session this should always be reviewed at the beginning of the next session. As clients learn to expect that their homework will always be reviewed, they will understand how valuable it is. If the clinician sets homework and fails to review it in the next session, the client will learn that it is unimportant, and noncompliance will likely follow. Once the agenda is set and homework is reviewed, new content is introduced and practiced before new homework consistent with the content is collaboratively set for the coming week. We routinely ask clients to reflect on three take-home messages at the end of the session to ensure a shared understanding of the key learning points of the session, to clarify any misunderstandings, and to consolidate learning. Much can happen in a session, and it is important that clients have some clarity regarding what has been meaningful and helpful to them. It is good practice always to ask clients how they feel the session went and whether they felt understood by the therapist. The client will learn that the therapist genuinely values the therapeutic relationship by taking the time to check in and ensure that the alliance remains strong. Remember that many clients with SAD will be worried about upsetting you and will not want you to think badly of them, so they may heavily edit their feedback. Look out for feedback that doesn't match their affect and gently allow them every opportunity to provide honest and open discussion.

Psychoeducation about SAD

It is often informative for the therapist to begin by asking clients what they understand about the main features of SAD. To start disentangling the different aspects of the client's experience, it can be helpful to frame this discussion around five columns headed with "common triggers," "thoughts/images," "behaviors," "body," and "feelings" on a whiteboard or sheet of paper. The clinician can then start to elicit common triggers for the client's social anxiety, cognitive themes, idiosyncratic safety behaviors and avoided situations, physical sensations, and emotional responses. To encourage engagement in the process, the client should be encouraged to write down her experiences in the columns as they are discussed, rather than the therapist taking charge of this process. The assessment of these aspects of the client's experience does not need to be exhaustive at this stage, and only a few examples in each column should be sufficient. More details will be elicited in each of these areas across the treatment. Some examples of Socratic questions to facilitate this process include:

- "What sorts of social situations do you find yourself feeling particularly anxious in?" [common triggers]
- "When you are expecting a situation like this, what do you imagine happening? When you've been in these situations in the past, what have you worried will occur, or what do you remember occurring? After social situations, what thoughts or images go through your mind about the situation?" [thoughts/images]
- "If you can't avoid a social situation, what do you do to try and prevent your social fears from coming true?" [safety and avoidant behaviors]
- "When you are in social situations, what feelings in your body are you most aware of?" [bodily sensations] And how do you feel emotionally? [feelings]

It can be helpful to spend a few minutes eliciting any feedback loops the client might notice between the thoughts/images, behaviors, and bodily sensations and feelings they experience. For example, the therapist might ask something like:

"I'm just curious. When you have that thought or image about what might happen, are you more or less likely to go to the party? And if you don't go to the party, what impact do you find that has on the strength of the thoughts/images over time? Does it strengthen them or weaken them? And if your belief that [something bad] will happen strengthens over time, what impact do you find this has on your anxiety? The more anxious you feel, what then happens to the sensations you experience in your body?"

You will notice that the therapist is taking a curious approach to encourage the client to really explore the links among his thoughts, behaviors, feelings, and physical symptoms. The therapist's aim at this point is just to start drawing the client's attention to how his responses to the thoughts and images might serve to maintain or exacerbate the thoughts and images and hence his social anxiety over time.

Many clients with SAD see their fear of evaluation as a weakness and generally as a negative trait that needs to be expunged from their personality. They are less aware of the positive qualities that often accompany a fear of negative evaluation, including empathy, caring, and sensitivity to others' needs, which are all attractive qualities that can facilitate relationships. It can therefore be helpful to discuss social anxiety and the underlying fear of evaluation as a continuum. Each of us can be placed anywhere along the continuum, from very low to very high. People who care little about being evaluated by others are at one end, those who care about being evaluated to some degree may be somewhere in the middle, and those who care too much may be at the upper end of the continuum.

We often find it useful to elicit from the client any negative characteristics she associates with people who have an extremely low fear of evaluation. Some clients might say that such people are "happy" or "relaxed," but after asking them to reflect on people they know who really don't care at all about what others think, most clients are able to identify negative characteristics (e.g., unempathic, selfish, arrogant, domineering). Asking clients how helpful these traits are for fostering quality relationships can often lead them to reconsider seeking to "not care at all" about what others think of them. We then ask clients to identify any positive characteristics of people who care a lot about being evaluated by others, and they start to appreciate that they might like to retain some of their positive qualities, such as empathy, caring, and a desire to form close relationships with others.

This exercise can be extremely helpful for destigmatizing social anxiety and to emphasize the fact that the aim of the treatment is to reduce the degree to which clients care about evaluation (i.e., shift down the continuum a bit), so that their lives are not dictated by social anxiety. The goal is not to change their personality so that they are the most gregarious person at parties, or so that they are aggressive and always must have their own way, but rather to learn skills so that their social anxiousness does not interfere with their life. This can be a relief to some clients, who fear that the treatment might turn them into the sort of person they currently find intimidating.

The next task when beginning treatment is to socialize clients to the treatment model. Handout 1, *What Is Social Anxiety Disorder?*, contains useful psychoeducation for clients about social anxiety and the model used to guide this treatment. Below we provide examples of how each specific component of the treatment model can be described to clients. It is useful to have a copy of the model (Worksheet 1, *My Model of Social Anxiety*; see the Appendix) in front of the client as each component is described. Although a sample script is provided below, it is important for the therapist to regularly check that the client understands each component and encourages discussion of relevant personal examples.

The Treatment Model

"This model provides an explanation for what maintains SAD, and is used to guide treatment. The shaded area on the left includes all the situations that trigger anxiety. A shaded arrow then leads to the 'perception of social threat.' This perception of social threat then activates the fear, or fight-or-flight, response."

Triggers

"We have already discussed several triggers earlier in the session. These included parties, interviews, eating or drinking in front of people, using public toilets, or just being observed by others. Are there any others you would add? For most people with SAD these triggers are virtually impossible to avoid completely—there are people everywhere! And usually when we try to avoid people it can affect our overall quality of life."

Perception of Social Threat

"When we encounter a trigger there is an automatic perception of threat—we think that (a) something bad is likely to happen and (b) it will be catastrophic when it does. We can consider the probability and cost of being evaluated by others as being separate but related beliefs. I might believe that it is highly likely that I will be negatively evaluated by someone, but if I don't think it matters very much (low cost), I'm unlikely to feel particularly anxious about it. If I believe it is unlikely that I will be evaluated, but it would be devastating if I were, then I might start feeling anxious in social situations because I believe that a catastrophe is possible. If I believe social evaluation is both highly likely and would be devastating, I am likely to feel very anxious because I believe that a catastrophe is probable. The trigger itself has not directly caused the fear because other people who encounter those same situations may not feel the same way. There must be something happening in between the trigger and the fear response. Our model suggests that it is our perceptions of the probability and cost of being negatively judged that determines the severity of our anxiety response."

The Fight, Flight, and Freeze Response

"The fear, or 'fight-or-flight,' response includes all the uncomfortable symptoms of anxiety you notice when in a social situation, such as the ones you mentioned before [i.e., sweating, shaking, heart racing]. Although the symptoms feel extremely uncomfortable, believe it or not they are designed to help us when we are under threat. What do you already understand about the fight-or-flight response? [Give clients an opportunity to discuss their current understanding.]

"The fight-or-flight response prepares our body for action, whether it be fighting a threat or fleeing from it. We start to overbreathe to increase the oxygen in our bodies, our muscles tense up in preparation for running or fighting, we sweat to help cool the body as we manage the threat, and so on. Actually, if we don't believe we can fight or flee from a threat our body is likely to freeze, which is also designed to protect us. Imagine if you are being chased by a lion in the African savannah at night and you know you can't run from the lion, and you certainly won't beat it in a fistfight. Your best chance of survival is to play dead or stay still so that it doesn't see you. If we perceive that we can't cope with a social situation our body might freeze in an attempt to avert a catastrophe. For this reason, this fear response is sometimes called the fight, flight, and freeze response. Our body's ability to manage threats in these ways has been critical to our survival.

"But what if we only 'think' there is a threat? It turns out that this is enough to trigger the fight, flight, and freeze response, even in the absence of a true threat. This is sometimes referred to as a 'false alarm,' and this is why we can experience severe anxiety even when objectively there is no actual threat. On these occasions, all the resources generated by the fight, flight, and freeze response (e.g., extra oxygen and adrenaline, tense muscles, sweating) are not used (unless we want to start fighting people at a party or in an interview—not a great idea because it will certainly lead to negative evaluation!), so we experience the symptoms as uncomfortable anxiety."

Maintenance of Social Anxiety

"The question is, what keeps this perception of social threat going? The white bubbles in the model represent six important maintaining factors that keep our perception of social threat going, and these will be the targets of treatment. The first is *negative social thoughts and images,* which may be from the past (i.e., past social events), the present (i.e., what is happening right now), or the future (i.e., what we expect to happen). The more negative thoughts and images you have, the greater the perception of social threat. What are some typical negative thoughts and images you have before, during, or after social situations?

"The second bubble is *avoidance*. Most people with significant anxiety avoid some of the triggers of their anxiety as a way of trying to avoid having their negative thoughts and images come true. [Elicit two to three situations the client avoids as well as an example of the feedback loop to perception of social threat.] What are some common situations you avoid for fear of evaluation from others? How might avoidance keep your perception of social threat going (e.g., don't get to test fears and find that they may be inaccurate)?

"The next bubble refers to what we call '*safety behaviors.*' Safety behaviors are those subtle avoidance behaviors we use when we can't actually avoid a situation. For example, I might go to a work meeting, but I won't say anything as a way of avoiding being criticized. So I haven't completely avoided the situation, but at the same time I have still protected myself from my fears coming true. Sometimes safety behaviors can be really hard to identify—for example, you might go to a party but not make very much eye contact with people so others won't try to start a conversation with you in case they find you uninteresting; or you might dress in really light clothes when you go out to reduce the chances that you will get hot and blush or sweat. [Elicit two to three examples of safety behaviors, as well as an example of the feedback loop to perception of social threat.] What are some of the safety behaviors that you recognize yourself using from time to time? How might these keep your perception of social threat going (e.g., I still don't get to test my fears—by not talking I don't learn that others are unlikely to criticize me)?

"The next bubble is the image of how you appear to others. [Elicit some examples of anxiety symptoms that the client believes are obvious to others, social performance that the client believes he is really bad at, and/or the client's perceptions of his physical attributes, imperfections, or attractiveness.] In your mind's eye, what do you imagine other people see when they are looking at you? When you have that image in mind, does it increase or decrease your perception of social threat? Often people with SAD can have a more negative image of themselves in their mind's eye than what other people actually see.

"The next bubble refers to self-focused and environment-focused attention. [Guide clients to recognize their tendency to be *self-focused* on physical sensations of anxiety, negative thoughts and images, and safety behaviors. Clients might often use the term 'self-conscious.' Also, elicit examples of negative *environment-focused* attention, such as looking for any sign of negative evaluation from other people in the area. Then guide the client to recognize that it would be most helpful to focus on the task at hand, such as the topic of the conversation, their own contributions, and what conversation leads they can take from what the other person is saying.] When you're in a social situation, what are you most aware of? What captures your attention most? What impact does focusing on these things have on your ability to focus on the task at hand? Where would be a more helpful place to focus your attention when socializing?

"Finally, the last bubble refers to *negative core beliefs,* which are very broad and general ways in which you see yourself, others, and the world. Core beliefs guide the specific negative thoughts and images you have in day-to-day social situations.

For example, if I hold the belief that I am boring, I'm more likely to have negative thoughts and images about others wanting to avoid me. I might then start to avoid social situations, regardless of whether my core belief is true or not. [Elicit one or two core beliefs if the client is readily able to do this, but don't dwell too much on them at this stage. Reassure the client that you will come back to this later in therapy.] What general conclusions have you come to about yourself, other people, or the world when it comes to socializing? These beliefs are important and we will come back to them later in treatment."

Once the client understands the model she should be encouraged to consider how each component relates to her own experience. Using Worksheet 1, *My Model of Social Anxiety,* the client can record examples from her experience as each component is described in session. The questions outlined in the treatment model section above, along with a range of self-report questionnaires, can help the therapist and client better understand how the components of the model relate to the client's experience. Below we briefly describe some questionnaires that could be used to complement the clinical assessment and help with case formulation. These measures can also be used to assess change during treatment and therefore the effectiveness of the intervention.

Measures to Aid Diagnosis, Case Formulation, and Outcome Evaluation

In this section we describe some measures that may help therapists to diagnose SAD and develop case formulations using Worksheet 1, *My Model of Social Anxiety* (in the Appendix). These measures can also be used to assess change during treatment and therefore the effectiveness of the intervention. Some therapists are hesitant to use psychometric measures because they feel that it disturbs the client rapport or burdens the client. In fact, most clients will see a thorough evaluation as very useful. It usually helps clients to feel that (1) the therapist is being very thorough and professional and has a complete understanding of his problem; and (2) he is not alone and that these sorts of problems and feelings are known and studied. After describing some examples of measures you could administer to your clients we illustrate how information can be integrated to create a personalized case formulation. Interested readers may want to consult the comprehensive review of SAD symptom and mechanism measures by Wong, Gregory, and McLellan (2016).

Establishing a Diagnosis: Structured Diagnostic Interviews

There are several structured diagnostic interviews that can help clinicians determine whether or not a client meets criteria for SAD. Unfortunately, most of these interviews are not in the public domain and need to be purchased. These costs can be prohibitive in some treatment settings such as community mental health clinics. The Anxiety Disorders Interview Schedule (ADIS-5; Brown & Barlow, 2014), published by Oxford University Press, comprehensively assesses DSM-5 criteria for anxiety, mood, obsessive–compulsive, trauma, and related disorders. The Structured Clinical Interview for DSM-5 (SCID-5; First, Williams, Karg, & Spitzer, 2016), published by the American Psychiatric Association, is a semistructured interview that can be used to establish DSM-5 diagnoses. Various versions of the SCID are published for different purposes (e.g., clinician version, research version, personality disorders, clinical trials), and the publishers will grant relatively cheap licenses to public and not-for-profit clinics. However, the ADIS-5 and SCID-5 are time-consuming to administer, and this level of detail is unlikely to be necessary in the majority of clinical settings.

A briefer and cheaper alternative is the MINI International Neuropsychiatric Assessment (MINI; Lecrubier et al., 1997; Sheehan et al., 1998). Clinicians may be able to obtain permission from the developers to make copies of the MINI for their own personal clinical and research use. We have used the MINI in our clinic, and in our experience it can be administered in around 20 minutes, or less if fewer modules are administered.

You may feel that a structured interview imposes too many constraints on your clinical intuition and is too detailed for your needs. The critically important issue as far as the treatment described in this book is concerned is that you are able to accurately identify that social anxiety is your client's primary problem. However, research evidence indicates that even experienced clinicians are less accurate in diagnoses when they rely on unstructured questioning rather than structured interviews. Even if you decide not to use structured interviews in the long run, we strongly urge you to read over one or more of these interviews to give yourself an appreciation for the sorts of questions that are asked and how they are structured and organized. Clear, systematic data collection is critical for an accurate diagnosis.

Triggers and Fear Response

Worksheet 2, *Personal Fear and Avoidance List* (in the Appendix), can be helpful in identifying triggers of social anxiety and obtaining baseline fear and avoidance ratings. We routinely readminister this worksheet at both the beginning and the end of treatment so that clients can fully appreciate the changes they have made. Anxiety and avoidance typically reduce for social situations clients have worked on in treatment, which reinforces the value of applying the treatment principles. It is often valuable for clients to also notice that they remain anxious in some situations they are still avoiding because it strengthens the rationale for reducing avoidance and provides some guidance about areas to continue working on after therapy.

In our clinic we use the Social Interaction Anxiety Scale (SIAS) and the Social Phobia Scale (SPS) as primary symptom and outcome measures (Mattick & Clarke, 1998). The SIAS and SPS are self-report questionnaires with 20 items each. They were designed as companion measures to assess two related but distinct facets of social anxiety. As the name suggests, the SIAS assesses anxiety during the initiation and maintenance of social interactions, such as making eye contact with others, speaking with authority figures, disagreeing with others, and meeting people at parties. The SPS measures performance anxiety in situations where an individual might be observed, such as eating, drinking, writing, and public speaking. SIAS scores of around 34–36 have been identified as clinical cutoffs in some studies (Heimberg, Mueller, Holt, Hope, & Liebowitz, 1992; Peters, 2000), although the average score for our clients in a community mental health clinic is around 55 (standard deviation around 12; Carleton et al., 2014; McEvoy et al., 2015). On average, clinical samples tend to score around 33 to 42 on the SPS (Carleton et al., 2014; Heimberg et al., 1992; Mattick & Clarke, 1998).

We use the full 20-item versions of both measures, but shorter versions have recently been published that reduce the burden on clients and are more practical in busy clinical practices. Nick Carleton and colleagues (2009) published a 14-item version called the Social Interaction Phobia Scale (SIPS), which comprised three factors: social interaction anxiety (five SIAS items), fear of overt valuation (six SPS items), and fear of attracting attention (three SPS items). Another three short versions have been developed, with 12 or 21 items (Fergus, Valentiner, McGrath, Gier-Lonsway, & Kim, 2012; Kupper & Denollet, 2012; Peters, Sunderland, Andrews, Rapee, & Mattick, 2012). The items vary considerably across the short versions. In a recent study Carleton and colleagues (2014) compared each of these short versions in terms of factor structure, sensitivity to change during cognitive-behavioral group therapy for SAD, and convergent validity with related measures. There was no clear winner psychometrically across the measures, although the SIPS (Carleton et al., 2009) and SPS–6 and SIAS–6 (Peters et al., 2012) performed consistently well. These measures are in the public domain and are freely available by contacting the authors or via a quick Internet search.

Negative Thoughts:
Fear of Evaluation and Repetitive Negative Thinking

Fear of negative evaluation (FNE) is a key theme of negative thoughts and images in SAD. A commonly used measure to assess FNE is the Brief Fear of Negative Evaluation Scale (BFNE), which has 12 items that were originally derived from the 30-item Fear of Negative Evaluation Scale (FNE) (Watson & Friend, 1969). The BFNE is faster to administer than the FNE, and its 5-point Likert scale (1 = not at all characteristic of me; 5 = extremely characteristic of me) is more sensitive to change than the FNE's dichotomous response format (true/false). One problem with the BFNE is that four items are reverse scored because they are negatively worded (i.e., a high rating means a *low* fear of negative evaluation). Negatively worded items can be confusing for respondents, and they tend to perform more poorly psychometrically. Rodebaugh and colleagues (2004) have evaluated the psychometrics of the eight positively worded items and have found evidence that these items alone are superior to the 12-item version (also see Weeks et al., 2005). This version, called the straightforwardly-worded Brief Fear of Negative

Evaluation Scale (BFNE-S), can be easily and quickly completed by clients to monitor changes in this core feature of SAD during treatment. The BFNE can easily be located using a web search. The negatively worded items (items 2, 4, 7, 10) are simply omitted if the 8-item version is desired.

Fear of positive evaluation has been defined as "feelings of apprehension about others' positive evaluations of oneself and distress over these evaluations" (Weeks & Howell, 2012, p. 83). Recent elaborations of cognitive-behavioral theory have incorporated fear of positive evaluation as a key maintaining factor of SAD (Heimberg et al., 2010, 2014), and recent evidence suggests that it predicts SAD symptoms above and beyond FNE (Weeks, Heimberg, Rodebaugh, & Norton, 2008). The idea is that people with SAD wish to be acceptable enough to avoid negative evaluation, hence they fear negative evaluation. On the other hand, they also do not wish to be so impressive that others feel threatened and therefore become critical and rejecting, hence they fear positive evaluation. The 10-item fear of positive evaluation (FPE) scale can be used to assess this construct during treatment. Sample items are "I am uncomfortable exhibiting my talents to others, even if I think my talents will impress them" and "It would make me anxious to receive a compliment from someone that I am attracted to." A clinical cutoff score of 22 has been identified. Mean scores (standard deviations) have been reported for clinical samples of 39.60 (*SD* = 14.92; Weeks, Heimberg, Rodebaugh, Goldin, & Gross, 2012). Again, a Web search will reveal the FPE scale.

Additional self-report measures of cognitive processes have been developed to assess repetitive negative thinking before social situations (anticipatory processing) and after social situations (postevent processing). The anticipatory event processing (AnEP) questionnaire developed by Laposa and Rector (2016) is a measure of anticipatory processing, but this is particular to a videotaped speech task. The Anticipatory Social Behaviors Questionnaire (ASBQ; Hinrichsen & Clark, 2003) is a 12-item measure of anticipatory processing that assesses negative thoughts about what might happen in a social situation, thoughts about how the individual would look to others, plans for escape or avoidance, and recollections of past failures. The Post-Event Processing Questionnaire (PEPQ; Rachman, Grüter-Andrew, & Shafran, 2000) was developed to measure rumination after social stressors, and recent refinements to the measure have resulted in a 7-item measure (Laposa & Rector, 2011). Anticipatory and postevent processing are closely related to each other (Laposa & Rector, 2016), so for many clinical settings a single measure of a client's tendency to engage in repetitive negative thinking in response to a stressor may be adequate to assess changes during treatment in vulnerability to both anticipatory and postevent processing. A brief measure we commonly use for this purpose is the 10-item Repetitive Thinking Questionnaire (McEvoy, Thibodeau, & Asmundson, 2014), which assesses engagement in thoughts and images.

Other measures have also been developed to assess negative thoughts during public speaking, such as the Self-Statements during Public Speaking Scale (Hofmann & DiBartolo, 2000) and the Performance Questionnaire (Rapee & Lim, 1992), or during social interactions, such as the Social Interaction Self-Statement Test (Glass, Merluzzi, Biever, & Larsen, 1982).

Imagery Content, Use, and Ability

The most comprehensive assessment of imagery in relation to SAD, the Waterloo Images and Memories Interview (WIMI), was developed by David Moscovitch and colleagues (Moscovitch et al., 2011) by modifying the Autobiographical Interview (Levine, Svoboda, Hay, Winocur, & Moscovitch, 2002). Interviewers examine mental images and associated autobiographical memories for positive (non-anxiety-provoking) and negative (anxiety-provoking) social situations. Respondents are first asked to spontaneously recall these images and memories, and then to elaborate on these recollections via probing questions. Administration of the WIMI requires training, and recording and transcribing of responses, so using it with fidelity is likely to be impractical in many clinical settings. However, interested readers may wish to read the original paper as a guide to some probing questions that may assist with accessing clients' images. We provide comprehensive examples of how to assess for mental imagery in Chapter 5 of this book, which is likely to be sufficient in most clinical contexts for assessing the content of distressing mental imagery including self-images.

Several measures of imagery ability are available that may be helpful in assessing the degree to which clients are tuned in to mental imagery. The Spontaneous Use of Imagery Scale (SUIS; Reisberg, Pearson, & Kosslyn, 2003) is a 12-item measure of an individual's awareness and habitual use of imagery in everyday life. Sample items are "when going to a new place, I prefer directions that included detailed descriptions of landmarks (such as the size, shape, and colour of a petrol station) in addition to their names." The Vividness of Visual Imagery Questionnaire (VVIQ; Marks, 1973) is a measure of imagery ability. The original VVIQ consists of 16 items assessing imagery ability across four scenarios, although a four-item version including only one of the scenarios has also been used (McEvoy et al., 2015). Each scenario is briefly described, and then respondents are asked to manipulate the scenario within imagery in four ways and to indicate the vividness of the imagery. Clinicians may wish to use the VVIQ as a quick assessment of clients' ability to engage with the imagery mode given its emphasis in this treatment, although it may be that this ability improves as clients become more "tuned in" to their imagery during treatment. A low score at pretreatment may therefore not preclude the use of imagery-based techniques.

Avoidance and Safety Behaviors

The Liebowitz Social Anxiety Scale (LSAS; Liebowitz, 1987) is the most common clinician-administered measure in clinical trials. An advantage of the 24-item LSAS is that it assesses both fear and avoidance of social situations, rather than just fear alone. Like the SPS and SIAS, the LSAS assesses the dimensions of social interaction anxiety and performance anxiety, resulting in four subscales: Fear of Social Interaction, Avoidance of Social Interaction, Fear of Performance, and Avoidance of Performance. Clinician-administered measures allow for a detailed exploration of situations that clients fear and avoid most, as well as discrepancies between fear and avoidance. Some highly feared situations might be rarely avoided if the task is highly valued by the client. For instance, a client whose career is fundamental to her identity might regularly speak at work meetings despite finding this highly anxiety provoking. Other tasks that are less anxiety provoking might nonetheless be more frequently avoided if they are perceived to be less important or are just more easily avoided (e.g., writing in front of others, returning goods to a store).

The Subtle Avoidance Frequency Examination (SAFE) is a 32-item measure of safety behaviors that was developed to assist with case formulation and assess for changes in this maintaining factor during treatment (Cuming et al., 2009). The SAFE has three subscales assessing the restriction or inhibition of behavior to avoid attracting attention, more active attempts to improve performance in social situations, and strategies that aim to reduce physical symptoms of blushing and sweating. Cuming and colleagues (2009) found that the SAFE was responsive to change during treatment. The SAFE is downloadable from the Centre of Emotional Health's website at Macquarie University (*www.mq.edu.au/__data/assets/pdf_file/0008/137078/SAFE_English_copyright_2015.pdf*).

Self- and Environment-Focused Attention

There are a few measures that can be used to assess focus of attention. The Focus of Attention Questionnaire (FAQ; Woody, Chambless, & Glass, 1997) was developed to assess focus of attention during a social interaction in particular. The FAQ consists of two, five-item subscales assessing self-focused attention or externally focused attention. The self-focused subscale assesses focus on what the individual will say or do next, the impression she is making on the other person, her level of anxiety, internal bodily reactions, and past failures. The external focus subscale includes items regarding aspects of the situation other than the client himself, including the other person's appearance or dress, the physical surroundings, what the other person might be feeling toward the client, thoughts about the other person, and what the other person was saying or doing (see Woody et al., 1997).

The Self-Consciousness Scale (SCS; Carver & Scheier, 1978; Fenigstein, Scheier, & Buss, 1975; Scheier & Carver, 1985) is another measure of self-focused attention. The SCS (revised version; Scheier & Carver, 1985) is a 22-item measure of the dispositional tendency to be aware of oneself privately or publically. Private self-consciousness includes hidden aspects of the self not observable to others such as beliefs, values, and feelings. Public self-consciousness includes aspects of the self that are observable to others, such as behavior, mannerisms, and expressions, and is especially relevant to social anxiety.

Negative Core Beliefs

The concept of core beliefs might be difficult for clients to grasp at this early stage, and so this can always be left blank in Worksheet 1, *My Model of Social* Anxiety, and explored in more detail later in treatment if necessary. Alternatively, self-report measures may be a useful adjunct to a clinical assessment. The 15-item Self-Beliefs Related to Social Anxiety (SBSA) Scale (Wong & Moulds, 2009; Wong et al., 2014) may be helpful for assessing three types of maladaptive beliefs related to social anxiety based on Clark and Wells's (1995) model (see Chapter 2): high standards, such as "I have to get everyone's approval" and "I need to be liked by everyone"; conditional beliefs, which take the form of "If . . . then . . ." statements such as "If I make mistakes, [then] others will reject me" and "If I don't say something interesting, [then] people won't like me"; and unconditional, broad, and global core beliefs such as "People think I am inferior." Other measures of core beliefs have also been developed, including the Social Thoughts and Beliefs Scale (STABS; Turner, Johnson, Beidel, Heiser, & Lydiard, 2003), Core Extrusion Schema (Rodebaugh, 2009), and the Maladaptive Interpersonal Belief Scale (Boden et al., 2012).

If the client is unable to readily provide personal examples for a particular component of the *My Model of Social Anxiety* case formulation, then the therapist can spend more time addressing this gap in his understanding. The gap can be resolved by administering a selection of the formal measures just reviewed and/or with the more detailed eliciting questions described in Chapters 5–9, which correspond to each maintaining factor in the model. Clients should be encouraged to ask questions about the model to seek clarification. Therapists should actively invite any queries and ask if there are any aspects clients believe are particularly relevant to them, or any elements they see as being less relevant.

Individualizing the Model: Jacquie's Case Formulation

If you recall Jacquie's story from the beginning of Chapter 1, we can now consider her case formulation. The therapist and Jacquie first worked through the section earlier in this chapter titled "The Treatment Model" to help Jacquie understand the maintaining factors of her social anxiety and better understand how each component relates to her own personal experiences. The therapist also asked Jacquie to complete Worksheet 2, *Personal Fear and Avoidance List,* for a baseline of how severe her anxiety was in a range of situations that were important to her and how frequently she avoided them. Jacquie also completed the SIAS as a general measure of the severity of her anxiety in social interaction situations and she scored 55, which is well within the clinical range for SAD. Jacquie's responses on the Fear of Negative Evaluation Scale (straightforwardly worded version) and Fear of Positive Evaluation Scale revealed that she had a severe fear of negative evaluation and she also felt very uncomfortable when others focused on her for positive reasons. Clinical assessment and her score on the Repetitive Thinking Questionnaire–10 revealed that Jacquie often experienced negative social thoughts and images before, during, and after social situations, which typically involved her anticipating or reflecting on perceived social catastrophes. Jacquie's ratings on the Vividness of Visual Imagery Questionnaire revealed high imagery ability, which suggested that she was likely to be able to engage well with the imagery aspects of the treatment with little prompting. Scores on the Subtle Avoidance Frequency Evaluation helped Jacquie to understand how frequently she relies on safety behaviors in social situations, and she was surprised to learn that some of the strategies she used to try and prevent her social fears may actually be maintaining her social anxiety. She reported that the behaviors are usually so automatic that she is not even aware she is using them. Ratings on the Focus of Attention Questionnaire showed that Jacquie's attention is predominantly focused on herself or unhelpful aspects of the environment that she perceives as indicative of social evaluation, rather than on the task at hand (i.e., the conversation). Finally, her scores on the Self-Beliefs Related to Social Anxiety Scale revealed that she strongly endorsed a range of extremely high social standards and negative core beliefs about her perceived inferiority. After considering all of the information collected from the clinical interview, discussions about the treatment model, and the self-report measures, Jacquie and her therapist included some examples in each component of Worksheet 1, *My Model of Social Anxiety,* to create her own personalized model of social anxiety (Figure 4.1). This model was then regularly referred to throughout treatment to ensure that each maintaining factor was being effectively modified.

Treatment Rationale

The treatment rationale follows directly from the model. The therapist can describe how the treatment is designed to modify the perception of threat by teaching skills to address each of the six maintaining factors described in the model. The client will learn strategies to (1) identify and challenge negative social thoughts and images, (2) gradually reduce avoidance, (3) reduce reliance on safety behaviors, (4) challenge negative self-images and discover how she actually appears to other people, (5) redirect attention to the task at hand, and (6) modify negative core beliefs. The therapist can then express curiosity about whether the client believes this approach could be helpful and why. This provides another opportunity to engage clients in the process of change as they hear themselves advocating for the value of addressing each of the target areas.

Looking Forward

Worksheet 3, *Looking Forward,* can be a helpful way of ending the initial phase of treatment. Successful treatment requires commitment and perseverance, and these qualities are going to be tested in our clients throughout the program. The Looking Forward exercise is an opportunity for clients to consider the potential costs and benefits of a future with and without change. For most clients thinking about a future without change is a depressing prospect, as they envision limited opportunities in their career and relationships and continued suffering. Envisaging a future with change is more optimistic and

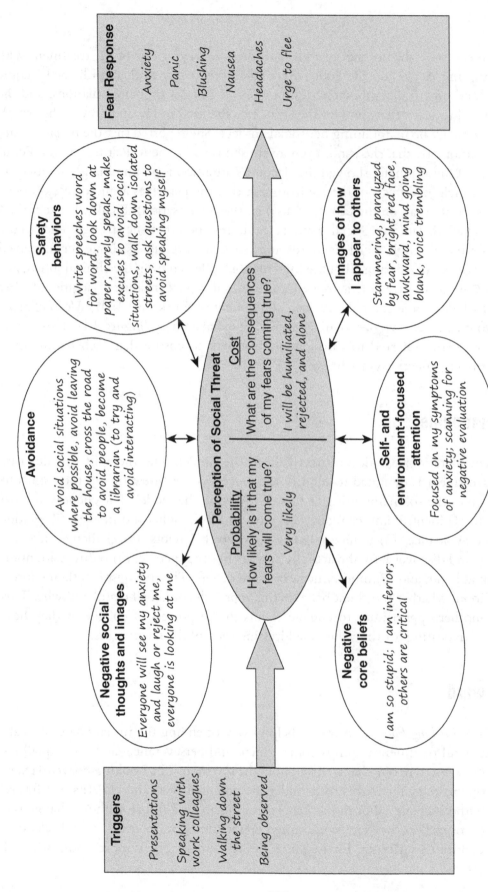

FIGURE 4.1. *My Model of Social Anxiety* (Worksheet 1), completed by Jacquie.

involves a more fulfilling and valued life. It is important for clients to elaborate both of these alternative futures to be clear about the importance of using treatment, right at this moment, to start working toward a more positive future. At this point the therapist can guide clients through an imagery exercise where they are first encouraged to imagine themselves in a social situation in the future with high social anxiety (e.g., work, social event, job interview, on a date). Clients can then reimagine the situation but this time seeing themselves as more confident. With these alternative futures vividly in mind, the value of changing sooner rather than later is clear.

The Looking Forward exercise also requires clients to consider potential obstacles to change that may threaten to derail their progress in therapy. These obstacles might include having to tolerate heightened anxiety in the short to medium term, difficulties maintaining motivation, having limited time to devote to homework, managing set-backs, and upsetting the status quo when other people expect them to be their agreeable and passive old selves. Some clients are also willing to admit that if they don't try and don't succeed, then at least they still have hope that if they do make a genuine attempt later on they could get better. The core fear is that if they genuinely engage with the treatment and it fails, then they could not cope with losing what they consider to be their "last hope."

The final aspect of the exercise is clients considering what they might lose by changing their social anxiety. Clients might report that they would become even less likable because they will become aggressive. Others acknowledge that if they no longer have social anxiety they will have to confront some difficult issues and tasks in their lives and therefore leave their "comfort zone," which they are currently able to avoid. If they begin the difficult process of change, they might be concerned that others will start to expect too much of them and then be disappointed.

We hope it is clear from these examples how critical it is to address these issues before clients commence the process of change. Time spent preempting and planning for identified obstacles is time well spent. Worksheet 3, *Looking Forward,* can be referred to when clients encounter these issues during therapy so they can remind themselves why they embarked on this difficult process (*for an alternative future*), to normalize the obstacles (*Ah, we thought this might come up at some stage, and here it is!*), and to plan helpful responses when they do arise (*Do you remember how you thought you might deal with this issue if it arose? Given that you thought it might come up, tell me about how you made the decision to persist with treatment anyway.*).

Summary

Socializing clients to the model and actively engaging them in the treatment rationale is where half the battle is won or lost. If a client understands the model, it fits with his experience, and he can articulate the potential benefits of modifying the maintaining factors, the value of fully engaging in the treatment strategies will be clear. Once clients understand what treatment involves, they will ideally feel a mix of excitement, anxiety, hope, dread, and enthusiasm (among many other emotions) as they embark on the course of therapy. These mixed emotions suggest that they understand they are going to find the process difficult, but also that the effort will be worthwhile and ultimately highly rewarding. It is critical that therapists pay close attention to the therapeutic alliance and client motivation throughout therapy. In the coming chapters we describe each maintaining factor in more depth, look more specifically at socializing clients to work on these factors, and introduce a range of treatment strategies that are designed to effectively target each maintaining factor in turn. It is the combination of these treatment strategies that will lead to a comprehensive and thorough therapy for SAD.

THERAPY SUMMARY GUIDE:
Socializing Clients to the Treatment Model

Therapy Aim: Establish rapport, hope, and expectations of change, provide psychoeducation about social anxiety disorder, and socialize clients to the treatment model.

Therapy Agenda Items:

▼ Setting the scene
- ◢ Building rapport
- ◢ The client is not alone
- ◢ There is hope
- ◢ Expectations of CBT and change
- ◢ CBT is collaborative
- ◢ The importance of homework
- ◢ Session structure

▼ Psychoeducation about SAD

▼ The treatment model
- ◢ Triggers
- ◢ Perception of social threat
- ◢ The fight, flight, and freeze response
- ◢ Maintenance of social anxiety (including measures to aid case formulation)

▼ Individualizing the model

▼ Treatment rationale

▼ Looking forward

Therapy Materials:

▼ Handouts
- ◢ Handout 1, *What Is Social Anxiety Disorder?*

▼ Worksheets
- ◢ Worksheet 1, *My Model of Social Anxiety*
- ◢ Worksheet 2, *Personal Fear and Avoidance List*
- ◢ Worksheet 3, *Looking Forward*

CHAPTER 5

Negative Thoughts and Images

THERAPIST: What makes social situations difficult for you?

CLIENT: Well, I feel like people are always judging, just waiting for me to slip up, it is like all eyes are on me and I don't like it.

THERAPIST: So, you have the thought "people are judging me, waiting for me to slip up," and you may even have an image that goes with that thought of everyone's eyes being focused on you, so understandably that makes the situation very intimidating?

CLIENT: But it doesn't feel like a thought or my imagination, it feels like the truth.

THERAPIST: Well, I guess one possibility is that you are absolutely right and people are judging and watching. Another possibility is that this isn't true and you just think and imagine that this is what is going on. We only need to think we will be judged for the fear response to be triggered, so we can't rely on our feelings as an accurate guide about whether we actually are being evaluated. We need to take a step back and see whether our feelings fit with what is actually happening. In therapy, we will have the opportunity to find out what you are thinking and imagining in social situations, and whether or not these thoughts and images are accurate.

About This Module: Addressing Negative Thoughts and Images in SAD

The first focus of SAD treatment is to assist clients to become more aware of and to question the specific negative beliefs (cognitions) that emerge for them on a regular basis in social situations that they typically find anxiety provoking. These situation-specific negative automatic cognitions may be verbal or imagery based in nature, and may reflect the past (i.e., recalling past social events), the present (i.e., what is occurring socially right now), or the future (i.e., what is expected to occur socially). This module covers the practicalities of targeting this level of cognition, including socializing clients to working within the imagery modality and methods for eliciting and modifying problematic thoughts and images.

As was previously mentioned in Chapter 3, another important cognitive component of the treatment model, negative core beliefs, is addressed much later in treatment. It is not uncommon for clients (and therapists) to question why core beliefs are not targeted first, given they are so influential in determining negative thoughts and images. The following rationale might be given should this issue arise:

"These negative core beliefs, which at the moment seem like core truths of who you are as a person, how other people are generally, and how the world is generally, can develop from our life experiences and how we have made sense of those experiences at the time. For example, we might interpret bad experiences as meaning something bad about ourselves or other people generally or the world generally, and therefore we might expect that bad stuff to occur again and again in life. In this way, the core beliefs color and taint what we expect here and now, acting like old baggage that we are carrying from the past into the present.

"We find that just talking about these core beliefs, trying to challenge them straight away 'head on,' just doesn't work and can be very frustrating for people. These beliefs are highly entrenched, so the best way to tackle them is by having many new experiences that don't fit with these core beliefs, showing that the core belief is outdated. The best way to get those new experiences is to start thinking and behaving in ways that give us the opportunity to learn something new in life—something new about ourselves, others, and the world. Tackling the other elements in the model will allow us to do this. For example, if we are entering social situations with an open mind, rather than avoiding and being preoccupied with negative thoughts and images, we may then have the opportunity to experience others not being judgmental, the social situation going OK, ourselves as being socially capable and coping when things don't go according to plan. Gathering these sorts of experiences is the best way to weaken your negative core beliefs. So when we are working on the other elements of the model first, we are still implicitly working on your core beliefs. When we have made some progress with these other elements, we will then be in a better position to return to the core beliefs toward the end of treatment and tackle them more directly."

The main message is that clients will need to start thinking in more open-minded and unbiased ways so they can enter rather than avoid social situations and process these experiences in a manner that allows the accuracy of their core beliefs to be tested. Addressing negative social thoughts and images is the first step in promoting the open-mindedness required for core belief change, and hence effective treatment.

Socializing Clients to Work with Imagery

Negative social images are a prominent cognitive feature in social anxiety; however, this can be an unfamiliar cognitive modality for many clients. People are generally more familiar with verbally based learning: talking, discussion, and being asked what they *think* about certain things (either in everyday life or by their therapist). "Tuning into" the pictures or multisensory images that flash through their consciousness is not something customarily asked of our clients. A client may have all manner of preconceptions about working with imagery, for example, ideas that it is an odd, magical, embarrassing, or foolish process, or that she "can't do it" because she perceives herself as not a very "visual person." She might believe that having images run through her mind is abnormal or a sign of insanity. Taking time to socialize clients to what imagery is, and the reasons for focusing treatment on identifying and modifying negative social images, not just verbally based cognition, is therefore important for engagement. The rationale for working with imagery is important for clients and therapists alike. With a solid rationale in place, therapists will have greater confidence working within this modality. The ways we go about introducing clients to imagery have been heavily informed by Hackmann and colleagues (2011).

Introducing Imagery

Imagery Discussion

It is important to set the expectation with clients that treatment will involve becoming aware of the negative social images they hold, not just negative verbal thoughts. One way of introducing the concept of imagery is by first asking clients about their understanding of what is meant by "image" or "imagery." During this discussion, therapists should look for any comments about visual or pictorial representations. In addition, they can ask, "What points in time can an image capture?" This can lead to the observation that images can be of experiences in the past (i.e., memories), the present (e.g., how I am coming across to others now), or the future (e.g., how I will come across to others). Imagery is best introduced as an experiential exercise, so feel free to keep verbal discussion brief.

The discussion can be extended by asking clients, "Do you think you are 'good' or 'not so good' at visualizing or thinking in pictures and images?" Encourage clients to be curious and to adopt a "let's find out" attitude. This can lead into the following experiential exercise.

House Imagery Exercise

"Would you be willing to try a simple imagery exercise where we try to bring a particular everyday image to mind to get a better sense of what imagery is all about?

Now, you may be able to form a clear image of the place I'm about to describe, or it may be fuzzy, more a 'felt sense' of the place (i.e., where you feel like you are in the place, but you don't have a vivid picture of it in your mind). Either is OK.

"If you feel comfortable doing so, just close your eyes for a minute while you imagine the front of your house. [pause] How many windows does it have? [pause] What color and texture are the walls? And what about the roof? What is the yard like? What does the front door look like? [pause] Now imagine yourself walking through the front door. [pause] Notice any ways in which you might be experiencing this image with your body or other senses. Open your eyes . . ." (elaborated from Hackmann et al., 2011, p. 62).

When debriefing the House Imagery Exercise, it is important to normalize varying experiences of imagery. Emphasize that there is no right or wrong. Give permission for fuzzy images, images that come in and out of awareness, or images that are predominantly experienced through nonvisual senses (e.g., auditory, tactile, olfactory, gustatory). The following prompts may be useful in facilitating discussion of client experiences:

- "Was the image clear or fuzzy? Was it more a 'felt sense' of being outside your house?"
- "Did the image take time to form or was it instant? Did the image drift in and out?"
- "Was it like a film or more like snapshots?"
- "Was it realistic or more fantasy-like?"
- "Was it just visual or were other senses involved? Touch (e.g., feeling the outside wind or sun on your skin, or the temperature shift when moving from outside to inside the house)? Sound (e.g., hearing the dog bark, or leaves in the yard rustle)? Smell (e.g., the fragrance of the flowers in the garden, the cooking aromas when you entered the house)? Taste (e.g., a sense of thirst and the urge to grab a drink of water as you entered the house)?"

If clients have difficulty accessing imagery, normalize their experience, for example:

"Difficulties are normal, and I can help you learn how to think in pictures . . . remember imagery is a mode we don't refer to a lot in everyday life. We use words all the time and are often asked what we think about something, but we rarely close our eyes to picture something, and we are rarely asked about images passing through our mind."

In summary, imagery can involve any sensory (e.g., visual, auditory, tactile, olfactory, gustatory) mental representation (e.g., an object, place, person, past event, current event, future event) that occupies our mind either very briefly or for more prolonged periods of time.

Free Association Exercise

To consolidate what the client has learned from the House Imagery Exercise, the Free Association Exercise can also be useful.

> "I will say a few words in a moment, and I just want you to notice what pops into your mind . . . car . . . summer . . . clown . . . Christmas . . . flower . . . beach . . . What did you notice? Was it words or images that arose in your mind?"

Typically, clients will be able to acknowledge that imagery of varying quality (brief, fuzzy, transitory, vivid, sustained, etc.) entered their mind with each word stimulus, rather than verbally based cognition. Thus, this exercise can help increase their general awareness of imagery-based cognition.

Negative Social Imagery Examples

Having introduced the concept of imagery more broadly, you can then narrow your discussion to exploring negative social images more specifically. For example:

> "Just as we have mental images to represent most things in life, it is likely that when we are socially anxious, we have images going through our minds that represent our social fears. People with social anxiety often say that they have pictures or snapshots of themselves behaving or appearing in a negative way; or of others reacting to them in a negative way; or even snapshots of past negative social experiences that seem like a scene frozen in time that keeps popping into their head in current social situations. Are you aware of what some of your common negative social images are?"

If clients are unable to access their negative social imagery early on from this more general discussion, again normalize this experience. It is likely that later use of Worksheet 5, *Thought and Imagery Record* (in the Appendix), to monitor their imagery in relation to specific social situations will assist in accessing their negative social imagery.

Rationale for Working with Imagery

Before embarking on further imagery work with clients, it is important to clarify why imagery is a central component of treatment. There are three key reasons why imagery is emphasized in treatment that can be discussed with clients, with each reason highlighting that the usefulness of imagery is not to be underestimated.

Imagery Promotes Cognitive Specificity

Many of the negative thoughts people have when they are socially anxious are catastrophic, abstract, and overgeneralized. For example, the most common response when a socially anxious client is asked, "What do you *think* will happen in a particular social situation?" is something like "I will look like an idiot" or "people will think I am an idiot." But what does looking like an "idiot" actually mean? These types of responses are so overgeneralized, it is unclear exactly what clients are predicting will happen in social situations. Vague predictions are a recipe for ineffective behavioral experiments (as will be addressed further in the next chapter). It is difficult to find effective ways to challenge and change vague and overgeneralized predictions.

Therapists can elicit specific details of social fears verbally by repeatedly asking clients for more specific descriptions. However, imagery immediately places clients within the feared situation, is associated with heightened negative affect, and is thus likely to activate the fear network more broadly and intensely. In our experience this process yields substantially richer and more specific details of feared outcomes. This then places clients in a much better position to effectively challenge and modify their predictions, hence facilitating effective treatment.

Rather than asking clients what they think might happen, we instead ask clients to "close your eyes and tell me what you *envision* happening in the social situation." To this a client might say, "I see myself shaking, stuttering, bright red, having nothing to say" (which is more specific than "I will look like an idiot"), or "I hear others laughing at me, criticizing me, they turn away and avoid speaking to me" (which is more specific than "they will think I am an idiot"). The process of envisaging social catastrophes thus provides specific and testable hypotheses (i.e., "Did you actually shake, stutter, go bright red, and have nothing to say like you had imagined? Did others actually laugh, criticize, turn away, and avoid you?").

Imagery Elicits Stronger Emotions

Research shows that imagery is more strongly linked to our emotional and physiological responses than words. You could use one or both of the following exercises to illustrate this concept with clients.

CHOCOLATE CAKE IMAGERY EXERCISE

"First silently say the words 'chocolate cake' to yourself a few times . . . notice how you feel. Now close your eyes and visualize a piece of chocolate cake in front of you. How do you feel? How does your mouth feel? Do you notice any physical sensations? Do you notice any urges? Open your eyes."

When debriefing this exercise, compare clients' emotional and physiological experiences between thinking in "word" mode versus "picture" mode. It is important to note that a client's reaction doesn't need to be positive for the exercise to have been useful. Aversive reactions are good too (e.g., "I feel sick because I hate chocolate cake, it's too rich"). Noticing a more intense emotional and/or physiological response in the picture mode compared to the word mode is the aim of the exercise. If the food is one the client neither loves nor hates, it will elicit limited emotional or physiological reactivity. If this is the case, you could redo the exercise, but first check you have a food the client is likely to be reactive to. Imagining eating a lemon (as suggested in Hackmann et al., 2011, p. 62) is another option you could try, as it is likely to generate an aversive physical reaction. A lack of difference in reaction could also occur if saying the word automatically generates an image (as in the Free Association Task), making the two conditions too similar to detect a difference. Likewise, if the client struggled to develop an image, then the two conditions may be too similar.

Following this exercise, you can discuss it with the client:

> "Given the aim of treatment is to overcome the emotional and physiological reaction of feeling anxious in social settings, it makes sense that we work in the 'mode' (i.e., imagery rather than words) that is most strongly connected to, and hence most likely to impact that emotion."

BRAIN INPUT AND OUTPUT EXERCISE

It can be useful to elaborate the concept that imagining something can have the same impact on our brain and body as if what we imagine were actually happening in reality. This concept can be expanded by using the following dialogue and the diagram in Figure 5.1, which are adapted from Gilbert (2009, p. 205).

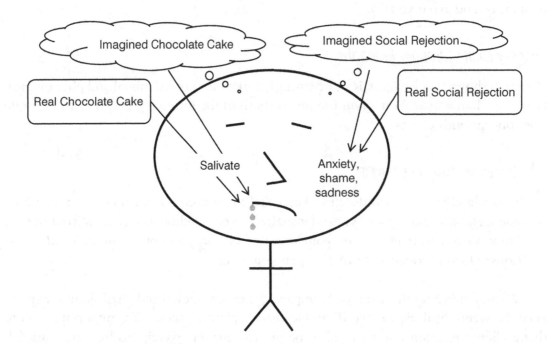

FIGURE 5.1. Schematic diagram of the equivalent physiological and emotional impacts of internal images and actual experiences.

Start by drawing a person's face (see Figure 5.1), and then discussing and adding in the following components:

> "If we have food we really like in front of us (e.g., a real-life chocolate cake) and it is processed by our brain, how does our body react? By salivating. Similarly, if we imagine the same food (i.e., an imagined chocolate cake), our body has the same reaction of salivating. Let's look at an example relevant to social anxiety. If we are rejected socially by someone, we may feel anxiety, shame, sadness. Equally, if we imagine being rejected socially, we are likely to have a similar reaction."

This concept could be used with other examples such as threat (i.e., a real danger versus an imagined danger can both generate the "fight-or-flight" response) or sexual arousal (i.e., sexual contact versus a sexual image can both generate sexual arousal). The idea is to show that the same emotional/physiological output from the processing of an external stimulus (i.e., the "real thing"), also occurs when an equivalent internal stimulus (i.e., the "imagined thing") is processed. It is important to check that clients understand this discussion.

> "The take-home message is that imagining something can be almost as powerful as the real thing. Our brains are not very good at distinguishing imagination from reality. Research shows that the same parts of the brain, the same neural processes, are involved in imagining doing something (e.g., lifting your arm) as actually doing it. This explains why images are more strongly linked to our emotions than words because our brain processes images as if what we are imagining is real."

It is important to relate all this information back to social anxiety treatment specifically.

> "So if we think about your social anxiety, the downside is that holding an image in mind of being rejected prior to going into a social situation can elicit the same feelings as actual rejection, and hence stop you from entering the social situation. But on the upside, if we can work together to develop more helpful images of being socially acceptable and competent, this can elicit the same feelings as actual social acceptance and competence, making you more inclined to give social situations a go."

Imagery Facilitates Exposure and New Learning

Helping clients to be more aware of their negative social imagery can also facilitate exposure. Following a client's negative social image from beginning to end is essentially a form of imaginal exposure. If clients can stick with and follow through their negative social imagery, rather than suppress it, they have the opportunity to run it on past the worst point of the feared situation, which is likely something they very rarely do. This imaginal exposure element can challenge their initial fears by leading to a reevaluation of the real cost and their true coping abilities should they face a social catastrophe.

The benefits of following negative social imagery past the worst point could be explained to clients in the following way:

"It is likely that when you have a negative social image pop into your head, you dwell on the worst part of it for a little bit, then when it becomes too distressing you suppress it, trying to push the image out of your mind. However, research shows that thought suppression often backfires, making you think even more about the thing you don't want to think about. So you get stuck in the worst part of the image as you think about it, then suppress it, think about it, then suppress it, and so on. Overall this keeps your anxiety and concerns about the situation very high. The alternative is to think about the negative social image fully from beginning to end, rather than suppressing it. By doing this you won't get stuck at the worst point. Instead you can run it on past this point and see what you discover about yourself and other people. You might be surprised to discover that your fears aren't as scary, or that you are able to cope better than you thought. It is likely that when you take this approach, your anxiety and concerns will be more like a wave, subsiding when you allow yourself to move past the worst point."

It is important to note that contemporary behavioral theory deemphasizes the need for anxiety reduction (i.e., habituation) during exposure tasks. Inhibitory learning theory (Craske et al., 2014) suggests that the most critical aspect of exposure is expectancy violation—whereby the client's negative expectations are directly tested and found to be highly discrepant from the actual outcome. This approach prioritizes the amount of "surprise" clients experience from their exposure tasks rather than anxiety reduction. From this perspective, the lack of constraints on imagery (any aspect of feared social situations can be imagined) compared to *in vivo* exposure (access to contexts and social situations is more limited) may enhance learning. More specific, elaborate, and vivid predictions can be generated in imagery, thereby potentially maximizing the number of "surprises" during either imaginal or *in vivo* exposure.

Identifying Negative Thoughts and Images

Thought/Image–Feeling Connection

The Thought/Image–Feeling Connection Exercise can be a useful way of socializing clients to the important role that thoughts and images have in eliciting emotion generally and, in particular, the role of negative social thoughts and images in eliciting anxious feelings. The exercise involves guiding clients through the completion of Worksheet 4, *Thought/Image-Feeling Connection* (in the Appendix). In this exercise a hypothetical trigger situation is provided (i.e., a friend is late meeting me at a café), as are four possible emotional reactions (i.e., angry, anxious, sad/depressed, neutral). Clients are asked to generate possible thoughts and images that might go through the protagonist's mind to generate each of these feelings. The exercise is used to illustrate the relationship between thoughts/images and emotions, and how different thoughts/images lead to different emotional reactions. Using a hypothetical example initially to facilitate this learning may help clients subsequently be more open to exploring their own problematic thoughts and images and the emotions these generate.

Eliciting Thoughts and Images

When identifying clients' own negative social thoughts and images, the two key themes for therapists to look for are:

1. Overestimation of the perceived likelihood or probability that negative events will happen in social situations, and
2. Overestimation of the cost or consequences of negative events occurring in social situations.

Therapists may be more familiar with eliciting verbally based negative social thoughts. Typically, this involves choosing a specific social anxiety trigger, which will often be an upcoming social situation clients anticipate going badly, but may also be a past social situation they perceive did not go well. Common questions used to elicit verbally based cognitions might include:

- "What concerns you the most about the situation?"
- "What are you worried about in this situation?"
- "What are you predicting will happen? What do you think happened?"
- "How do you think people will react? How do you think people reacted?"
- "How do you think you will come across? How do you think you came across?"
- "What do you think people will think about you? What do you think people thought of you?"
- "What's the worst part of the situation for you?"
- "What's bad about that?"
- "What does that mean to you?"
- "What does that mean about you?"

Given that recent theory and evidence suggest that people with SAD may be fearful of both negative and positive evaluation, it might be worthwhile asking clients, "How do you feel when you receive positive attention?" If they report feeling uncomfortable, the questions above are likely to elicit the idiosyncratic negative meanings of positive evaluation.

Some typical SAD thoughts that may be revealed by these questions include:

- "They will judge me."
- "They won't want to know me."
- "I made a bad impression."
- "I said the wrong thing."
- "They think I am an idiot, stupid, weird, weak, boring."
- "I won't know what to say, or I'll say something stupid."
- "I looked awkward, anxious, foolish."
- "I will do something embarrassing."
- "I will be humiliated."
- "I won't be able to cope."
- "They will laugh at me."
- "They might think I'm a snob."

When it comes to eliciting negative social images, as with eliciting verbal thinking, it is useful to start with a specific social anxiety trigger. Once a specific trigger has been identified, clients can then be asked to imagine the scenario, and during this experience the therapist asks questions to uncover negative social images. The imagined social situation may be in the future, or a memory of a past social situation that they perceive went badly. The following questions can be used as a guide to facilitate this process:

"Close your eyes and imagine being in that situation as if you are there right now experiencing it firsthand. So, looking through your own eyes out at the situation . . ."

- "Where are you?"
- "What are you doing? What is happening?"
- "What can you see? Are there any other sensations of note (sounds, smells, sensations on your body/skin)?"
- "Who is there?"
- "What are other people doing? How are other people responding to you? What are other people noticing about you?"
- "What happens next?"
- "What are you thinking?"
- "How are you feeling? Where do you feel that in your body? What physical sensations go with that feeling?"
- "How are you handling the situation? How are you coping?"
- "What part of this situation bothers you most?"

These questions are a guide only. Depending on the scenario being explored, therapists will need to judge which questions are most helpful to use, how many questions to use, and how circular the line of questioning needs to be (i.e., "what is happening . . . what are people doing . . . what are you thinking . . . what are you feeling . . . what happens next . . . now what are you doing . . . how are other people reacting now . . . what are you thinking now . . . how do you feel now . . . now what is happening . . . , and so on."). When uncovering negative social images, clients are initially encouraged to adopt a first-person, present-tense, field perspective (i.e., "looking through your own eyes out at the situation . . ."). During the course of eliciting imagery, clients may naturally switch to an observer perspective, identifying imagery about how they are appearing and performing socially from others' perspectives. This can be considered a specific subtype of negative social imagery, that is, the negative self-image. Images of this nature will be addressed more explicitly in Chapter 7.

The negative social images clients report will generally be richer elaborations of the previous themes uncovered when eliciting verbal thoughts. The imagery may be literal or more metaphorical in nature. Common images might include:

- "I am alone in the corner of the room, separate from everyone else. Everyone else is talking and having a good time, and I am not part of it."
- "I say something stupid and others laugh and turn away, not wanting to hang around me anymore."
- "I trip and drop my things. I look like a bumbling fool, and others laugh or stare at me strangely."
- "Other people are talking about me behind my back, sniggering and pointing at me."
- "I see myself trembling, shaking, and looking as bright red as a beetroot."
- "I can hear my voice, it sounds squeaky, stuttery, unstable, like my voice is breaking."
- "I have this sensation of being hot, under a spotlight, all eyes zeroing in on me."
- "Specific past memories of being bullied or humiliated at school flash through my mind."

Thought and Imagery Record

Self-monitoring outside of therapy sessions can be a useful method of identifying thoughts and images. Discuss with clients the usefulness of Worksheet 5, *Thought and Imagery Record* (and see Handout 2, *Recording Thoughts and Images*—both are in the Appendix) as a means of "catching" or "tuning in" to their negative social thoughts and images, which typically have been very automatic and unconscious for some time. Explain that paying more attention to these thoughts and images and writing them down will give us the best opportunity to do something about them.

The record can be completed anytime between sessions (and also within session) when clients feel socially anxious, using anxiety as the cue to complete the record. When clients notice this cue, the *Thought and Imagery Record* prompts them to note the trigger situation, trying to be specific regarding the "where," "what," and "who" of the social situation that is bothering them. They then reflect on what thoughts are going through their mind about the situation. Separate from the verbal thoughts they identify, clients should then try to notice any specific visual images that arise from or with these thoughts. They can also note if there are any other sensory qualities aside from the visual domain that accompany the image (i.e., sensations of sound, body/touch, tastes, or smells that may be part of the image). Finally, they must note how they feel emotionally, which will likely be some variant of an anxiety/fear response but may also include other emotions such as shame or humiliation. The Subjective Units of Distress Scale (SUDS) is used to rate from 0 to 10 the intensity of their emotional reaction.

Complete a full example in the *Thought and Imagery Record* collaboratively in session with clients first to increase their confidence that they can complete the form independently for homework. Generally, clients would use this monitoring form for one week as a homework exercise, with the aim of increasing their awareness of negative social thoughts and images and the impact of these cognitions on their emotions. Doing this will lay the foundation for subsequent cognition modification strategies (i.e., imagery challenging and behavioral experiments).

Difficulties Accessing Negative Thoughts and Images

Some clients may be able to readily identify and monitor their negative social thoughts and images, while others may struggle with accessing thoughts, images, or both. Common difficulties may include the following:

Cognitive Avoidance

Negative social thoughts and images are going to be anxiety provoking, with negative social images likely to be more anxiety provoking than thoughts. In either case, avoidance of thoughts and/or imagery may be a client's habitual coping strategy. If clients are particularly anxious and avoidant of imagery, ensure that the rationale for working with imagery to enhance the effectiveness of the treatment has been adequately addressed. Normalize any elevation in anxiety that occurs from identifying negative thoughts and images, reassuring clients that this is likely to be temporary, and even reframing this as a positive sign that they are challenging their anxiety. Clients need to appreciate that rather than avoiding these thoughts or images they need to start paying attention to them, so they can then do something about them. The following metaphor may be useful in communicating this concept.

> "It is a bit like boxing with a blindfold on, it is pretty hard to do when you can't see your opponent. If you take off the blindfold your opponent may initially look scary, but you will be in a much better position to plan a strategy for how to overcome them once you can actually see them."

Behavioral Avoidance

Some clients may not be experiencing much day-to-day social anxiety due to pervasive social avoidance, which limits opportunities to catch their negative social images and thoughts. Clients may need to purposely confront social situations, or use imaginal social scenarios to activate thoughts and imagery that can then be used for monitoring. It may be useful to engage clients in real or imagined social situations within the session, so the therapist can assist them both in reversing avoidant behavior and accessing their cognitions.

Limited Cognitive Awareness

If clients report no awareness of mental images or thoughts, you could try the following, which all rely on the notion that when affect is activated, cognitions will be more easily accessible.

• Identify a very specific recent example of when a client has felt socially anxious, and then imaginally reexperience the scenario (e.g., "Close your eyes and pretend to be back in the supermarket line about to approach the cashier"). You can then question what thoughts or images are going through his mind, being back in the scenario experiencing it firsthand as if it were happening now (e.g., "I'm thinking I don't know what to say—get me out of here," "I am awkward, I'm stuttering, I can't string a sentence together," "everyone is staring at me"). If that line of questioning is unproductive, you could stay with his recollection of the scenario and ask what he concludes from it now (e.g., "I looked like a bumbling fool, I just have no social skills"). Again, if this leads nowhere ask him to guess "What do you think could go wrong here?" Alternatively, you could pose the likely opposite expectation, such as "are you thinking that talking to this person will be really easy and go really smoothly?" These questions should help to elicit the client's negative expectation, even if it hasn't been labeled as an actual thought or image.

• Identify an upcoming anxiety-provoking social situation (e.g., attending a work party) and encourage clients to imaginally visualize how they predict the scenario will play out. For example:

THERAPIST: Close your eyes and imagine you are entering the party right now, what do you see?

CLIENT: Everyone is having a good time—laughing, chatting.

THERAPIST: Where are you in the picture?

CLIENT: I am all alone, no one is talking to me.

THERAPIST: What happens next?

CLIENT: People are staring at me.

THERAPIST: How are you feeling?

CLIENT: Really nervous.

THERAPIST: What concerns you about people staring?

CLIENT: They are probably thinking "Oh no, what's he doing here?"

- Create an anxiety-provoking situation that can be completed within the therapy session (e.g., the client dropping paperwork on the floor of the waiting area). The questions previously outlined to elicit cognitive content can be used prior to, during, or after the task. Even if clients are too anxious to follow through on the task, elevated anxiety is a sign that negative social thoughts and images are activated, and therapists can focus their efforts on accessing these.

Fear of Negative Evaluation

Fear of negative evaluation may present itself in the therapeutic relationship and interfere with identifying negative thoughts and images. Clients may perceive their thoughts and images to be stupid or illogical, or may question whether the thoughts and images they are identifying are "right." Thus, they may be reluctant to disclose their thoughts and images because they feel embarrassed and may fear being judged by the therapist. It is important to explicitly communicate that whatever thoughts or images arise for clients, there are no right, wrong, or stupid examples, again reinforcing the importance of awareness to facilitate change. To normalize cognitions about negative evaluation, clinicians might describe some examples from past clients, or even some of their own thoughts and images in social situations.

When it comes to accessing social imagery in particular, clients may find the process of closing their eyes in front of the therapist embarrassing and anxiety provoking. They may become distracted by concerns over what the therapist is seeing and thinking. This issue can usually be solved by the therapist agreeing to drop his gaze to the floor, turning therapist and client chairs back to back, or having clients start with their eyes open and dropping their gaze to the ground, working up to eyes-closed imagery work. This reluctance can be framed as an opportunity for in-session graded exposure or behavioral experimentation.

Tips for Accessing Negative Thoughts and Images

Using Thoughts to Identify Imagery

Clients may be able to identify thoughts readily but struggle with associated imagery. If this is the case, the following questions can be useful:

- "What does that thought (e.g., 'I'll look like an idiot'), look like as a picture?"
- "When you think (e.g., 'I'll look like an idiot'), what do you see or hear happening? What do you envisage playing out? What do you imagine? If this were playing out like a movie, describe to me what would be happening in the scene."
- "If I were there (e.g., when you were looking like an 'idiot'), what would I be seeing and hearing?"
- "Sit with the feelings, sensations, and thoughts this situation brings up for you and see if you can allow an image to emerge that represents how you feel. It might not

be an image of a real thing. It could be a fantasy or purely imaginary representation of your fear (e.g., an image of being a lot smaller in stature than the other person you're interacting with, or an image of being onstage under a spot light with a hundred eyes on you)."

Using Imagery to Identify Thoughts

Conversely, clients may be able to identify images readily but struggle with associated verbal meaning. If this is the case, the following can be useful questions:

- "How would you summarize what is happening in that picture?"
- "What does the image mean to you?"
- "What does the image mean about you?"
- "What does the image mean about other people?"
- "What is that picture overall suggesting about how you are coming across, performing, or appearing, or the observability of your anxiety?"
- "What is that picture overall suggesting about other people, their reactions to you, or their evaluations of you?"
- "What is that image suggesting about other social interactions you may encounter?"

A client in one of our social anxiety groups experienced severe anticipatory anxiety about making phone calls, which resulted in almost wholesale avoidance of using the telephone. Despite extensive and varied questioning from her therapist, she was having great difficulty identifying any specific concerns about making phone calls. The therapist eventually asked her to imagine that she was involved in a conversation and that this was playing out on the television screen. She was encouraged to see herself and the other person on the screen, separated by a diagonal line as depicted in the old TV shows in the 1960s. The therapist then asked how the other person was looking on the screen. The client described the other person as looking irritated for being kept from other activities she would prefer to be doing. In this example, the imagery enabled the client to identify the predictions that friends would be inconvenienced and irritated by her calling them and that they did not want to speak to her, which explained her anxiety and avoidance of phone calls.

Modifying Negative Thoughts and Images

Once clients can identify their negative social thoughts and images using the *Thought and Imagery Record,* the next step is to work on challenging and modifying these cognitions using Worksheet 6, the *Imagery Challenging Record* (in the Appendix). While clients' awareness of their cognitions is necessary for the modification process, it is important to move to the task of modifying cognitions as soon as possible. Identifying negative thoughts and images is the first important step toward cognitive change, but awareness is not enough to produce enduring emotional change. It is important that clients have an early experience of success or change in therapy, so don't delay moving to the challenging process unless the client is really stuck on basic cognitive awareness.

The *Imagery Challenging Record* assists clients to make more accurate judgments about perceived social danger by challenging the overestimation of both the probability and consequences of social catastrophe. The notion of cognitive challenging can be introduced to clients in the following manner.

"Now that we are more aware of some of your typical negative social thoughts and images, we are in a good position to take a step back and look at how accurate they are. Previously these thoughts and images have been so quick and automatic, that understandably you have just accepted them without question. Up until now, you haven't had the opportunity to question them, to be curious about them, to check them out further. The Imagery Challenging Record will be the tool we will use to do this. When we do this, it will be a bit like taking the stance of a lawyer or detective, putting the negative thoughts and images on trial and looking at the factual evidence that does or does not support them, to see how they 'hold up.' If we get to the end of the process and find out that your negative social thoughts and images are valid, then this means there is a real problem going on for you that needs to be addressed, and we could then use problem-solving strategies to do this. However, if we get to the end of the process and discover that your negative social thoughts and images may be inaccurate in some way, then we can update them to better reflect reality, which should in turn have an impact on how fearful you are in social situations."

Notice that the stance that is taken in this explanation is one of curiosity about the accuracy of client's cognitions, rather than a presumption that her cognitions are "wrong." It is important for therapists to adopt this genuinely agnostic attitude during the cognitive challenging process, and to instill this same attitude in their clients. Cognitive challenging is not intended to be a process of interrogation, persuasion, or entrapment. It is an invitation for clients to curiously explore the accuracy of their ideas.

It is often helpful to socialize clients to the challenging process by completing an *Imagery Challenging Record* on a hypothetical example that is unrelated to their primary concerns (see Handout 3, *Challenging Negative Thoughts and Images,* in the Appendix for a completed example). Clients typically find it easier to familiarize themselves with the process of cognitive restructuring when they are unencumbered by their own emotion-laden examples. Once clients are familiar with this process, they can then use the *Imagery Challenging Record* to tackle their own real-life examples. Their first attempt at this should be done with the therapist in session. Depending on how well they apply this new skill, they can then try doing this independently as a homework exercise any time they feel socially anxious. Highly avoidant clients who are unable to identify specific thoughts or images will need to imaginally or behaviorally expose themselves to social scenarios so they have some "grist for the mill."

When using the *Imagery Challenging Record* there are eight steps involved in the modification process. The first three steps should be familiar to clients, as they center on identifying negative social thoughts and images, and are essentially a streamlined version of the *Thought and Imagery Record* they have already been using. The remaining five steps will be new to clients and may require greater discussion.

How to Challenge Negative Social Images

The eight steps of imagery challenging as explained to clients are outlined below, and are also included in Handout 3, *Challenging Negative Thoughts and Images*. The handout can be provided to clients as psychoeducational reading material to assist them when acquiring this new skill. As you will see, imagery features specifically at steps 2, 6, and 7 of the imagery challenging process. Essentially the only deviation from standard cognitive therapy is to put more emphasis on ensuring the initial negative automatic thought is accessed in the imagery modality, and the new balanced or helpful thought at the end of the restructuring process is also in the imagery modality and accessed as such. This is not a radical shift from other forms of cognitive restructuring. However, this simple adjustment is intended to enhance an already tried and true technique by increasing the intensity of the emotional connection. As will be discussed later, imagery can also be incorporated in other ways during the restructuring process when the therapist judges this to be useful.

Step 1: Trigger Situation

"What is the social situation concerning you? Briefly and objectively describe the situation (e.g., where it is, what is happening, who is there). This might be a past situation that you are reflecting on or a future situation that you are anticipating."

Step 2: Negative Image

"Describe the negative visual images and thoughts going through your mind about the trigger situation. Also, describe any other senses that are part of the image (i.e., sounds, body/touch sensations, tastes, smells). If thoughts in the form of words are most prominent, try to close your eyes and see what picture arises that represents those thoughts."

Step 3: Emotion

"Describe the emotions you are feeling in relation to the trigger situation, and indicate their intensity using the Subjective Units of Distress (SUDS) rating (0–10)."

Step 4: Contrary Evidence

"Look for contrary evidence that suggests these thoughts and images may not be entirely accurate, and consider alternative ways the situation could play out. The focus on contrary evidence is because people tend to be very good at remembering experiences that confirm their fears but find it more difficult to recall contrary experiences. The best way to counteract this bias is to think about evidence that does not support your negative thoughts and images. It is important to recognize that your initial negative thoughts and images portray just one of many possible outcomes, so it can be useful to entertain alternative perspectives. Asking the following questions can assist in uncovering contrary evidence and alternative views."

- "Have I had any experiences that show that this image is not completely true all of the time?"
- "Are there any small things that contradict my image that I might be ignoring?"
- "Have I been in this type of situation before? What happened? Is there anything different between this situation and previous ones? What have I learned from prior experiences that could help me now?"
- "Is my image based on facts, or am I 'mind reading'? What evidence do I really have?"
- "Am I jumping to conclusions that are not completely justified by the evidence?"
- "If someone who loves me knew I was having this image, what would they say to me? What evidence would they point out that would suggest that my image was not 100% true?"
- "Are there other ways of looking at this situation?"
- "What are all the possible explanations in this situation? Are there any alternatives to mine?"
- "What's the best that could happen?"
- "What's the worst that could happen? What's so bad about that? Could I cope with this? Would life go on? What could I do that would help?"
- "Will this still bother me in 1 week/month/year?"
- "If the roles were reversed, how might I judge the situation/other person?"
- "Regardless of whether the image is true, is it helpful to think this way? What are the negative consequences of thinking this way? What would be a more helpful way to think or a more helpful image to hold?"

Step 5: Realistic Probability and Consequences

"Given the contrary evidence and alternative perspectives, now consider the most realistic probability and consequences. If you are completing the record regarding a past social situation, you might want to think about the true probability that your interpretation of events was entirely accurate. If you are certain that your interpretation is accurate (based on good evidence), you might want to spend more time focusing on the true consequences in a balanced way."

PROBABILITY

"What is the most likely outcome? If the situation is in the future, how likely is it that your negative image will actually occur? If the situation is in the past, how likely is it that your negative image is an accurate and balanced picture of the whole situation? You might want to also consider how likely it is that a negative outcome would occur in the same situation in the future."

CONSEQUENCE

"What are the most likely consequences? If something bad happened, then so what? Is it really a catastrophe? What can you do to cope? If you anticipate something bad happening, how bad would it really be? Will you still be thinking about it a day, week, a year, or 10 years down the line? If not, can you let it go now?"

Step 6: Helpful Image

"Given what you have learned for steps 4 and 5, now develop a more helpful or realistic image of the situation. In as much detail as you can, create a new picture of how things are likely to go. If this is about a situation that has already happened, then create a more helpful image that incorporates your contrary evidence and realistic consequences."

Step 7: Visualize Helpful Image

"Now spend a few moments visualizing the helpful image. Spend at least 2 minutes bringing this new image to mind. Doing this is important, as it will allow you to experience the full emotional impact of your new more helpful and/or realistic image."

Step 8: Rerate Emotion

"Describe and rate the strength of how you feel visualizing the helpful image. Use the SUDS rating (0–10)."

The Contrary Evidence and Realistic Probability and Consequences sections of the *Imagery Challenging Record* are essentially standard verbally based cognitive challenging techniques. One could use the questions strictly in this manner and then summarize the findings from this line of questioning by developing a more helpful image (i.e., step

6), and then activating the image by visualizing it (i.e., step 7). The addition of steps 6 and 7, which are not standard in traditional thought records, is intended to enhance the emotional connectedness of any cognitive shifts that have been achieved. Having a new cognitive perspective represented in an imagery format, and then activating that image by purposely bringing it to mind, should elicit a stronger emotional impact than keeping the new cognitive perspective purely in a verbal format.

Therapists can also encourage clients to find ways to work in imagery mode throughout the whole thought-challenging process, not just when prompted at steps 2, 6, and 7. For example, at step 5, when encouraging clients to consider the true consequences of social mishap, encouraging them to imagine things going wrong and running this image on past the worst point may help shed light on the severity and longevity of social catastrophe. In addition, at step 4 when clients recall experiences that provide contrary evidence to their negative social images, the therapist can ask them to imaginally reexperience these events to give the evidence more emotional weight. The following dialogue illustrates how this might be done:

THERAPIST: Are there any experiences you have had, no matter how small, that don't quite fit with the image that people at your office party are going to stare, not talk to you, and be wishing you weren't there?

CLIENT: I don't know . . . I guess the other day one of my coworkers asked me if I was going to the party, and when I said yes she seemed pleased.

THERAPIST: How did that make you feel?

CLIENT: Good, I guess . . . at the time.

THERAPIST: It might be useful to get a bit more in touch with that "good" feeling. I am wondering if you could take a moment right now to close your eyes and imagine being back in the situation when your colleague spoke to you, as if it is happening right now. So looking out of your own eyes at the situation . . . what's happening?

CLIENT: I am at the coffee machine, I'm almost done with getting my coffee, and I turn around and see Tania heading for the machine after me. She says hi and smiles . . . I say hi back. I turn to leave, and she says, "So are you going to the party?" I say, "Yeah, I think so." Tania says "Great, I'll see you there." Again she is smiling and cheery.

THERAPIST: How are you feeling now?

CLIENT: Positive, happy, it feels nice to have someone being friendly and seeming to want me around . . . but she was probably just being polite.

THERAPIST: For now, I want you to stay with the positive feeling, rather than allowing your mind to steer you away from that. How do you know you feel happy? Where do you feel it in your body?

CLIENT: In my chest.

THERAPIST: What do you feel in your chest?

CLIENT: Lightness, energy, warmth.

THERAPIST: What about your body posture and facial expression, what are they doing as you feel this sense of happiness?

CLIENT: I am smiling, head up, shoulders back as I walk away.

THERAPIST: Can you do that now . . . smile with your head up and shoulders back . . . See if you can stay with that feeling a little bit longer . . . when you are ready you can open your eyes. So, Tania seeming happy about you attending the party, is that contrary evidence that we can jot down?

At step 7, when clients are encouraged to visualize the more helpful and/or realistic image, therapists may need to prompt them to engage and persist with this process, revisiting the rationale that this will generate a greater emotional impact than just looking at the words on the paper. Therapists can facilitate this process with some combination of the following prompts, depending on what seems appropriate for the image being explored. In group treatment, therapists can follow the prompts exactly. In individual treatment, clients will be able to give verbal feedback in response to the prompt questions, and their feedback will guide the prompts selected:

"Close your eyes and spend a few moments visualizing this new more helpful and realistic image as if you are experiencing it firsthand right now."

- "What do you see, hear, sense?"
- "What is happening?"
- "Where are you?"
- "Who is there?"
- "What are you doing?"
- "What is your posture like?"
- "What is your facial expression like?"
- "How do you feel?"
- "Where do you feel it in your body?"
- "What physical sensations do you notice?"
- "What are you thinking?"
- "What happens next?"

The final step of the *Imagery Challenging Record* allows client and therapist to reflect on the experience of visualizing the more helpful image, particularly exploring the emotional impact of the visualization. Aside from emotional impact, it can be useful to take the impact of the imagery challenging one step further, discussing any effect on the client's preparedness to enter the social situation in the future. This can provide a nice bridge into the behavioral experiments to come.

The helpful image developed from the imagery challenging process can then be called to mind anytime clients notice they feel anxious regarding the event in question. It is important that clients realize this is not a guarantee of how things will occur in reality. This is not a case of imagine it and it will come true. Nor is the image to be misused as a safety behavior, with clients feeling compelled to hold these helpful images in mind constantly to prevent their fears coming true and enable them to cope. Instead the image is a shorthand reminder of a more realistic and helpful perspective, and elicits the feelings associated with this perspective. Some mental rehearsal of the image may be appropriate, as is calling it to mind briefly before, during, or following the social event, with the overall aim of the image being to assist clients to more flexibly consider alternative helpful and realistic images, and hence engage and persist with much-needed social behavior change.

Tips for Challenging Negative Thoughts and Images

The most common material worked with in imagery challenging for social anxiety centers on anticipatory anxiety about an upcoming social situation. The thoughts and images identified often reflect a fairly literal but negative conception of how clients imagine social scenarios will play out. After looking at contrary evidence and realistic probabilities and consequences, the client will create a new image that will reflect a more realistic and literal version of events. However, sometimes the material worked on in imagery challenging may be more fantasy or metaphorically based (e.g., "I am walking a tightrope as onlookers jeer and shout at me"). In this case, the new image may be metaphorical in nature too, conveying a more helpful perspective (e.g., "People aren't really interested in watching me on the tightrope, they are caught up watching some other performer, so I just start playing around, trying a few jumps and flips, and there is a net underneath to catch me, so there isn't any real danger"). We have therefore referred to this image in the *Imagery Challenging Record* as the "Helpful Image" to accommodate images that might be realistic or metaphorical in nature. To prompt for a new metaphorical image after the client has considered contrary evidence and realistic probabilities and consequences, the therapist might ask, "What needs to change in your original negative image, so the image better reflects this information we have just uncovered?"

If the initial negative image is literal in nature, it is OK if the more realistic image happens to take on a more fantasy-based or metaphorical tone, provided it is capturing the more helpful perspectives gained from filling out the Contrary Evidence and Realistic Probabilities and Consequences sections of the worksheet and has a helpful emotional impact. For example, the initial negative image may be of one's peers being nasty and openly critical, and the new helpful image may be of these peers being the size of mice to convey the perspective that their opinions aren't that important. With this principle in mind (i.e., that the content of the new image is irrelevant, it is the meaning represented that is most important), there may be some therapeutic credibility to the old lay advice for performance anxiety given to many of us by well-meaning relatives, that of imagining one's audience in their underwear. This type of image communicates the sentiment that the audience is not superior, judgmental, or any real threat to us. However, it is important that the new helpful image be the client's own creation, communicating helpful meaning in an idiosyncratic way, rather than a prescription from the therapist, like a glib old uncle telling us, "Just imagine everyone is in their underwear and you'll be all right!"

An *Imagery Challenging Record* may also be applied to social situations that have already occurred that clients judge have gone badly. In these circumstances, it is important to remember that the negative image they hold is still a representation of the event that is laden with meanings they have attached to it, even if the event was objectively negative (e.g., someone openly being rude and calling them "weird" in front of other people). In these circumstances, all the questions of step 4 designed to elicit contrary evidence and alternative perspectives are still relevant, except for "What's the best that could happen?" and "What's the worst that could happen," as the event has already transpired. However, these questions could be asked about whether there are likely to be ongoing consequences into the future. When it comes to examining realistic probabilities and consequences, focusing more on the consequences may be particularly helpful in these instances, using questions like:

- "Was it really as bad as the negative image I'm holding?"
- "How biased is the negative image?"
- "What was the real cost or the consequences?"
- "Did I cope? Survive? Get through it?"
- "What could I do now to cope with it?"
- "Will this still matter in 1 week/one month/one year/etc.?"

The helpful image will then incorporate the alternative perspectives that have been generated. For example, the image may include people staring at the other person for being so rude, and may also include other people encountered at the same event who were pleasant. Playing out the whole image from beginning to end will reduce the risk of getting stuck at the most distressing aspect of the situation, and instead will involve moving past that point to focus on how clients coped with the rest of the event. It might also be helpful to fast-forward the image to a year later, imagining what clients might be doing and how much they will care about the negative event or negative person with the passage of time.

A common difficulty during imagery challenging is a lack of contrary evidence. This can either be the result of clients having endured an unusually large number of negative social experiences due to exposure to a specific negative environment (e.g., highly critical family members) and/or a pervasive and long-standing pattern of avoidance that leaves clients with limited social experiences to draw on. It may be necessary in these instances to design behavioral experiments (see Chapter 6) in generally "safe" environments as a means of gathering new evidence. As new evidence is collected in the here-and-how, clients will become more aware that their negative experiences were specific to a certain time and place, and may not hold true now or in other environments. Behavioral experiments then become the means of gathering contrary evidence.

Another difficulty encountered in standard thought challenging work is the disconnect between rational knowledge (i.e., the "head") and emotion (i.e., the "gut"). This is usually captured by clients saying at the end of thought challenging, "I know logically that my thoughts aren't true, but I still feel like they are." The use of imagery in the cognitive challenging process is designed to bridge the gap between head and gut, connecting emotion to cognitive change, and hopefully minimizing this common discrepancy. However, if the disconnect persists, you can explain to clients that together you will "check out" whether their thoughts and images are true later by using behavioral experiments, which will help them to really believe their new evidence at an emotional level.

A final difficulty that can emerge regarding imagery challenging is the sheer effort involved in developing this skill. Early in treatment clients will need to formally complete the *Imagery Challenging Record* to get the maximum benefit, which may seem an onerous task. It must be acknowledged that applying this skill does take some effort, but is a means to an end, the end being to retrain the mind to become more flexible and produce more realistic and helpful thoughts and images. Reassure clients that with practice and persistence, entertaining more helpful perspectives will become a more automatic and less effortful cognitive process.

Clinical Case: Modifying Negative Imagery

A client who was extremely fearful of walking along a populated café strip had the negative image of many people along the street and in the cafés staring at him as he walked past, frowning and sneering at him, with their dirty looks indicating that they were thinking he wasn't "good enough." After considering the contrary evidence and the realistic probabilities and consequences, he could logically accept that it was unlikely people would be paying him much attention, as they would likely be caught up in their own world. When constructing a new image that captured this knowledge, a more fantasy-based metaphorical image came to mind of the people being replaced by dogs and cats. We played around with the image, imagining dogs and cats dressed in human clothes going about human business, for example the barista dog making the client's coffee. We had a good laugh at this together. We discussed that it didn't necessarily matter that the new image wasn't reality based, it was the meaning it represented that was important. When asked about its meaning the client said, "Well, dogs love you unconditionally, and cats don't give a s___ about you." Hence, the new image represented the meaning we were looking for, that there was no need to fear negative judgment because people are mostly accepting and nice, or couldn't care less about you.

THERAPY SUMMARY GUIDE: Negative Thoughts and Images

Therapy Aim: Identify and modify negative social thoughts and images reflecting a high probability and cost of social catastrophe.

Therapy Agenda Items:

▼ Introduce imagery:

◢ Imagery discussion

◢ House Imagery Exercise

◢ Free Association Exercise

◢ Negative social imagery examples

▼ Provide a rationale for working with imagery:

◢ Imagery promotes cognitive specificity

◢ Imagery elicits stronger emotions, as illustrated by the Chocolate Cake Imagery Exercise and the Brain Input and Output Exercise

◢ Imagery facilitates exposure and new learning

▼ Identify negative thoughts and images:

◢ Worksheet 4, *Thought/Image–Feeling Connection*

◢ Worksheet 5, *Thought and Imagery Record*—review hypothetical examples, then apply to client examples with therapist assistance, then complete independently for homework when social anxiety is triggered

▼ Modify negative thoughts and images:

◢ Worksheet 6, *Imagery Challenging Record*—review hypothetical examples, apply to client examples with therapist assistance, client completes the record independently for homework when social anxiety is triggered, and later in therapy as preparation for behavioral experiments

Therapy Materials:

▼ Handouts

◢ Handout 2, *Recording Thoughts and Images*—includes Thought and Imagery Record Example

◢ Handout 3, *Challenging Negative Thoughts and Images*—includes Imagery Challenging Record Example

▼ Worksheets

◢ Worksheet 4, *Thought/Image–Feeling Connection*

◢ Worksheet 5, *Thought and Imagery Record*

◢ Worksheet 6, *Imagery Challenging Record*

CHAPTER 6

Avoidance and Safety Behaviors

THERAPIST: So, how have you usually tried to manage your social anxiety?

CLIENT: Mostly I just stay away from people. I can't be judged if there is no one around to judge me.

THERAPIST: So, avoiding people is one way you cope. Are there ever situations that you just can't avoid and you have to suffer through them?

CLIENT: It is hard to avoid people completely, so yes. You know I have to go to work, grocery shop, those sorts of things that I need to do just to live. I can't completely avoid people.

THERAPIST: In these sorts of situations what do you do to control your anxiety or avoid others judging you?

CLIENT: At work I don't say much to people, just keep to myself and make sure I always look too busy to be chatting with others. At the shops, I only go really late at night when there is hardly anyone there, and I am in and out really quick, I don't hang around.

THERAPIST: So, it sounds like when you can't outright avoid a situation you do other things to try to keep yourself safe, like stay quiet, look busy, be strategic about the time you go, or rush through the experience. These are what we call "safety behaviors." Safety behaviors are subtle forms of avoidance. Do you think avoiding people and using these sorts of safety behaviors have been helpful ways to cope with the problem?

CLIENT: Well, it keeps the anxiety at bay, otherwise it would be completely unbearable.

THERAPIST: In therapy, we will have the opportunity to look at these avoidance and safety behaviors in more detail. On the surface or in the short term it might feel like they are helping, it might feel like you are managing the problem. But we need to be curious and look at the impact of these behaviors in the long term, to see if they might be making the problem worse in some way.

About This Module:
Addressing Avoidance and Safety Behaviors in SAD

Most people with significant anxiety avoid some or all the triggers of their anxiety. People with SAD often avoid any situation in which they perceive that social threat is likely and costly. While on the surface it may be clear that clients are avoiding particular trigger situations, what they are more specifically avoiding is the possibility of their negative social thoughts and images coming true in these situations.

Some social situations will be completely avoided, whereas others may be endured with distress, at least until escape is possible. In these situations, it is likely that some form of safety behavior will be at work. Safety behaviors are subtle covert avoidance behaviors that are used when overt avoidance is not possible. For example, an individual might attend an obligatory work meeting while using the safety behavior of not speaking to prevent feared images of being criticized by colleagues from coming to fruition. On the surface safety behaviors look different from avoidance, but they serve exactly the same function. Wholesale avoidance and safety behaviors are both methods of trying to prevent feared social thoughts and images from becoming a reality.

Successful treatment of SAD depends on identifying all forms of avoidance and safety behaviors, helping clients understand how these overt and subtle forms of avoidance play an important maintaining role in their SAD, helping to instill a willingness to drop avoidance and safety behaviors, and using these behavioral changes as an opportunity to experientially test the validity of clients' feared thoughts and images. This module covers the practicalities of getting clients on board with and appropriately implementing this part of treatment, with behavioral experiments being the central strategy for addressing avoidance and safety behaviors. All other components covered in this chapter (e.g., behavioral experiment hierarchies, coping imagery) are implemented in the service of behavioral experiment engagement and effectiveness. In our experience, behavioral experiments are the most effective component of treatment, occupy the most time and attention during therapy, and are usually the most challenging aspect of treatment for both clients and therapists.

Socializing Clients to Modify Avoidance and Safety Behaviors

Identifying Avoidance and Safety Behaviors

The first step in motivating clients to target their avoidance and safety behaviors is to identify the behaviors most relevant to them. The following questions may be useful for eliciting avoidance behaviors.

- "What are some common situations you avoid for fear of . . . [negative evaluation from others/people thinking badly of you/others judging you/being the focus of attention/being noticed/standing out/interacting with others/performing badly in front of others/others observing you]?"
- "What situations make you feel socially anxious? Do you avoid these situations or suffer through them?"
- "Is there anything you are not currently doing that you would like to be doing? Why aren't you doing these things? Are you avoiding these things because of social anxiety?"

Avoided situations can be pervasive, varied, or quite select. Some clients may avoid all forms of interpersonal interaction, while others may steer clear of particular types of interactions. Some clients might cope very well in situations generally considered to be more challenging (e.g., performing in public), yet avoid seemingly easier situations (e.g., a one-on-one conversation). Professional actors with SAD, like our case-study subject Max from Chapter 1, for example, often feel quite at home performing from a script on camera or in front of a large audience, but they find the prospect of interacting socially with others offstage terrifying. It is important to remember that it is not so much the type of situation that determines if someone has social anxiety, but that the avoidance is driven by the perception of social threat. Humans are social creatures, and it is very difficult to avoid people in most modern societies. The potential triggers for social anxiety are therefore many and varied. Box 6.1 lists a range of possible situations that socially anxious people may avoid. As you will see, many of these involve simple tasks of daily living.

When identifying safety behaviors in particular, the following questions may be useful:

- "When you can't avoid a situation, do you do anything to prevent your . . . [fears/predictions/negative social images] from coming true?"
- "When you can't avoid a situation, do you do anything to make yourself feel . . . [safer/less anxious/more at ease]?"
- "When you feel anxious in a social situation, do you do anything to . . . [hide your anxiety/stop your anxiety/conceal yourself/not draw attention to yourself/come across better to others]?"

When exploring the common safety behaviors clients use in social situations, be aware that they might use different safety behaviors in different situations. For example, they might rely on alcohol at casual social events, overpreparation at work, mental rehearsal of what they are going to say before conversations, scripting what they will say during presentations, and wearing sunglasses or pretending to use a mobile phone while walking down the street. Therefore, encourage clients to first think about some of the different social situations that trigger their anxiety, and then record all the strategies identified (beside outright avoidance) to try and prevent their negative social thoughts and images from coming true.

BOX 6.1. Possible Social Anxiety Triggers

- One-on-one interactions
- Small-group interactions
- Large-group interactions
- Initiating conversation
- Maintaining conversation
- Contributing to discussions
- Meetings, classes
- Public transportation
- Shopping
- Leaving the house
- Public toilets
- Parties
- Interacting with strangers/unfamiliar people
- Interacting with acquaintances
- Interacting with close/familiar people

- Eating out or in front of others
- Public speaking, presentations
- Expressing an opinion
- Speaking to authority figures
- Being in a public place (e.g., walking down the street, getting in a crowded elevator)
- Performing a task in front of others
- Writing in front of others (e.g., signing one's name)
- Attending appointments (e.g., doctors, hairdressers)
- Drawing attention to oneself (e.g., different hairstyle, bright clothing)
- Handing money to a cashier
- Joining hobby or sporting groups

Normalizing the Function of Avoidance and Safety Behaviors

Some clients will feel embarrassed by or ashamed of their avoidant coping strategies. It is important to normalize the use of these behaviors for clients by acknowledging that avoidance and safety behaviors have an intended purpose or function, typically aimed at protecting and keeping them safe. They are in fact very understandable, and in some ways they have been valuable to clients. It can be useful to link avoidance and safety behaviors to negative social imagery, so clients can explicitly see what these behaviors are designed to prevent. A useful question in this regard is "What do you imagine happening if you didn't avoid the situation or didn't use this safety behavior?"

You could record this information using two columns noting what the avoidance or safety behavior is, and what negative image it is designed to prevent. Table 6.1 provides some common examples.

Obvious avoidance behaviors are usually easier to detect than safety behaviors. Therapists can sometimes be unsure if a behavior qualifies as a safety behavior. It is important to remember that the *function* of the behavior, rather than the behavior itself, determines if it is a safety behavior. If the primary aim of the behavior is to prevent feared negative social thoughts and images from coming true, then it is serving an avoidant function (just like outright avoidance) and can be classified as a safety behavior. For example, one socially anxious client always wore headphones for his portable music player on public transport. Around the same time the therapist was seeing him for treatment, she also regularly caught the bus to work and was doing the exact same thing. The therapist and client talked about how they both listened to music on public transportation, but that

TABLE 6.1. Common Examples of Avoidance and Safety Behaviors and Their Intended Function

Avoidance of . . .	Aimed at preventing . . .
Parties	Being alone with no one to talk to
Public places	All eyes on me, looking awkward and out of place
Shopping	People getting angry as I hold everyone up in line while I fumble for my wallet
Dating	Saying the wrong thing and offending my date
Work	Not performing my duties properly and people saying behind my back that I am useless
Conversations	Having nothing to say, long awkward silences, and other people getting annoyed with me

Safety behavior is . . .	Aimed at preventing . . .
Avoiding eye contact	Someone starting a conversation with me and me not knowing what to say back
Wearing sunglasses	Others noticing my anxiety and looking at me like I am weak
Alcohol/drugs	People at a party finding me boring and moving away
Using my cell phone	Appearing awkward and anxious, not knowing where to put my arms
Overrehearsing conversations	Long silences with nothing to contribute, making the other person feel uncomfortable and want to get away
Not contributing to conversations	Saying something stupid and being criticized; looking awkward if I'm the focus of attention
Overpreparing speeches	Stuttering, umming, going blank, long pauses, making no sense, people being confused or laughing
Hair covering my face	Bright-red blushing cheeks being noticed
Makeup	Bright-red blushing cheeks being noticed
Inconspicuous clothing	People noticing me, looking, and judging
Keeping hands in pocket	People noticing my hands shaking and thinking I am a weirdo

the reasons behind their behaviors differed. For the therapist, it was because she enjoyed listening to music on the journey to and from work, and if for some reason the battery ran out or she forgot her music player that day she felt disappointed but could still get on the bus, and it had no impact on her anxiety. However, the client used this behavior to reduce the likelihood that someone would start a conversation with him and he would appear awkward and not know what to say. For him, to not have his music device would mean a huge increase in his anxiety and a strong likelihood he would avoid using public transportation altogether. So, when it comes to safety behaviors, it is not what you do, but *why* you are doing it that is the primary issue. When it is being used in an attempt to stop feared negative social thoughts and images from coming to fruition, and hence to reduce anxiety, it is unhelpful in the context of effective SAD treatment and needs to be addressed.

Useful questions to determine if a behavior is indeed a safety behavior are:

- If you couldn't do the behavior, what would happen?
- What would happen to your anxiety?
- What would happen to your ability to be in that situation?

Highlighting the Maintaining Role of Avoidance and Safety Behaviors

Once relevant avoidance and safety behaviors have been identified, it is important to normalize their occurrence, but then start instilling a sense of curiosity regarding their helpfulness. Clients can be introduced to the vicious cycle of avoidance using Socratically guided psychoeducation as follows (which is also described in Handout 4, *The Cycle of Avoidance and Anxiety,* in the Appendix):

"People with social anxiety often rely on avoidance. Avoidance might take the form of complete avoidance of particular situations or, when situations can't be avoided, subtler forms of avoidance called safety behaviors. Safety behaviors like [insert client examples] are often used because people believe they will help to prevent their fears from coming true. On the one hand, avoidance seems like a very sensible strategy. It makes sense to avoid things that we think are dangerous to us. On the other hand, avoidance is the main reason that social anxiety persists.

"In what way do you think avoidance is a problem? What have been the negative consequences of continuing to avoid social situations? Although avoidance brings some relief of anxiety in the immediate short term, what has it done to your anxiety over the long term? How might avoiding social situations be keeping your social anxiety going? How might avoidance keep your perception of social threat going?"

The following concepts should be covered during this discussion about the consequences of avoidance.

We Never Get to Test Our Negative Images

"When we avoid a social situation, we are assuming that our negative images are accurate reflections of reality. However, avoidance never gives us an opportunity to directly test our fears. If we did, we might discover that our images are actually inaccurate. We might learn that in fact what we fear rarely occurs and instead that things often turn out pretty well. We might also find that even if social experiences don't go according to plan sometimes, we can cope with this as well. So avoidance prevents us from getting an accurate impression of the true probability and cost of our fears coming true."

We Never Get Opportunities for Positive Experiences

"If we avoid social situations, we have no chance of having positive social experiences that would motivate us to socialize more."

Loss of Self-Esteem

"Because people with social anxiety aren't doing what they would really like to do, they tend to be very self-critical and can have low self-esteem. They may ruminate a lot about aspects of life that are passing them by, which leaves them more vulnerable to further anxiety and depressed mood. In fact, people with social anxiety can often use their avoidance as just another reason to criticize themselves."

Avoidance and Anxiety Can Generalize

"As we avoid situations and lose confidence in one area of our lives (e.g., relationships with peers), our anxiety can start to generalize to more and more domains of life (e.g., work, family relationships).

"The vicious cycle of avoidance and anxiety that captures all of these long-term problems might look something like this . . . [Draw Figure 6.1 collaboratively with the client on a whiteboard or piece of paper.] In social anxiety we can get very stuck in this cycle, as avoidance keeps our negative social images in place, hence maintaining our anxiety and narrowing our quality of life.

"To overcome social anxiety, we need to break or reverse this cycle, and the most tangible place we can start is with our behavior (i.e., avoidance). We need to drop our avoidance behaviors, and instead gradually place ourselves in situations that bother us. We also need to do this without the precautions of using our safety behaviors because we need to find out what happens when we allow ourselves to just *be* in the situation. Now, of course we will initially feel anxious when we do this. But as someone with social anxiety living in what is a very social world, you are kind of used to that feeling. So if we persist with the situation, and ride through that initial anxiety, what might happen? What might we have the opportunity to discover? [Draw Figure 6.2 collaboratively with the client to illustrate reversing the cycle.]

"What do you see as the take-home message of our discussions? How helpful do you think your avoidance is now that we have had the chance to think about it more? . . . The key message is that by no longer avoiding or using safety behaviors, we have the opportunity to test the validity of our negative social thoughts and images, an opportunity that avoidance has robbed us of for so long. These new social experiences may then update these images to be more realistic, which in turn will

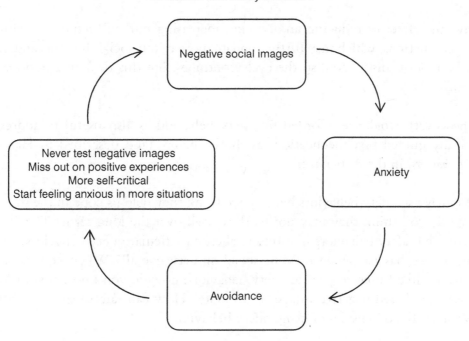

FIGURE 6.1. The vicious cycle of avoidance and anxiety.

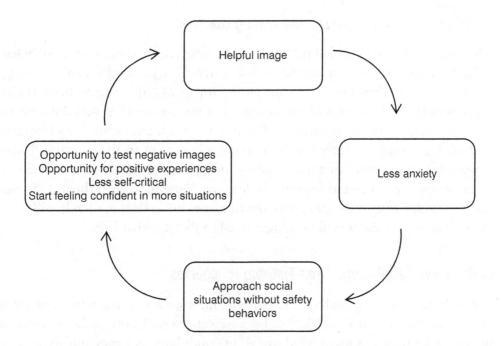

FIGURE 6.2. The positive cycle of approach and reduced anxiety.

have the effect of reducing anxiety and increasing our willingness to try further social situations, which may further update more of our social thoughts and imagery to be more realistic. And so the cycle continues, but this time in a positive direction."

The covert avoidance afforded by safety behaviors is also useful to address with Socratically guided psychoeducation, as shown below (and described in Handout 5, *Safety Behaviors,* in the Appendix).

"We may use safety behaviors because we think they help us cope in the short term; how do you think they may not work so well over the long term? The more you have used safety behaviors like [insert client's particular safety behaviors], what do you notice has happened to your social anxiety overall? When you use a safety behavior like [insert a specific safety behavior], how do you know if your fear that [insert predicted negative image] is accurate? How can safety behaviors backfire? What are the downsides of using safety behaviors?"

The following concepts should be covered during this discussion about the consequences of using safety behaviors.

Safety Behaviors Stop Us from Directly Testing Our Fears

"Although we haven't avoided the situation completely, by using our safety behaviors we are not directly testing our fears. For instance, if I attend a work meeting but don't contribute, then I never get to test my image of 'saying something stupid and other people laughing or looking confused at my answers.' When the next meeting comes along the same image will come to mind, and again I will be gripped by fear. If I directly test my fear by making a comment in the meeting, I have an opportunity to discover that my negative image may be inaccurate. After I test the image numerous times and find that it does not come true, then the negative image can be seen for what it is—just an image that does not reflect reality. It will have less emotional impact and it will no longer need to dictate what I do."

Safety Behaviors Can Become "Self-Fulfilling Prophecies"

"Safety behaviors can actually cause the outcomes we are trying to prevent by using them. For instance, if I use alcohol because otherwise I don't believe that I could interact with people, I might find myself overindulging at times and acting in ways that result in negative evaluation from others (e.g., drunken behavior). So the "safety behavior" has increased the chance of negative evaluation rather than reduced it. Similarly, my boss might be more frustrated with me for not contributing in meetings than if I did contribute from time to time."

If Our Fears Don't Come True, We Mistakenly "Thank" the Safety Behavior

"If we use our safety behaviors and our fears don't come true, we might believe that the safety behaviors 'prevented' our fears from happening. As a result, we never feel less anxious about the situation, as we still think it was dangerous if not for the safety behavior. We can become very dependent upon our safety behaviors and start to feel even more anxious if they can't be used (e.g., no alcohol available, being 'put on the spot' to speak at a meeting). The truth may be that our fears were unlikely to have come true even without the safety behavior, but we never discover this as long as we continue relying on them."

Safety Behaviors Increase Our Self-Focused Attention

"When people use safety behaviors they often scrutinize themselves very closely (what they are doing, how they are doing it, monitoring their thoughts), which can be very distracting. Self-focused attention hijacks attention from the 'task at hand' (e.g., the conversation), which can make it even more difficult to keep up with conversations and contribute.

"So, for all these reasons safety behaviors maintain social anxiety in the longer term. If anxiety remains high after repeatedly confronting a social situation, chances are you are using safety behaviors that are preventing you from directly testing your fears."

Using Imagery to Understand the Impact of Safety Behaviors

An imagery exercise could be used to encourage clients to evaluate the impact of using the safety behaviors they have identified, as a means of enhancing motivation to drop these behaviors. This may be useful for clients who recognize that their outright avoidance behaviors are unhelpful, but view their safety behaviors as harmless and more of a helpful "coping strategy." Of course this point could be made during a verbal discussion. However, using imagery may allow clients to *feel* the impact of using safety behaviors and may also serve as an opportunity to mentally rehearse dropping safety behaviors, making it easier to do so in reality. The following instructions are a guide to help clients experience the impact of using safety behaviors.

Impact of Safety Behaviors Imagery Exercise

IMAGE 1

"First I would like you to choose one situation in which you use safety behaviors . . . If you feel comfortable doing so, close your eyes and spend 2–3 minutes imagining yourself in that situation and using all of your safety behaviors . . . What is happening? What are you doing? What are you most aware of? Where is your attention?

What do you notice about your posture? How is the other person responding? What are they noticing about you? How do you feel? Where do you feel this in your body?"

IMAGE 2

"Now I would like you to rewind and imagine the same situation again, but this time with no safety behaviors and instead in a more open, assertive, relaxed manner . . . What is happening? What are you doing instead of using safety behaviors? How is your posture now? What are you focusing your attention on? How is the conversation flowing or the situation progressing? What are you now able to notice about the situation that you missed before while using your safety behaviors? How is the other person responding? What are they noticing about you? How do you feel? Where do you feel this in your body?"

In group treatment, these scripts are read verbatim and experiences are then elicited and debriefed at the end. In individual treatment, as clients are guided through this exercise they will be able to respond to therapist-prompted questions, and therapists can record their responses for use in the debrief discussion. During the debrief, it is important to contrast client experiences whilst envisioning the alternative images. Differences that may be discussed include how anxiety provoking each image was, other feelings that may have arisen, body sensations, posture, self-consciousness, social performance, and other people's responses.

Some clients might report that the image of using safety behaviors was *more* anxiety provoking. Therapists should prompt clients to identify specifically what was different in the image. Clients may mention that they appeared more confident and relaxed in the image without the safety behaviors. These outcomes can lead to a discussion about the true value of continuing to use safety behaviors, which can be further tested with an actual behavioral experiment (see the section on safety behavior experiments later in this chapter).

Other clients might report that the image of using safety behaviors was *less* anxiety provoking. This possibility can be entertained as a hypothesis that might be valuable to "test out" (i.e., "Your imagination tells you that using safety behaviors is better, how can we be sure? How can we test this out in reality?"). Encourage curiosity about which image is most accurate, which again would lead into the *Safety Behavior Experiments* outlined later in this chapter. It may also be useful to separate client feelings from what the other person within each image is seeing and how they are responding (e.g., "although you may feel less anxious in the short term using your safety behaviors, what may be some of the consequences in terms of how the other person relates to you?"). Clients might be able to take the "observer perspective" and report that they appear more confident when they are not using their safety behaviors. Another approach might be to normalize the fact that given their habitual use of safety behaviors, it may not be surprising that this felt more comfortable. However, given all the other potential problems with safety behaviors (discussed previously), the pros and cons of relying on them can be further discussed.

Behavioral Experiments: Modifying Behavior to Challenge Negative Thoughts and Images

Avoidance and safety behaviors maintain SAD because they limit opportunities to face feared situations and experientially discover if the negative social thoughts and images fueling these fears are valid. As such, avoidance and safety behaviors keep social-anxiety-related cognitions firmly in place, robbing clients of the natural cognitive challenging process that comes with behavioral exposure.

Behavioral experiments are a powerful method of changing avoidance and safety behaviors, with the primary purpose of challenging the thoughts and imagery that maintain social threat perception. Behavioral experiments are essentially tasks that clients undertake, within and outside therapy sessions, with the purpose of directly testing their cognitions. The form that behavioral experiments take can vary, such as modifying behavior within social situations to observe the consequences or conducting surveys, and they are a common transdiagnostic CBT strategy with numerous applications (for more detail, see the *Oxford Guide to Behavioural Experiments in Cognitive Therapy*; Bennett-Levy et al., 2004). In the area of SAD, behavioral experiments will typically involve clients stepping out of their comfort zone by gradually reversing avoidance behaviors and dropping safety behaviors in social situations, and being curious about whether or not the actual outcome matches their a priori negative social thoughts and images.

Behavioral experiments therefore focus on testing cognition via experiential learning. Identifying key cognitions of interest is the central focus, followed by devising behavioral methods of testing these cognitions, specifying evidence to observe during the experiment that would either confirm or disconfirm the cognition being tested, conducting the experiment and noting the outcome, and reflecting on how the outcome relates to the cognition under examination. It may be useful to query anticipated SUDS when planning the task, to get a sense of how challenging the task is for the client and hence the likelihood of task completion, but monitoring SUDS during the task is not essential in behavioral experiments (unless one of the key predictions to be tested is the client's anticipated severity of anxiety and its trajectory), as habituation of anxiety is not the primary focus. Behavioral experiments are often graded to assist with engagement in what is a challenging process for clients, but this is not essential for a successful behavioral experiment. The experiment task only needs to be conducted for as long as it takes for the cognition in question to be tested, and therefore may not need to be prolonged. Likewise, repetition only needs to occur until the client and therapist are satisfied the cognition has been fully tested and they can be confident in the validity of the information they have gathered. Clients may need to replicate an experiment several times and in several contexts before the strength of a belief sufficiently diminishes (e.g., < 5%). Thus, some experiments may be repeated many times and others may only need to be done once. The critical condition is a "prediction error"—a discrepancy between the client's expectancies of the social situation and the actual outcome. The larger the prediction error, the more powerful and enduring the learning will be.

Introducing Behavioral Experiments

Behavioral experiments are typically the most emphasized, powerful, and challenging part of treatment for clients with SAD. Much of the time in therapy is devoted to setting up, conducting, and debriefing repeated behavioral experiments to recalibrate clients' social expectations. Therefore, socializing clients to this component of treatment is particularly important to increase engagement in this crucial part of therapy. Based on the rationale already provided to clients regarding the importance of tackling avoidance and safety behaviors, behavioral experiments can be introduced as a powerful technique for reducing reliance on avoidance and increasing self-efficacy. The following pointers provide some ideas that may also be helpful:

Curious Scientist

Conducting behavioral experiments can be likened to adopting the role of a curious scientist. That is, the client has a specific hypothesis in mind regarding social situations, and the challenge is to find ways to test that hypothesis. Introducing this concept can introduce some objectivity and hence emotional distance toward the behavioral task and its outcome.

Next Logical Step

Framing behavioral experiments as the next logical step onward from the imagery challenging work already done can be helpful.

"We have done a lot of work questioning your negative thoughts and images, looking at the contrary evidence, and developing more realistic and helpful thoughts and images . . . but how are we going to know for sure which is correct—your old negative images or your new helpful images? What would need to happen to find out once and for all?"

The aim is to help clients acknowledge that action (behavioral experiments) rather than speculation (imagery challenging) is ultimately the best method for challenging their social fears.

Previous Success

It can be helpful to elicit examples of when clients have completed a task out of their "comfort zone" only to find that it did not go in the negative way they had expected. If they are able to recall such an experience, you can then frame it as a behavioral experiment. Focus clients on what the experience was like for them, how they felt before and after, and what they gained from it. You can then summarize that they already know how to do a behavioral experiment, and that the behavioral experiments completed in therapy will just be a bit more strategic and planned.

The Most Active Ingredient in Therapy

Acknowledge that while the idea of changing their behavior may initially sound challenging or scary, at the end of treatment other clients have reported that this is the most powerful and effective part of treatment, and that the short-term "pain" was worth the longer-term "gain." It can be helpful to communicate that this is the most effective way you know as a therapist to overcome social anxiety. Emphasizing the old adage that "we must do something differently if we want a different outcome" may focus clients on behavior change rather than continued avoidance.

The Graded Nature of Behavioral Experiments

It may be reassuring for clients to give them permission to start with easier experiments that might initially be like "dipping a toe in the water" before moving to harder experiments as confidence builds, so that eventually they might be willing to "take the plunge." Reassure clients that the guiding principle will be to set up experiments that are "manageable challenges." If experiments aren't challenging, then clients aren't doing anything therapeutic that challenges their social anxiety, and so nothing will change. If clients do find an experiment more challenging than they expected, this can also be an important learning opportunity. The clinician can focus on any discrepancy between perceived versus actual coping during the experiment. These challenging experiences can be particularly helpful for reducing relapse when clients encounter any negative social experiences after therapy.

Therapist Support

Reassure clients that you (the therapist) are willing, where practical, to participate in the behavioral experiments too, so they are not alone in this process. Therapists may need to model some of the experiments as a first step to engaging clients in the process. From a cognitive perspective, clients can learn about the likelihood of negative evaluation by observing others. Therapists can also be useful allies during behavioral experiments, prompting clients *in vivo* to focus their attention in the service of gathering evidence against their feared outcomes. However, clients will need to complete experiments themselves so that they learn that they too can cope with the possibility of negative evaluation, or with actual negative evaluation should this occur.

Preparation before Action

If clients are still resistant to the idea, encourage them to go through the process of setting up a behavioral experiment with no expectation that they have to do it. This may warm them up to the idea and increase their willingness to try it out eventually. Ideally, this would be an experiment that can be done during the therapy session, and possibly one that the therapist could do first to model the process (e.g., dropping some papers in the reception area of the clinic, having a conversation with the therapist about a common topic like movies or travel). You may even be able to turn the behavior of declining to do behavioral experiments into a behavioral experiment. What did they envision would happen if they said no, compared to what actually happened?

A Note about Therapist Anxiety

Therapists don't need to cover all the ideas above with their clients with SAD. Often therapists' anxiety about behavioral experiments can lead to excessive justifications to convince clients to "get on board." Sometimes this need can be about convincing the client, but other times it is about convincing ourselves as therapists to neutralize our own anxiety. Sometimes therapist anxiety can steer us away from promoting the use of behavioral experiments with our clients altogether.

Therapist anxiety regarding behavioral experiments will often relate to some negative thoughts and imagery we hold about clients not coping with their anxiety or the behavioral experiment turning out badly (i.e., the client's negative thoughts and images coming true!). Such images may then activate our own core beliefs regarding what it means to be a "good therapist" (e.g., "a good therapist must always make her clients feel good, take away client distress, and ensure all therapy tasks are always a positive experience"). As such, therapist anxiety may arise because, although we may intellectually know that behavioral experiments are highly therapeutic, they can also make us feel that we are treading a little too close to the brink of potentially being a "bad therapist." This is a common experience many therapists face. If this applies to you, you may need to do your own imagery challenging and behavioral experiments to explore further your predictions about behavioral experiments and your beliefs about what it means to be a "good therapist," particularly if some of your beliefs are interfering with using behavioral experiments in therapy.

Excessively long discussions and justifications for behavioral experiments with clients, rather than just doing them, can exacerbate client anxiety as they have more time to worry about the process. Unless there is obvious reluctance, it may be worth getting right into the behavioral experiment process and giving clients some credit for being able to handle more than we imagine. We believe it is critical that therapists assume that their clients are more robust and capable than clients believe themselves to be. If therapists believe their clients are fragile and that anxiety is unacceptable and must be avoided, it will be difficult for clients to believe otherwise.

It may be worth reminding ourselves that tolerating anxiety is a valuable skill for everybody to learn. In addition, while positive and neutral outcomes from behavioral experiments are helpful for challenging beliefs about the probability of social catastrophes, negative outcomes can also be therapeutic. Negative experiences offer clients the opportunity to discover that the true cost or consequences when things don't go smoothly may not be as bad as first thought, and that they can cope with those consequences. Resilience will come from coping with negative outcomes, not just from believing negative outcomes are unlikely. Therefore, whether the behavioral experiment outcome is positive or negative, it is a "win–win" situation when it comes to therapy.

As an example of this "win–win" philosophy in action, in one memorable behavioral experiment, one of our clients entered a bookstore while simulating extreme and clearly observable shaking to test his belief that it is unacceptable to appear nervous. He dutifully and vigorously shook his whole body while reading magazines within the store for some time. As he was leaving the store a staff member called out to him, "Excuse me sir, you've left your medication on the counter." The medication was not his. Needless to say, the therapist was initially concerned about how the client would respond to this apparently clear evidence that others had noticed his shaking. During the debrief the therapist asked the client what he learned from the experience, and he was very balanced in his appraisal. He reported learning that others seemed to just get on with their own business, and his usual shaking, which is far less obvious compared to what he displayed during this experiment, was therefore unlikely to draw negative attention in the future. The therapist, noticing that he appeared to be ignoring the medication issue, took a breath and then asked directly what he thought about that. The client simply answered with indifference, "Well, it wasn't mine." This was an important experience for the therapist, who learned not to catastrophize when unexpected things occur during behavioral experiments!

The Process of Behavioral Experiments

Once clients understand the rationale for behavioral experiments, the therapist can review the eight steps involved in conducting a behavioral experiment. A handout outlining these steps can be provided to clients for psychoeducational purposes (see Handout 6, *Behavioral Experiments,* in the Appendix). When setting up behavioral experiments with clients for the first time, it may be useful to first describe the process of using Worksheet 7, the *Behavioral Experiment Record* (in the Appendix) by referring to a hypothetical example (see the example included in Handout 6). Completion of all eight behavioral experiment steps should initially be done within therapy sessions with the guidance of the therapist, including conducting the behavioral experiment itself. Once clients are familiar with the process, the next step is to set up experiments in session (steps 1–4), conduct the experiments outside of session (step 5), and then return to debrief the findings in subsequent sessions (step 6–8). The final aim would be for clients to do all eight steps independently as homework exercises.

Step 1: Negative Image

This involves identifying a specific social situation that triggers anxiety and bringing to mind an image of what clients envision will happen in the situation. Clients should have already developed some skill in this area from using Worksheet 5, the *Thought and Imagery Record* and Worksheet 6, the *Imagery Challenging Record*. Clients should spend a couple of minutes running the image through their head in detail from start to finish, as if it were a show on TV. They can then write a description (in words or pictures) of this image. Helpful prompts to guide clients through the image are:

- "What is happening?"
- "What are you seeing, hearing, smelling, tasting, touching?"
- "What are you doing?"
- "What are other people doing?"
- "How are they responding to you?"
- "How will they respond to you in the future as a consequence?"
- "What happens next?"
- "How does the image start and end?"

Step 2: SUDS

Clients then rate the intensity of their anxiety about this situation (SUDS: 0 = no anxiety, 10 = maximum anxiety). That is, how anxious do they feel as they think about and envision the situation? Clients may have some predictions about how anxious they will be when they are actually in the situation, and this would be part of the negative image to be tested (e.g., "I will be so uncontrollably anxious I won't be able to speak").

Step 3: Experiment

The next step is to plan an experiment to test the negative image. What could clients do to find out how accurate their image is? What situation could they put themselves in or create to test the accuracy of their image? It is important to plan the experiment as specifically as possible to increase the likelihood of appropriate completion. Specify *what* needs to be done, *where* it will take place, *when* it will take place, and *who* will be involved in the experiment.

When planning the experiment, particular attention should be paid to safety behaviors that would typically be used during the situation in question. That is, aside from avoiding the situation altogether, what other things might clients do with the aim of preventing negative imagery from coming true? Help clients understand how these behaviors will contaminate the results of the experiment, preventing them from truly testing the cognition in question. If the experiment goes well, the client will attribute it to the safety behavior, rather than learning that the situation is safe. Make sure it is clear what safety behaviors need to be dropped (e.g., hunched posture and not making eye contact to avoid attention) and what needs to be done instead (e.g., standing up straight, head up, shoulders back, making general eye contact).

Step 4: Evidence to Observe

Before doing the experiment, it is very important to specify what evidence clients need to look for to confirm or disconfirm the negative image. This evidence must be *unambiguous* (i.e., clear, observable, objective evidence). A useful approach is to consider whether the evidence would hold up in a court of law, or if the judge would "throw it out of court" because it was too subjective. Discuss some examples of ambiguous social cues that can be easily misinterpreted (e.g., a yawn or looking at one's watch being a sign of boredom). Clients should also explicitly consider where their attention needs to be placed during the experiment (see Chapter 8 for more information).

Step 5: Do the Experiment

Step 6: Results

Now it is time to reflect on what actually happened. Ensure clients stick to the facts. Specifically, what evidence either for or against the negative image was observed?

Step 7: Conclusion

Encourage clients to reflect on the following questions and draw some conclusions from the experiment.

- "How do the results compare to the negative image?"
- "What do the results tell us about the accuracy of the initial negative image?"
- "What did you learn from the experiment?"

The conclusions clients develop may be about the discrepancy between the:

- Imagined threat versus actual threat.
- Imagined cost of something going wrong versus the actual cost.
- Imagined reactions of others versus actual reactions.
- Imagined social abilities versus actual social abilities.
- Imagined coping versus actual coping.
- Imagined anxiety versus actual anxiety.

Step 8: Update Imagery

Clients are then encouraged to close their eyes and spend a few minutes re-creating the image in their mind, but this time incorporating what they have learned from the experiment. This step essentially involves reliving the experiment and observing the situation as it was, rather than how they initially envisioned it would be. The prompt questions used in Step 1 are equally useful for this imagery exercise. The following questions are useful if clients automatically revert back to the initial negative image:

- "How does the image need to change to better reflect reality?"
- "How can you update the image to be more realistic/more in tune with reality/ incorporate what you now know/better reflect or represent what you discovered from your experiment?"

Once clients have fully accessed this new updated image, the therapist can help them reflect on the experience of this new image compared to the initial negative image. How is it different? What does the new image mean to them? How does the new image make them feel?

A Note about Imagery Enhancements for Behavioral Experiments

The use of imagery in Steps 1 and 8, which is not a standard feature of behavioral experiments, has been included to enhance the behavioral experiment process in a number of ways. First, traditional behavioral experiments that are set up in a more verbal manner require clients to develop a *prediction* of what they *think* will happen. Requesting that clients develop an *image* of what they *envision* will happen instead is designed primarily to increase the specificity of client predictions. This places the therapist and client in a stronger position to devise an appropriate and effective experiment, as the prediction being tested should have greater detail, richness, and clarity by being in imagery format. The specificity of the imagery-based prediction then makes it more obvious what evidence needs to be observed for the image to hold true, as essentially we would have to see that exact image play out for the prediction to be confirmed.

The addition of updating the negative image to better reflect reality at Step 8 is intended to enhance the emotional impact and memorability of the experiment. Behavioral experiments, unlike thought records, are already an experiential mode of learning, generating large emotional shifts even without the use of imagery. Adding imagery to this technique may then be thought of as a way of "supercharging" an already emotionally powerful therapy tool. Also, if clients have held one view for so long (e.g., that they are socially unacceptable), and their behavioral experiments contradict this view, they may be too quick to move on from these experiences as a form of minimization to preserve their old world view. Sitting a little longer with the experience and emotions associated with it via the imagery updating section may therefore prolong the experience and increase the chance of this experience being fully processed and consolidated.

As previously mentioned in Chapter 3, Brewin's (2006) retrieval competition theory suggests that how we feel about any given situation is governed by the memory representations we retrieve about that situation. That is, we hold positive and negative memory representations for most aspects of our life (e.g., social, work, relationships, self) that compete for retrieval. More accessible memories will win out and govern how we feel about the situation at hand. Clients with SAD may have an absence of positive memory representations of social situations or very accessible negative memory representations of social situations. Therefore, asking them to relive a positive social experience they have had during behavioral experiments may help increase the memorability and accessibility of the experience, thereby increasing the chances that it may win out during retrieval competition in the future.

Different Types of Behavioral Experiments

Standard Future-Focused Experiments

Most experiments that clients will complete in SAD treatment will fit into this category. Clients will have certain types of social situations that bother them (e.g., going to parties, interacting with a checkout clerk, spontaneous social chitchat with colleagues, speaking in classes). Linked to these situations will be negative imagery representing what they predict will happen (e.g., "I am stuttering and not getting my words out right, people are looking at me confused and others are laughing at me, people now turn away from me and find other people to talk to with, I am alone and look awkward and out of place"). Upcoming situations (i.e., the next party or class session) or purposely constructed situations (i.e., having a social conversation with a therapist's colleague, giving a talk to any people the therapist can recruit from their building to listen) can then be used as opportunities to test clients' negative social images. These types of experiments will typically require repetition, as one positive experience will generally not be enough to modify clients' default negative social thoughts and images. Experiments should be repeated until clients' expectations of the relevant social domain (e.g., walking down a crowded street, speaking to work colleagues in the lunchroom) have been updated to incorporate their behavioral experiment findings. As a result, clients' predicted imagery when entering the social domain in question on new occasions should better align with reality. When this is achieved, they can progress to more challenging behavioral experiments.

Standard future-focused experiments typically involve attempting to engage in a social situation in a fairly standard manner without using any safety behaviors that may inhibit standard social engagement. For example, instead of using typical safety behaviors such as looking down and staying quiet, clients may be more conscious of making eye contact, speaking up, asking questions, and making a personal contribution to the discussion. It is probably useful to start SAD treatment with this standard type of behavioral experiment. Some examples of common SAD behavioral experiments are listed in Box 6.2. The choice of experiment will be guided by the situations that are bothersome to clients and the specific negative imagery associated with those situations that requires testing.

BOX 6.2. Examples of Common SAD Behavioral Experiments

- Talking to a checkout cashier
- Making social conversation with work colleagues or classmates
- Speaking in meetings or classes
- Speaking to people in authority (e.g., manager, teacher)
- Spending time in public places (e.g., public transport, shopping centers)
- Speaking to someone attractive

- Attending group gatherings
- Ordering food or coffee at a restaurant or café
- Starting a conversation with a stranger
- Asking for information from someone in a customer service role
- Making a phone call
- Joining an interest or sporting group/club

Once clients have had the opportunity to complete their own behavioral experiments under the therapist's supervision and the therapist is confident that they are familiar with the experience of a properly conducted behavioral experiment, clients can then start to regularly engage in these types of experiments as homework exercises between sessions. These experiments will predominantly test the likelihood of social catastrophe occurring. Generally, clients find that their engagement in social interactions goes better than expected, thereby reducing the estimated probability of social threat. On the rare occasion that it does go poorly, they then have an opportunity to test the true cost of things not going smoothly and their ability to cope when this occurs.

Shame-Attacking Experiments

Standard behavioral experiments effectively adjust the perceived *likelihood* of social catastrophe because the overwhelming majority of client fears will not come true. This may be a great relief to our clients, but one risk is that the perceived *costs* of social catastrophes will remain unchanged. If clients leave therapy believing that their fears are unlikely to come true, but that if they did the consequences would be intolerable, then they will remain vulnerable to anxiety. Most of us encounter socially awkward situations at times, and future faux pas could trigger a relapse for clients if they catastrophize the consequences. Therefore, it is important to construct experiments that are specifically designed to test the cost of breaking social norms. These types of experiments are known as "shame-attacking" experiments because we are purposely trying to draw attention to ourselves by doing something that is socially unconventional. The idea of purposely doing something embarrassing can be quite threatening for our socially anxious clients, so it is important to spend time providing a strong rationale regarding the purpose and usefulness of these exercises. Completing experiments with the therapist, at least initially, can provide much-needed moral support and a bond-strengthening shared experience. Eventually clients will need to conduct these experiments alone to ensure that the therapist's company does not become a safety behavior. The following points can be discussed with clients to emphasize the therapeutic value of shame-attacking experiments:

1% LIKELIHOOD VERSUS 100% COST

"So far our behavioral experiments have mostly tested the likelihood of something going wrong socially, and we have mostly found that things go better than expected. However (remembering the social anxiety model), it is also important to test the cost, not just the likelihood, as both determine our sense of social threat. Even if you believed that the likelihood of things going wrong socially was only 1%, if you still thought the cost would be really bad if it did go wrong—100% bad—you would still be really anxious, worrying about when that 1% is going to happen, hence leaving you feeling socially vulnerable."

BANDWIDTH AND TIGHTROPE METAPHOR

"People with social anxiety often have a very narrow 'bandwidth' for what they believe other people will accept when it comes to social behavior and what they believe they can cope with. In terms of what they think is socially acceptable in life, it is as if they have been walking a tightrope, and if they put a foot wrong they are 'a goner.' They are socializing under a lot of stress and pressure because of this. But what if these experiments provided an opportunity to discover that what is considered socially acceptable behavior is not as narrow as a tightrope, but in fact more like a wide plank or even a secure and wide bridge, and that there is a lot more leeway— then how would you feel when socializing? Safer because there is less pressure, less of a precarious 'life-and-death' situation."

Once clients are socialized to the concept of shame-attacking behavioral experiments, the therapist can present them with a menu of behavioral experiment options to choose from (see Handout 7, *Behavioral Experiment Menu*). In group therapy, we ask clients to vote on their preferred experiment from the menu options and choose the top two for the whole group to complete in the session. You can always collaboratively construct your own set of shame-attacking experiments, and tailor them more specifically to the client's areas of concern. This is particularly relevant if clients' anxiety relates to specific concerns about how other people may react to anxiety symptoms they believe are obvious to others, such as blushing, shaking and sweating. In these circumstances, shame-attacking experiments may involve going out in public and purposely exaggerating the symptom of concern (e.g., putting on excessive red blush, or purposely shaking profusely, or putting water under their armpits and on their forehead). This may be quite radical for clients, as they have typically spent much time trying to conceal such symptoms, and they are now being encouraged to manufacture and magnify the symptoms to discover the true cost of drawing attention to these areas.

Shame-attacking experiments are set up in a similar manner to standard behavioral experiments. The *Behavioral Experiment Record* (Worksheet 7) is completed (i.e., Steps 1–4), although in many instances the experiment is already known, particularly if the client has chosen it from the menu. Thus the focus is not on thinking of an experiment, but on identifying the negative image of what the client envisions will happen when she does the selected experiment, and hence the evidence to observe. In terms of evidence, clients may say things like "people will look, laugh, and yell abuse." It is important that clients be very specific about these predictions. For example, in their image what *proportion* of people are looking, laughing, yelling? In what manner are they doing these things (e.g., how long do they look, what expression is on their face, what specifically do they yell)? When planning the experiment ensure safety behaviors are dropped, particularly those that interfere with gathering evidence (e.g., looking down). Therapists then complete the task with clients (i.e., Step 5). Before they embark on the experiment, remind clients that the aim is not to feel calm and relaxed, possibly self-disclosing that you find these tasks somewhat embarrassing too. The aim is to test if feeling embarrassed is the worst thing that happens, if they are able to tolerate and cope with feelings of embarrassment, and to experience the transient nature of these feelings.

Following the experiment, the therapist and client return to the therapy room to complete the remainder of the *Behavioral Experiment Record* (i.e., Steps 6–8). The debriefing process should particularly focus on the impact of the experiment on "broadening the bandwidth" of the client's perception of socially acceptable behavior. Conclusions that are typically drawn from these experiments are:

- "People are focused on themselves and their own activity rather than caring very much about what I am doing."
- "People seem to accept other people doing unusual things."
- "People are less hostile than I initially thought."
- "It can actually be fun to do silly things sometimes."
- "The worst consequence is feeling embarrassed—I can cope with feelings of embarrassment and the feelings pass."

Many clients may be reluctant to engage in shame-attacking experiments as they involve really taking the plunge, and some may not be willing to do this at all. This can occur in individual treatment and group treatment settings alike. Our experience is that although most clients find these tasks highly anxiety provoking and challenging, the positive peer pressure available in group treatment settings helps with motivation to engage in the tasks, particularly if the group has a critical number of particularly enthusiastic members. Regardless of whether the reluctance is occurring in an individual or group treatment context, it can be handled in the same manner. Therapists should take the stance that they are not forcing clients to do something against their will, they are just providing the opportunity to do something that other clients have found very helpful in the treatment of their social anxiety. If they don't wish to participate, the experiment can still be done as an observational experiment in the hope that they will learn from seeing how people react to someone else engaging in unusual social behavior. This modeling experience can be provided by either the therapist alone in an individual treatment setting or the therapist and other group members in a group treatment setting. Above all, it is about clients making an informed choice in treatment once they are aware of the value of shame-attacking experiments in fully treating their social anxiety by challenging the cost of social mishaps.

As already mentioned in Chapter 3, therapists who are highly socially anxious themselves and unwilling to challenge social norms may not be well equipped to effectively treat individuals with SAD. It is important that clinicians who themselves are overly fearful of negative evaluation conduct their own shame-attacking exercises prior to treating clients with SAD, or the therapist's anxiety will compromise client engagement in shame-attacking behavioral experiments. In addition, when initially observing their therapist breaking social norms some clients may overempathize with the therapist, feeling embarrassed and anxious *for* the therapist. In these instances, it is important that the therapist redirect clients' attention to the actual consequences observed, rather than allowing clients to become preoccupied with their own emotions. Unfettered "anxiety by proxy" may strengthen social fears via the same in-situation processing biases that have maintained the problem in the past (e.g., self-focused attention preventing clients from observing that strangers accept or completely ignore the therapist's unusual behavior).

Past-Oriented Behavioral Experiments

On most occasions the *Behavioral Experiment Record* will be used to plan for future social situations, but at times a past social situation will be bothersome and may then become the platform for a subsequent behavioral experiment. For example, clients may report a social situation they perceive went poorly (e.g., "I tried saying hello to a work colleague and he walked straight past me, he clearly thinks I am an idiot and doesn't want to know me"; "my in-class presentation was awful, I spoke gibberish and made no sense"). An experiment can then be constructed to test if their interpretation or imagery representation of what happened is valid or distorted (e.g., say hi to the same colleague and ask two questions to see if the same response occurs, or wait for their grade and feedback from the instructor as a more objective indicator of their public speaking performance). Under these circumstances, Worksheet 6, the *Imagery Challenging Record,* is also useful in dealing with perceived or actual negative outcomes. For example, if the colleague doesn't respond again or the instructor's grade and comments are poor, then finding a helpful way to make sense of these experiences that is not solely based on clients' social acceptability will be important, as will developing a more helpful image to capture this perspective.

Safety Behavior Experiments

The need to drop safety behaviors is an important consideration when planning all behavioral experiments. It is important for clients to appreciate the importance of dropping the various "crutches" they have developed to cope with their SAD, and a behavioral experiment that specifically tests the true value of using safety behaviors can be useful for this purpose.

Safety behavior experiments involve manipulating the use of safety behaviors, that is, contrasting using safety behaviors with not using them and observing the difference. This could be done in several ways, and it is preferable to initially complete these experiments with the therapist. A regular and easily repeated situation in which clients typically use safety behaviors could be used (e.g., traveling on public transportation, buying groceries, eating in the lunchroom), or a situation could be constructed. In group therapy, we ask clients to choose a relatively unknown group member with whom they will have two 5-minute conversations on a topic of their choosing (e.g., places they've been, jobs they've had, places in the world they'd like to visit, music/TV shows/books/movies they like). In individual treatment, this can be done with one of the therapist's colleagues or with the therapist. During the first 5-minute conversation clients use as many of their safety behaviors as they can for the whole conversation. In the second conversation they use no safety behaviors. We find the contrast of the two conversations useful, as it tends to be a good illustration that focusing so much attention on using safety behaviors leaves little attention for effective engagement in the conversation, making the interaction far more taxing and unnatural.

Regardless of what situation is used to compare the use and nonuse of safety behaviors, Worksheet 8, the *Safety Behaviors Experiment,* can be used to guide the experiment. Once a situation or task has been designed, the next step is for the client to close her eyes and picture the worst possible outcome she fears in this type of situation. Once she has a clear image, she can then use it to pay attention to what safety behaviors she would normally use to prevent her worst outcome from occurring. Ensure that the feared image and typical safety behaviors are clearly recorded on the worksheet. It is important that the safety behaviors be clear and specific, so the client knows what she needs to be focused on during the first phase of the experiment (e.g., while having a 5-minute conversation I must keep my sunglasses on and my head down the whole time; I must mentally rehearse everything I say before I say it; and I must ask lots of questions to keep the spotlight off me by not having to say anything personal).

The client is now ready to engage in the social task for 5 minutes while using all her safety behaviors. After completing the task, she can then rate her anxiety, self-consciousness, perceived observability of anxiety, and perceived social performance.

The second phase of the experiment involves repeating the same task, this time under the condition of using no safety behaviors. Before doing this, encourage the client to close her eyes and imagine herself engaging in the situation again without any safety behaviors. Ask her to imagine this in as much detail as possible, taking note of what she is doing, her posture, eye contact, what she is focusing her attention on, how she is feeling in her body. Based on this image, the client clearly records what she will actually do instead of using safety behaviors, so she knows what to do in the second phase of the experiment (e.g., while having the 5-minute conversation I will keep my head up, shoulders back, and look at the other person the majority of the time; I will really listen to what the other person is saying, and just allow my responses to naturally follow from what they have said).

The client is now ready to engage in the social task for 5 minutes while using no safety behaviors. After completing the task, she again completes ratings of anxiety, self-consciousness, perceived observability of anxiety, and perceived social performance. As well as self-ratings, where possible at the very end of the experiment, the client could elicit feedback from the other party she was interacting with, getting their impression of the impact safety behaviors had on the interaction. It can be very helpful within groups for participants to reflect on whether their conversational partner looked more or less comfortable with or without their safety behaviors. Almost invariably clients say the conversation flowed better, the person seemed more engaged, and they could focus on the content of the conversation when their conversational partner was not using safety behaviors.

The final step is to debrief any discrepancies in ratings across the two conditions, and from these observations draw some conclusions about what clients have learned about the impact of safety behaviors. It is hoped that one of two outcomes occurs. Clients typically find that safety behaviors inhibit social performance, increase self-consciousness, prolong anxiety, and can generate the very outcome they are trying to avoid (i.e., a less favorable evaluation from others because they seem disinterested or distracted during social interactions when focused so much on their safety behaviors). This outcome usually facilitates a willingness to drop safety behaviors. While dropping safety behaviors may have initially generated more anxiety during the experiment, clients may discover that this increase in anxiety is short-lived, as they are better able to absorb themselves in the social task at hand. Equally, if clients find little difference between the two conditions, then safety behaviors can be abandoned in the knowledge that they bring no added value.

If clients continue to perceive safety behaviors as helpful and of no detrimental impact after the experiment, the case for dropping them in other behavioral experiments still needs to be made. As a way of reducing the chance of an impasse between the client and therapist, it can sometimes be helpful for therapists to express some surprise about the possible value of using safety behaviors given the model that is being used to guide treatment and past experiences with other clients. Therapists might say something like "Well, this is very interesting to me. I'm now wondering whether safety behaviors might actually be of some value. If so, the model we're using to guide treatment might be wrong, and I might need to start suggesting this to my other clients, and to start using them myself in some situations. But before I do, how could we continue to gather evidence to test out this possibility?" Therapist and client can then collaboratively develop a range of additional behavioral experiments to repeatedly test the perceived benefits of safety behaviors in different contexts. Therapists might also agree to conduct their own behavioral experiments during the week and gather evidence to present feedback on in therapy. They can offer a guarantee that if they both consistently find evidence for the benefit of safety behaviors, then they will change the model and start using them more often. To present this in a therapeutic manner, therapists need to maintain a stance of genuine curiosity.

Behavioral Experiment Hierarchies

Behavioral experiments (particularly standard future-focused experiments and shame-attacking experiments) are typically graded to increase client engagement and confidence in confronting difficult situations. Once clients are familiar with the behavioral experiment process, a hierarchy of likely behavioral experiments of increasing difficulty is collaboratively devised. Developing a hierarchy ensures that each behavioral experiment, which should still be thoroughly planned using Worksheet 7, the *Behavioral Experiment Record,* is working toward an overall valued goal. The hierarchy provides an overall plan, guide, or direction regarding a succession of behavioral experiments for clients to attempt.

Practically, it can be challenging to complete a hierarchy of social situations in a stepwise manner, given that social interactions are not entirely controllable or predictable, and sometimes clients will be concerned that there is too big a "jump" between steps on their hierarchy. It is not imperative that experiments always be completed in a linear fashion. The critical aspect of a behavioral experiment is that there is a discrepancy between the client's expectancies and the actual outcome (prediction error). Generally speaking, larger prediction errors lead to more powerful learning and better long-term outcomes. Grading behavioral experiments, and even reductions in anxiety during behavioral experiments, are not necessarily related to longer-term outcomes. In fact, if grading behavioral experiments, reduces the magnitude of the client's prediction error because he sees the outcome as being safer and more predictable, then learning and long-term benefits may be reduced.

Nonetheless, the process of developing a hierarchy will help clients to plan very specific tasks and will prime them to apply their behavioral experiment skills in a range of situations. If clients come across situations that they could not imagine confronting at this stage, the use of hierarchies allows them to at least start contemplating them for the future. By the time they reach those steps, the situation will seem much more achievable.

There are four key steps involved in grading behavioral experiments to develop a hierarchy or "stepladder." These steps are outlined in Handout 8, *Behavioral Experiment Hierarchies,* with sample hierarchies included for therapist and client reference. The outcome of working through these four steps with clients can be recorded in their own personal *Behavioral Experiment Hierarchy* (Worksheet 9).

Step 1

Start by helping clients identify an area of their life that they want to start working on. Useful questions may be:

- "What would you like to be different?"
- "How would you like things to be?"
- "What would you like to be doing that you aren't currently doing now?"
- "In what area of your life are you having difficulties that you would most like to change?"

Common examples are meeting new people, socializing more, speaking in public, initiating conversations, dating, and being assertive. There may be more than one area clients wish to change, and this may mean that they will need to develop more than one hierarchy. It is best to initially focus on one area of the client's choosing. This decision may be based on an area the client believes will be easiest to change, or the area that is most important.

Step 2

Identify negative images of situations that reflect the area of life clients want to change. These images can be elicited by saying:

> "Close your eyes and imagine yourself in this type of situation (e.g., meeting new people), as if you are experiencing it right now. Where are you? What is happening? What are you doing? What are others doing? What do you feel or sense?"

This image will tie all of the behavioral experiments together, as they will all provide opportunities to challenge it across a variety of contexts.

Step 3

Set a specific behavioral goal related to the area clients would like to change. This involves specifying what they would like to be able to do (or not do) and provides an end point to aim for. Again an imagery exercise can be used to assist clients in generating this goal.

> "Close your eyes and imagine this type of situation (e.g., meeting new people) is no longer a problem for you. Imagine that anxiety isn't a problem. Shoot for the stars! What would you be doing that you currently find extremely difficult? How would you like it to be? Where are you? What is happening? What are you doing? What are others doing? What do you feel or sense?"

Make sure there is consistency between the goal and life area chosen to work on, and that the goal reflects something of importance and value to clients.

Step 4

Brainstorm with clients a variety of situations around this theme that would give them the opportunity to test their negative images and work toward their goal. Ensure clients make a SUDS rating (0–10) for each experiment. The idea is to produce some relevant experiments that generate mild anxiety (i.e., 3–4 out of 10) at the bottom of the hierarchy, some experiments that generate moderate anxiety (i.e., 5–7 out of 10) in the middle of the hierarchy, and some experiments that generate high anxiety (i.e., 8–10 out of 10) at the top of the hierarchy. When developing the experiments, consider with clients what would make it harder or easier for them to complete the experiment, so that they can start to generate stepladders of social tasks that reflect a range of difficulty. Useful prompts for grading are:

- *What* are you going to do? (e.g., just say hello, or sustain a 10-minute conversation)
- *Where* will you do it? (e.g., How familiar or unfamiliar is the place?)
- *When* will you do it? (e.g., How busy or quiet will it be? What day and time?)
- *Who* will be involved? (e.g., How many people will be involved? How familiar or unfamiliar are the people?)

By manipulating these variables, you can create behavioral experiment steps that are harder or easier to complete.

Just as dropping safety behaviors is considered when planning specific behavioral experiments, safety behaviors must also be considered when planning the broader behavioral experiment hierarchy. There are two approaches clinicians can take in this regard. The preferred approach is that clients use no safety behaviors within their hierarchy. While clients may be able to accomplish harder steps with the use of safety behaviors (e.g., accepting a party invitation if they can take a friend rather than going alone), dropping safety behaviors in their hierarchy may mean they need to start with easier steps (e.g., accepting an invitation to a friend's house for dinner and going alone). Starting lower on the hierarchy with no safety behaviors is preferred for all the reasons described earlier, most notably that safety behaviors prevent clients from directly testing their social fears, hence often making the behavioral experiment a less useful learning experience. However, if clients are unwilling to start any experiment without the use of safety behaviors, then the progressive dropping of safety behaviors would need to be explicitly incorporated into the steps of the hierarchy, so that the steps involve a gradual abandoning of various safety behaviors (e.g., the first step is going to the gym with a friend, the next step is going to the gym alone).

Tolerating Anxiety: Coping Imagery

Conducting behavioral experiments while dropping safety behaviors and working up a hierarchy is the most anxiety-provoking component of SAD treatment. However, it is also the most crucial and effective component. Therefore, attention needs to be paid to helping clients tolerate or "surf" the anxiety that is likely to occur when conducting behavioral experiments. The idea of anxiety as something that is tolerable, rather than something to be escaped from, will likely be foreign to most clients, and they will require strategies to help them adopt this attitude. Just to clarify, when we use the word "tolerate," which can hold different meanings for different people, we mean fostering an attitude of learning to cope *with* anxious feelings, rather than trying to get rid of them.

There are various methods a therapist could teach clients to assist their ability to handle anxious feelings (e.g., helpful coping statements, flash cards, mindfulness-based attention training, or focusing attention on the task at hand). Worksheet 6, the *Imagery Challenging Record,* is also good preparation for engaging in behavioral experiments, as clients can use this process to arrive at a more helpful or realistic image that increases their willingness to engage in the challenging behavioral experiment situation. Regardless of what methods are used, the aim is to help clients persist with behavioral experiments, even in the face of emotional discomfort. We focus on one particular additional method, that of developing metaphorical imagery, or the more client-friendly term, "coping imagery."

Client Rationale

The aim of coping imagery is to develop an individualized metaphorical image that assists clients to cope with their anxiety during behavioral experiments. You might introduce this concept by asking clients, "What is a metaphor?" In discussing this, you can say, "A metaphor is a symbol/object/concept that represents our experiences or feelings, as opposed to being something real or literal." Perhaps normalize metaphors by saying that we often talk or think in them without realizing it (e.g., "I felt like a fish out of water"; "I was being put through the wringer"; "I nearly jumped out of my skin"). Discuss the fact that putting our feelings into words can be hard and metaphors seem to be a really good way of capturing how we are feeling emotionally. Also, metaphorical images seem to connect to our feelings more strongly than words. The following imagery exercise may provide an illustration of this concept.

Metaphorical Imagery Exercise

"Say to yourself a few times (in your mind) the word "hope," "hope," "hope"— notice how that feels within you physically and emotionally . . . now close your eyes and visualize something, someone, or somewhere that for you represents "hope" . . . If nothing comes to mind immediately, that's OK. Just sit with the idea of hope for a while and see what emerges. Notice how that feels within you physically and emotionally."

Discuss any differences in emotional and physical experiences between the literal word and the metaphorical image. Conclude that if metaphorical images can effectively capture what we are feeling, and also elicit our feelings, then if we can develop a metaphorical image that represents us coping with our anxiety, this could be a helpful tool to enable us to tolerate our anxious feelings during behavioral experiments.

Developing Coping Imagery

When developing an individualized coping image with clients, normalize that some people find it hard at first, and the image they initially develop may not necessarily be the image they end up using in the long run. They can consider it a creative "work in progress." It can be useful to give clients some examples of coping images that past clients have used to represent coping with their anxiety. This can help give them a feel for the sort of images that may be appropriate. Table 6.2 provides some of the coping images our clients have developed over the years:

Coping Imagery Instructions

There are three phases to developing a coping image, which we have elaborated from Hackmann and colleagues' (2011, p. 154) guidelines on metaphorical imagery. The first phase involves eliciting an anxious image, followed by developing a metaphorical image to represent the activated anxious feelings, and then finally developing a coping image by making appropriate changes to the metaphorical image. The following script can be used as a guide to help clients through this three-stage process:

Eliciting an Anxious Image

"If you feel comfortable doing so, close your eyes, sitting comfortably . . . bring to mind a situation in which you typically experience strong anxiety . . . try to visualize a specific recent example of this situation . . . imagine this difficult situation as if you are there right now, experiencing it firsthand . . . let's explore this situation as if it's happening right now . . ."

- "Where are you? What is going on? What can you see, hear, taste, smell or touch?"
- "What are you thinking?"
- "What do you feel in your body? What sensations do you notice?"
- "What are you feeling emotionally?"

TABLE 6.2. Client Examples of Coping Imagery

Anxious image	Coping image
Drowning in a giant ocean wave	Surfing the wave in to shore
Hiding in a dark cave	Stepping out of the cave into the light of a beautiful sunny garden
Being trapped under a cage	A loved one lifting the cage and freeing me
A big rock weighing down on my chest	Pushing the rock off my chest, standing up, and taking a breath
A big red disgusting oozy mass	Widening out my perspective to see it as a volcano that is just part of a wider beautiful landscape
Being in a dark jungle with a tiger circling	The jungle turns bright and sunny, and it is no longer a tiger but my cat, which I am holding and petting

Eliciting a Metaphorical Image

"Having tuned in to how this situation makes you feel physically and emotionally, let the image go and allow an image to arise that represents this feeling . . . let an image arise that symbolizes how you feel . . . this may take some time . . . stay with it even if it seems strange . . . you may or may not be in the image, it doesn't matter as long as it represents the anxiety you feel . . . if several images occur, pick the strongest.

"Now that you have an image that represents your anxiety . . . let's explore it using whatever senses seem most appropriate for the image. First . . ."

- "How it looks . . . (notice the size, color, lighting, how it looks from different angles or distances)"
- "Is there anything of note in terms of its texture, weight, temperature, the feel of it to touch . . ."
- "Any sounds of note . . ."
- "Any smells or tastes of note . . ."
- "What does this image mean about you or your anxiety? What is the image trying to convey?"
- "How does the image make you feel emotionally? And what body sensations go with that feeling?"

Eliciting a Coping Image (Changing the Metaphorical Image)

"Now, what would need to change in the image to make you feel better or resolve the problem that is going on there? It may involve introducing some new action, or person, or object, or seeing the image from a different vantage point or manipulating the image in some other way. Think about what is needed to change the image for the better.

"Now that you know what needs to change, try to see these changes taking place now. Find ways of making these changes happen in the image. It may take a number of tries, but keep persisting until the problem in the image has a satisfactory resolution.

"Now, notice how this new image makes you feel emotionally. And in your body what sensations do you now notice, and where do you feel them? . . . When you are ready you can let go of the image and open your eyes."

Coping Imagery Debrief

Worksheet 10, *Coping Imagery,* provides a guide for debriefing and recording client learnings from the exercise, as well as describing how to strengthen the image and apply it in the future. The debrief should focus on how the coping image (i.e., the transformed metaphorical image, not the initial metaphorical image) made clients feel emotionally and physically, and what the coping image means about them and their anxiety. Generally, useful coping imagery will be associated with feelings of warmth, lightness, calm, and soothing, and clients often report experiencing these feelings in their chest region. Meanings of the image will often relate to themes of strength, fortitude, persistence, confidence, safety, security, or stability. If clients are not satisfied with the coping image that arises, or the feelings and meanings derived from the image do not appear to serve the purpose of coping with anxious feelings, feel free to rewind the image and try again.

It is important to discuss methods for strengthening this image so it becomes easily retrievable from memory in high-anxiety situations. This could simply involve regular imaginal rehearsal of the image, or other methods such as creating or finding drawings, pictures, music, poetry, or objects that represent the image. These can serve as reminders of the image and may themselves become associated with the same feelings and meanings that the coping image generates. For example, one client had his coping image of being unshackled from handcuffs illustrated, and he then used illustration as the background picture on his cell phone. The client reported using the image as a regular reminder of the increasing freedom he felt from persevering with his behavioral experiments. Assist clients to consider how they will apply the image to help them cope with behavioral experiments. For instance, they could bring the image to mind prior to a behavioral experiment, during a behavioral experiment if the urge to escape is present, or after a behavioral experiment to self-soothe back to baseline. Handout 9, *Coping (Metaphorical) Imagery,* can be provided to clients as useful psychoeducation on the development and use of coping imagery.

Coping Imagery: A Caution

Watch out for the misuse of coping imagery as a safety behavior, and ensure clients are clear about when it is helpful to use coping imagery to persist with behavioral experiments versus when it is unhelpful because it undermines learning from a behavioral experiment. Using glimpses of the image to approach and fully engage with a difficult situation is helpful. Needing to sustain the image and use it to avoid anxiety is problematic. This distinction can be subtle at times, and assessing the attitude adopted by clients when using coping imagery is important. Ensure clients' intention is to use it as a tool to tolerate anxiety, rather than as a safety behavior aimed at removing anxiety. Directly asking clients why they are using the coping image may give you an insight into their motives. Another option is to ask clients to rehearse out loud how they would use the coping image when anxious (i.e., verbalizing their internal self-talk and imagery), or when anxious in the presence of the therapist get them to report out loud how they are using their coping image. The words they use, their tone and volume, and the rapidity of their speech will give you some insight into whether they are using their coping image to genuinely "ride the wave of anxiety" or whether they are using it to attempt to "get the hell off the wave!"

The ultimate aim of coping imagery is to convey the sentiment "this is just anxiety, just sensations—I can cope with this." This could obviously be provided to clients as a helpful coping statement on a flash card. However, coping imagery can be a nice short-hand method of conveying this same meaning, yet in a far more emotionally evocative way. It may be less cumbersome than a flash card, more memorable and accessible than having to spontaneously remember a series of coping statements, and ideally more emotionally and physically impactful. Therefore, coping imagery can become a useful tool to facilitate anxiety tolerance, and thus help clients to persist with the challenges of much-needed social behavior change.

Clinical Case: Behavioral Experiments

We just couldn't stop at one clinical anecdote when it comes to behavioral experiments, as we have shared some very memorable experiences with our clients! However, we don't want the following clinical anecdotes to misrepresent the nature of behavioral experiments undertaken in SAD treatment. Most behavioral experiments conducted in treatment will involve engaging clients in fairly standard social contexts in fairly conventional ways (e.g., walking into a busy shopping area to test the fear that everyone will look at me, or saying hi to a work colleague to test the fear that I'll saying the wrong name). Shame-attacking exercises usually form an essential minority of the behavioral experiments conducted with clients. They are perhaps overrepresented in our clinical anecdotes because they tend to be so memorable and powerful, both for clients and therapists.

The culmination of numerous standard and shame-attacking behavioral experiments for one client was skipping down a main café strip with a party hat on and blowing a whistle. It was amazing to see the big smile on this client's face and the sheer look of liberation as she truly discovered experientially that "even if I do something that's crazy and attracts attention, there is no real tangible negative cost." In fact, several bystanders who were unsure what it was all about cheered her on anyway. This freed her from the "tightrope" of what is socially acceptable behavior, as she recognized that "if I can do this and suffer no real tangible consequence, then I can handle usual everyday social interactions."

Another client who had struggled over many group sessions to really engage with any of the strategies either within or between sessions had a noticeable shift when he took part in a shame-attacking exercise of walking around a crowded place with toilet paper purposely hanging out the back of his pants. He was depressed because of his social isolation and was caught in the trap of his depression interfering with his engagement with social anxiety treatment. However, after many weeks with little progress, this one experiment made a significant impression on him. It was the first time we had seen him smile as he said, "No one seems to care what I do, so maybe I shouldn't care so much either."

The following story is especially for therapists who worry about behavioral experiments going wrong (i.e., the client's prediction coming true). In a group session where the clients and therapists were embarking on a strange procession in single file through a public area, one client's biggest fear was that he would see someone he knew and be ridiculed. The client was a young male who reported that many of his friends socialized in the area, so for him this feared situation was likely and highly costly. From past experience the therapists were pretty confident that the likelihood of this occurring was actually very slim, but a brief discussion followed about strategies for managing this situation should it arise. Some group members suggested that he say the strange behavior in the group was part of an acting course. Others suggested that he tell them that it was none of their business! Armed with these potential responses the clients and therapists set off to complete the behavioral experiment. Well, what do you know . . . the client did see a friend (another young male) who came up and asked, "What are you doing?" During the debrief the therapists held their breath as they anticipated the outcome of the conversation. The client reported that he was shocked to see his friend, and rather than lie he decided to tell him the truth, "I am doing a social anxiety course." Again, the therapists held their breath. The friend's response was astounding to the client and to the whole group. His friend said, "I think I might need to do something like that too." This experience was pivotal for this client and provided an important corrective experience for the whole group, including the therapists.

In another group therapy session, one of the shame-attacking experiments we did as a group was to walk down a public street with each of us dragging an object on a string as if we were taking it for a walk. I (LS) had a paper coffee cup at the end of mine, some people had pens or toilet paper rolls. So, we walked in a rough line with one cotherapist (PM) guiding the front, and me at the back. Being at the back was interesting. People's reactions to our group were initially a lack of attention, then eventual surprise, and then curiosity. My colleague, being at the front, often went unnoticed, as people only tuned in to this unusual behavior after several people walked past them with strange objects on strings. At the end of the line another client and I therefore attracted the most interest and attention of all, none of it malicious, all just genuine curiosity. The climax came when we were stopped by a bunch of foreign tourists, not to ask what we were doing, but instead to ask if they could take a photo with us. The client consented, and so we had our photo taken with about five other tourists, who all flashed big happy smiles and peace signs, and were extremely grateful to us. They never bothered to ask what we were doing or why. The client walked away exclaiming, "That was actually fun!" I have always wondered how those tourists made sense of those pictures when they returned home.

THERAPY SUMMARY GUIDE: Avoidance and Safety Behaviors

Therapy Aim: Identify avoidance and safety behaviors, and use behavioral experimentation methods to reverse avoidance and drop safety behaviors. These methods are intended to challenge and modify the negative social thoughts and images that avoidance and safety behaviors serve to perpetuate.

Therapy Agenda Items:

▼ Socialize clients to changing avoidance and safety behaviors:

   ◢ Identify avoidance and safety behaviors

   ◢ Normalize the function of avoidance and safety behaviors by linking them to the feared negative imagery these behaviors are designed to prevent

   ◢ Highlight the maintaining role of avoidance and safety behaviors via Socratically guided psychoeducation, including the vicious cycle of avoidance and anxiety and positive cycle of approach and reduced anxiety

   ◢ Discuss the impact of the Safety Behaviors Imagery Exercise

▼ Develop strategies for coping with anxiety during behavioral experiments. Imagery Challenging is one method already available from Chapter 5, with another option being the development of metaphorical coping imagery

▼ Modify behavior to challenge cognitions via behavioral experiments:

   ◢ Introduce behavioral experiments with a focus on increasing client motivation

   ◢ Worksheet 7, *Behavioral Experiment Record*—review hypothetical examples, apply to client examples within therapy sessions (conducting the behavioral experiment in session), plan and debrief experiments in session that are conducted by clients outside session, and then have clients independently complete multiple experiments as ongoing weekly homework

   ◢ Develop a behavioral experiment hierarchy to guide the direction and planning of behavioral experiments over the course of treatment

   ◢ Conduct a safety behaviors experiment, if necessary, to increase client commitment to dropping safety behaviors during behavioral experiments

   ◢ As early as clients are willing, conduct shame-attacking experiments to ensure the cost of social mishaps is tested during treatment

Therapy Materials:

▼ Handouts

   ◢ Handout 4, *The Cycle of Avoidance and Anxiety*

   ◢ Handout 5, *Safety Behaviors*

   ◢ Handout 6, *Behavioral Experiments*—includes behavioral experiment record example

▲ Handout 7, *Behavioral Experiment Menu*

▲ Handout 8, *Behavioral Experiment Hierarchies*—including four behavioral experiment hierarchy examples

▲ Handout 9, *Coping (Metaphorical) Imagery*

▼ Worksheets

▲ Worksheet 7, *Behavioral Experiment Record*

▲ Worksheet 8, *Safety Behaviors Experiment*

▲ Worksheet 9, *Behavioral Experiment Hierarchy*

▲ Worksheet 10, *Coping Imagery*

CHAPTER 7

Negative Self-Image

THERAPIST: What do you envision happening if you went to the party instead of avoiding it?

CLIENT: It would be a disaster!

THERAPIST: How so?

CLIENT: Well, I wouldn't know what to say, I wouldn't be able to keep a conversation going, people will find me boring or annoying. They will think I am weird because I look so anxious.

THERAPIST: Is there an image that comes to mind that captures the thought that people are going to be bored or annoyed by you?

CLIENT: I guess the other person's eyes sort of glaze over; they look at their watch a lot and search the room for someone else to talk to as an escape from me. They make some weak excuse and walk away as soon as they can. They roll their eyes and keep looking back at me as they talk to their "savior," and you can just tell that they are talking about me.

THERAPIST: What about the part where you said, "They will think I am weird because I look so anxious"—how exactly would they be able to pick up on your anxiety? What would they be seeing in you that would indicate you were anxious?

CLIENT: Well, I would be bright red in the face, sweating, shaking, I would "umm and ahh" a lot, I would just look like a fool, so of course they will think "What's their problem?"

THERAPIST: That prediction of being bright red, sweating, shaking, does that ever enter your mind like a photo or video of yourself looking that way?

CLIENT: Sort of, I guess I am always conscious that my anxiety is pretty obvious.

THERAPIST: It sounds like there are two kinds of negative social images you might hold. Those that are about how others are reacting to you, and those that are about how you are appearing to others, that is, how anxious you look and how you are performing socially. So far we have mostly focused on challenging and experimenting with images regarding other people's reactions to you. I would also like to turn our attention specifically to the negative self-image that you hold, that picture of how you imagine you are appearing to others, and see if we can challenge and experiment with this type of image too.

CLIENT: But I am red, I am sweating and shaking, all that is true. It isn't imagined.

THERAPIST: You are absolutely right. You are feeling anxious, and when we are anxious we do feel all those symptoms in our body of things like flushing, sweating, shaking. But what I would like you to be curious about is whether those symptoms are as observable to others as you think. So the issue is not whether or not these symptoms are occurring, but are they as observable to others as you think, and is the image you have of yourself completely accurate?

About This Module: Addressing Self-Imagery in SAD

Clients with SAD often underestimate their social performance and overestimate the observability of their anxiety. This is a form of emotional reasoning—"because I feel anxious and I am very aware of it, everyone else must also be aware of it and I must look like a fool." Therapists can have similar biases about their clients. Therapists might assume that because clients with SAD have typically been avoidant for some time they must have a social skills deficit, either because they have not acquired appropriate skills earlier in life or because of a lack of practice. Therapists may therefore share clients' fears of negative evaluation from others, assuming clients are not able to socialize in a conventional manner. However, research and clinical experience suggest that a skills deficit in SAD is not the norm, and that clients with SAD often have perfectly adequate social skills and performance. The problem is usually that anxiety and safety behaviors *inhibit* social skills. Once anxiety is successfully treated, our clients' natural social skills often become apparent.

Clients' underestimation of performance and overestimation of the observability of their anxiety often manifests cognitively via negative self-imagery. Many clients will hold a negative image from an "observer perspective," that is, how they appear to others, as if they were observing themselves through the other person's eyes. This means that when anticipating, participating in, or reflecting on social occasions, clients' negative social imagery may be intermixed with snippets that occur from a field perspective (i.e., looking out at the situation through their own eyes to see other people's reactions) and snippets that occur from an observer perspective (i.e., seeing themselves from others' perspectives). The problem is that the self-image formed in the client's "mind's eye" is guided by internal cues (e.g., anxiety symptoms) and ambiguous external cues (e.g., seeing someone yawn or look away), rather than objective feedback. The self-image can therefore be highly biased. This module covers the practicalities of identifying self-imagery and effectively engaging clients in the challenging behavioral experiments that are required to correct biased self-imagery, with a particular focus on using video feedback as a corrective tool.

Identifying Negative Self-Images

Negative self-images are a subset of negative social imagery and hence can be targeted via similar challenging and experimentation principles that have already been discussed in Chapters 5 and 6. When eliciting negative social images more broadly (see Chapter 5), which is usually done by asking clients to adopt a field perspective, it is likely that they will spontaneously shift into an observer perspective, and therefore negative self-imagery will emerge. Thus, the prompt questions and Worksheet 5, *Thought and Imagery Record,* already introduced for eliciting negative social images generally, will likely reveal some negative self-imagery too. However, if this spontaneous shift does not occur, then clients may need more specific prompting to adopt an observer perspective:

"It is very common for people with social anxiety to have negative images not just of people judging them and reacting to them negatively, but also of themselves appearing in some way that will generate negative judgment from others. We will call this a negative self-image, where you have a negative image of how you appear to others, as if you were one of them observing yourself.

"When you are in a social situation and feeling anxious, how do you imagine you look to others? How do you imagine you are performing? If I were there what would I be noticing about you? [Client gives general examples.]

"Close your eyes and imagine being in [a social situation] as if you are there right now experiencing it firsthand. This time take the perspective of the other person looking at and observing you. What are they seeing? What are they noticing about you? How are you appearing? How are you performing socially?"

As with any aspect of treatment, the rationale for targeting self-imagery must be clear to our clients. A convincing rationale is particularly important given that clients typically find the main recommended experiment for modifying negative self–imagery (i.e., video feedback) very challenging. Before clients are likely to willingly engage in video feedback they must first be convinced of the positive impact that challenging their negative self-image will have on their treatment outcome. Handout 10, *Self-Image: How I Really Appear to Others,* can be helpful to provide to clients as psychoeducation, and the following are important points to discuss with clients to reinforce the rationale for tackling negative self-imagery.

- Negative self-imagery *promotes self-focused attention* rather than task-focused attention, which can reduce clients' ability to fully engage in the social encounter and negatively impact social performance.
- Negative self-imagery *increases perceived threat* in social situations as it heightens awareness of anxiety symptoms and exaggerates the presumption that these symptoms are obvious to others.
- *More negative images follow from the self-image* regarding negative evaluation from others that will result from observable anxiety and poor performance.
- Negative self-imagery *increases the urge to avoid or escape* if we perceive that the image we are presenting to others is inadequate.

The following are potentially useful questions to Socratically elicit each point from clients.

- "How do you think these negative images of yourself contribute to your social anxiety?"
- "Does the image increase or decrease your self-focused attention? What impact does self-focused attention have on you? What impact does it have on your anxiety? What impact does it have on your social performance? Are you able to fully participate in the social situation when this negative self-image is at the forefront of your mind? If you can't participate fully, then what happens? Do you find that the image can be very distracting, increasing your awareness of your anxiety and focusing your attention inward on trying to control the anxiety? Is it possible that all of this takes attention away from the task and might interfere with your social performance?"
- "In what ways might the negative self-image increase or decrease your sense of social danger? If your negative self-image suggests that your anxiety symptoms are noticeable, and you believe that others seeing your anxiety will lead to negative evaluation, then what impact does the self-image have on your sense of danger in social situations?"
- "What images do you have about how others will react to seeing your anxiety or poor social performance? And how do you then see yourself reacting to this? It sounds like the negative images about yourself can start to snowball into other negative images."
- "When you have these self-images, are you more or less likely to stay in the social situation? Are you more or less likely to want to go into similar social situations in the future? How might this avoidance prevent you from ever testing your image of the obviousness of your anxiety symptoms (i.e., the true likelihood of others noticing)? Even if some people do notice your anxiety, how does avoidance prevent you from directly testing how much this really needs to matter (i.e., the true cost of others noticing)?

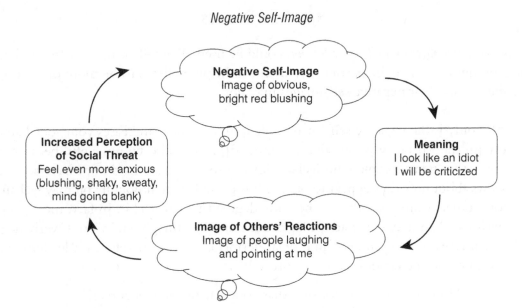

FIGURE 7.1. The vicious cycle of negative self-imagery and social threat.

In addition to discussion of these points, the vicious cycle diagram shown in Figure 7.1 can be drawn collaboratively with clients. The diagram illustrates how the negative self-image leads to the beliefs that anxiety is obvious and performance is poor (e.g., I look like an idiot), and that negative judgment and reactions from others will follow (e.g., I will be criticized). These beliefs then lead to further negative imagery of other people's negative responses. The perception of social threat then escalates because negative evaluation seems even more likely, and so further anxiety is generated in response to this threat. The anxiety symptoms that feature in the negative self-image then become more intense, and are then presumed to be even more observable. This process strengthens the negative self-image and the cycle continues.

Modifying Negative Self-Images

As with the negative images discussed in Chapters 5 and 6, negative self-images can be modified via challenging and experimentation methods. The role of the therapist is to cast doubt on the accuracy of clients' negative self-images, cultivate a curiosity within clients to discover how they truly appear when anxious, and provide opportunities to gather this evidence.

Challenging Self-Images

Many of the questions used for general imagery challenging in Chapter 5 can be applied here to assist with identifying and challenging the accuracy of self-images, and Worksheet

6, the formal *Imagery Challenging Record,* could be used. The following concepts and disputation questions may be particularly useful in helping clients to be more open to the possibility that their negative self-images may not be valid:

"Not only is the negative self-image unhelpful because it increases your social anxiety [in the various ways previously outlined], it may also be unhelpful because we know that many people who feel anxious in social situations do not have accurate views about how they appear to others. It is possible that although you may feel anxious, others cannot see this to the same degree that you feel it. In fact, most people with social anxiety come across far better than they imagine they do. Overly negative images of your anxiety and social performance can therefore mislead you and increase your perception of social threat."

- "How do you know for sure that your self-image is accurate?"
- "How do you really know how you appear to others?"
- "How often do you get an objective picture or reliable feedback?"
- "What do you base your self-image on? Is this good, solid, reliable evidence?"
- "What evidence or experiences support your self-image being true?"
- "Have you had any experiences that show that this self-image is not completely true?"
- "Is your self-image based on unambiguous facts, or are you using emotional reasoning (i.e., because I feel anxious therefore I must look anxious to others)? What evidence do you really have?"
- "Is it possible that the symptoms you are concerned about may be less obvious than you think? Because they are happening within you, is it possible that they seem magnified to you? To an outsider who is not specifically looking for these things, is it possible that they may be less obvious and go unnoticed?"

Often clients will recognize that they have no clear evidence to support their negative self-image other than the anxiety they feel. If this is the case, it is important that they realize they are jumping to the conclusion that an internal emotional and physiological experience is very observable externally. It might be useful to question if they have ever heard other people say "I was so nervous," yet their perception was that the person didn't look nervous, or if they did it was quite minor and understandable given the task.

Sometimes clients will be able to recall experiences where people have noticed their anxiety and commented. If this is the case, then it may be useful to place this feedback within a broader context by asking the following:

- "How many times have you been anxious in your life, and how many comments have you had, exactly?"
- "What specifically was the feedback you received? While your anxiety may at times be noticeable to others, have you had reliable feedback about the intensity of all the specific things you are concerned are noticeable?"

- "Was it your anxiety symptoms or your safety behaviors that others were noticing? If it was your safety behaviors, it sounds like using them might be increasing the risk of negative evaluation. That's interesting, what do you make of this?"
- "When someone has made a comment, then what? What happened next? What was the true cost or consequence when someone noticed? Did you cope? How could you cope?"
- "What does it say about the other person who would make a comment about someone else feeling uncomfortable? What do you think other people would think of their behavior?"
- "When you notice that someone is looking uncomfortable, how do you feel toward them? Do you tend to be highly critical or more compassionate?"

Behavioral Experiments for Negative Self-Images

Challenging self-images cognitively may not necessarily shift clients' self-imagery significantly. However, the aim of this line of questioning is to start undermining the validity of self-imagery, generate curiosity about alternative self-images, and prepare clients for behavioral experiments that will more reliably and powerfully test the accuracy of their self-images. Regardless of whether the self-imagery challenging process has been "successful," therapists should move to questioning what would need to be done to gain more valid information regarding their appearance by asking, "So how could we go about getting a more accurate image of how you are coming across to others when you're feeling anxious?"

Feedback from Others

Clients might bring up the possibility of getting feedback from others. While a behavioral experiment could achieve this, the problem is ensuring that the feedback is objective, constructive, and believable. Discuss with clients how they might obtain feedback that meets these criteria. Clients would need to be able to identify who they trust to give accurate and constructive feedback that is not unduly biased in a negative or positive way. This might include friends, family, a boss, a tutor, or a job interview panel. Friends and family could always be drawn on to give very general feedback (e.g., "do I look anxious when I am talking to people I don't know well?"), but more specific feedback will have a greater impact. This would involve identifying a specific situation within which clients will be observed and identifying beforehand the specific aspects of appearance they are concerned about, so the person providing feedback can comment specifically on each. Worksheet 7 (*Behavioral Experiment Record*), discussed in Chapter 6, could be used to assist with planning the specific details of a feedback experiment.

Consideration should be given to whether to cue the observer in to the client's specific appearance concerns prior to the observation task. One option is not to tell the observer the client's appearance concerns and see if the observer notices them. If they go unnoticed and cannot be specifically identified, then this is important information about the likelihood of the symptoms being noticed. The observer can then be prompted retrospectively for feedback on the specific appearance concerns for further confirmation. This approach is most naturalistic because people generally do not closely scrutinize others' performance or appearance, and therefore the risk of minor symptoms being magnified by excessive attentional focus is reduced.

However, if the client has strong concerns about a particular aspect of his appearance and performance, it may be valuable for him to learn that even when someone was specifically paying attention, the symptom wasn't obvious or as intense as imagined. In these instances, it may be helpful to ask the observer to focus on particular symptoms before engaging in the task. After receiving feedback from others, as we do in all behavioral experiments, this information is used to update the negative self-image into a more helpful, realistic self-image.

Video Feedback

Using feedback from other people as a means of updating negative self-images still runs the risk of not providing objective and believable evidence. There is potential for clients to dismiss positive feedback as being disingenuous. Instead, the therapist could encourage clients to consider the option of obtaining video feedback by asking questions like "How could you find out once and for all, in a way that would be convincing to you, how you come across when you're feeling anxious, without having to rely on other people's feedback?"

Ideally clients will generate the idea of video feedback themselves, which the therapist can endorse as a "great idea!" Video feedback offers clients the best opportunity to gather objective evidence about their appearance that is *most likely to be convincing to the client*. Video feedback experiments involve videotaping clients when they are anxious and then having them repeatedly view this video in a strategic manner. The aim is for clients to directly compare their self-image to the video image. The typical task used to generate anxiety in group therapy is a 2-minute impromptu speech given in front of the group. Therapists offer clients the option of giving the speech on a topic of their choosing or a topic randomly chosen for them. After discussing the rationale for challenging self-images, if clients are willing, it might be preferable to move immediately to the video feedback task prior to extensive thought and imagery challenging to maximize the impact. The therapist must be careful to keep the thought and imagery challenging from providing too much reassurance or removing any of the surprise the client might experience from observing the discrepancy between her self-image and video-recorded image.

In individual therapy the same speech task could be used, and the therapist's colleagues could be recruited as an audience. Having the therapist alone as an audience may be enough to generate sufficient anxiety for some clients. The size of the audience is unimportant, but the task must generate anxiety (a SUDSs rating of at least 5 out of 10). Clients need to feel anxious when being taped, so they have the opportunity to observe how they appear when in an anxious state. If they don't feel anxious when being taped, the experiment is useless. If they report that the task is not anxiety provoking, question what they could do to make it anxiety provoking, for example altering the type of task, type of audience, number of people, length of time, and where the task is completed. You may need to get creative! If clients are concerned because they will be anxious, the therapist should respond with enthusiasm.

> "Great! If you weren't anxious it would be a waste of time. The whole purpose is to feel anxious and to then observe once and for all how obvious those symptoms really are."

If clients still express reluctance it might be worth Socratically eliciting the potential payoff from the task.

- "What would it be like, after all these years, to discover that although you might feel anxious these symptoms are nowhere near as obvious as you thought they were?"
- Why might this be useful to know?"
- What impact would this knowledge have on your ability to make genuine choices about what you would like to do and not do in your life, without this unfair and inaccurate negative self-image dictating these choices for you?"

Video Experiment Setup

Worksheet 11, the *Speech Form,* provides a useful guide through the steps involved in setting and conducting a video feedback experiment. The *Speech Form* can be amended if the task being used to elicit anxiety during videotaping is a different social task such as a social interaction. Prior to the taping, clients are prompted to close their eyes and create a mental image of how they think they will appear to others while giving the speech. They then write a brief description or draw a picture of this image. Following this they complete Worksheet 12, the *Speech Rating Form,* rating how anxious they predict they will feel, how anxious they predict they will look, identifying any specific symptoms they predict will be obvious based on the mental image they created, and rating how observable they predict each symptom will be on the recording. Before embarking on the task, it is important to remind clients to drop their usual safety behaviors because these may also impair performance (e.g., looking down, not making eye contact, speaking quietly, overrehearsing), increasing the likelihood of a more negative video image. Alternatively, if their anxiety symptoms are not obvious on the tape, they might attribute this to the use of their safety behaviors. In addition, clients should not use their coping image prior to the task, again because the aim of the task is to be as anxious as possible.

As with all behavioral experiments, other than ensuring the experiment is clearly planned, too much discussion beforehand can be a potential form of avoidance, so it is usually helpful to get straight into the speech task. In a group setting we ask who is prepared to go first and continue until all clients who have chosen to participate have completed a speech. If clients are reluctant to participate because they feel anxious, remind them that the aim of the task is not to feel calm, but to purposely do a task that makes them feel anxious so that they can test whether the video recording matches their mental image of how they come across when anxious. If they think they will be most anxious if they go last, then they can do this. If they think they will be most anxious if they are first, then they should be encouraged to do this. As with all experiments, you are not forcing clients to do something against their will, but rather providing the opportunity to learn something new that may have a significant impact on how they see themselves and hence how socially anxious they feel.

After completing their speech, clients then close their eyes and form a clear image of how they think they came across during the speech, constructing an "internal video" of how they think they will appear on the recording. They then write a brief description or draw a picture of this image. Clients then revisit the *Speech Rating Form,* rating how anxious they felt, how anxious they think they looked, and how observable they think each previously identified symptom was.

On a practical note, obviously this exercise requires having access to a recording device, and ideally some way of replaying the recording immediately after the task is done. Replaying should be on a screen of sufficient size for the client to see themselves clearly. Ideally, the recording should be in a format that the client can take away for repeated viewing for homework.

Watching the Video

Now for the moment of truth, watching the video! The video is typically watched four times (at least once in session and the other times for homework). The therapist may decide that all four viewings should be done in his presence, if particular clients need extensive prompting to facilitate viewing the recording in an unbiased manner. The rationale for viewing the video on more than one occasion is that most people initially dislike seeing themselves and hearing their voice on video, and this can adversely impact perception. Clients often need to desensitize to this initial discomfort before they can make objective judgments about what they are seeing. Watching the video is usually anxiety provoking for clients and also for some therapists, with both parties concerned that the self-image will be confirmed in the video feedback. It is important for therapists to have some clear strategies for ensuring the video feedback is viewed in an unbiased manner by clients, and that the experiment is a therapeutic experience.

Therapists may need to work hard to counteract attention and interpretation biases during the video viewing. The following points are important to cover with clients prior to watching the video, and may need to be reinforced during or after the viewing. Each point assists in setting the tone for processing the video in a helpful manner:

• *Distinguish between how one feels versus how one looks.* Ask clients to pay attention to how they look in the video rather than how they felt during the speech (or are feeling while watching themselves on video). Normalize the "yuck" factor we all get when watching ourselves on video, and request that they don't let that interfere with being able to objectively look at whether the video matches their original negative self-image. Mention that viewing it four times is designed to help them put their emotions to the side so they can look at the video more objectively.

- *Encourage maximum objectivity.* Ask clients to watch the video as if watching a friend or someone else they care about. Request that they observe the whole picture, rather than homing in on a particular aspect they dislike. To do this they will need to make sure they are not using safety behaviors such as hiding their face, averting their gaze, or only intermittently looking at the video recording.

- *Identify unrealistic expectations.* Preempt any double standards clients may hold for themselves by encouraging them to apply the same expectations they would have of others doing the task. Unrealistic expectations often involve the idea that they should not say "um," pause, stumble on any words, fidget, or move. Encourage them to consider if their expectations of themselves are reasonable given the task demands. Are they reasonable given their level of experience in public speaking or the impromptu nature of the task? Would they be willing to abandon their double standards temporarily for the purpose of this exercise, and rate themselves based on the standards they would apply to others in the same situation?

- *Prepare for clients noticing negative aspects they hadn't predicted.* Decatastrophize any aspect of their performance clients would like to change. Frame this as a learning opportunity. There may be things they want to improve with their public speaking, and this is fine. Remind them that the aim is to test the predicted image of what they look like when anxious, not to evaluate their public speaking ability, which is a skill that can be developed. Request that they focus on discrepancies between the predicted image and the actual image. Acknowledge that they will be good at finding things they don't like, but ask them to also look for things that were better than they expected.

Following the first viewing of the video, the *Speech Rating Form* should again be completed, to gather ratings of how anxious they actually looked and how observable each previously identified symptom was. Again, a new internal video of how they really appeared should be brought to mind, and a brief description or picture drawn to represent this. The same is then done after watching the video three more times to see if their perception changes with repeated viewing. When the final more realistic self-image is recalled by the client, it can be inserted into a variety of contexts within the client's life within imagery to further consolidate and generalize the learning.

Video Experiment Debrief

The video feedback experiment should be debriefed and some helpful conclusions drawn after the first viewing and again after the additional three viewings. Therapists should focus on any discrepancies from early to later ratings, and hence any differences between the negative self-image and the video image. Be aware of getting sidetracked by clients wanting to focus on anything they perceive as negative. Always try to redirect them to discrepancies between the predicted image and predicted symptom ratings, as compared to the actual image and actual obviousness of symptoms.

If the client's unrealistic expectations become evident (e.g., you shouldn't say "um"), you might ask the following:

- "Are you watching yourself in the same way others would watch you in an interaction, or are you over scrutinizing/being critical/holding higher expectations/ looking for a specific symptom rather than taking in the whole person?"
- "How obvious do you think the symptom would be if you weren't purposely looking for it?"
- "If you saw someone else displaying [the symptom], what would you think? How would you feel toward them?"
- "What would be acceptable if someone else was speaking (e.g., how many "um's" would be OK)?

The video could be watched again with the therapist, and the perceived "symptoms" can be counted to see how they compare to what is acceptable for others.

If clients also hold unrealistically high expectations of what is acceptable for other people, they may need to do some observational experiments watching everyday people do a similar task (e.g., work colleagues presenting at meetings, the therapist doing a videoed impromptu speech, wedding speeches, everyday people giving media interviews). Ensure the source of their observational experiments is not an experienced public speaker. One of our clients compared his social performance to Barack Obama and, perhaps unsurprisingly, believed he came up short every time! Another client declared that she just wanted to speak like a newscaster, after which the therapist encouraged the whole therapy group to have a conversation sounding like newscasters. It became apparent very quickly that this rule generated some very awkward conversations.

If clients are harsh in their appraisals of themselves and you are working in a group context, group feedback can be sought to challenge their appraisals. If you are working in individual therapy, identifying other people in the client's life (i.e., friends or family) who could watch the video and provide fair and genuine feedback may be an option. Alternatively, the therapist could provide feedback, or with client consent the therapist could show the tape to colleagues and survey their feedback. However, as previously discussed, the feedback needs to be considered by clients as objective, constructive, and believable. If feedback is being sought from other people, then after watching the tape they should make the same symptom ratings that the client has been completing.

The following questions are used in group therapy when drawing on other people's feedback to moderate clients' harsh appraisals of their performance. These questions can be adapted when feedback is sought from friends, family, the therapist, or the therapist's colleagues:

- "How do you explain the difference between your observations of yourself versus the group's observations? Do you think they are just being nice? What could be other reasons? Who's likely to be more objective?"
- "If the rest of the group couldn't pick it up (even though they were specifically looking for signs of anxiety), would someone not looking for it notice?"
- "Do you think anyone else in the group has been harsh in how they have seen themselves on the video? Is it possible that this might be happening for you too?"

If clients find the video feedback particularly helpful and meaningful because they appear much better than they anticipated, then it is important that they develop and regularly mentally rehearse a new self-image of how they really appear when anxious, as a way of consolidating this learning. If these new self-images are well practiced, then clients will have a better chance of retrieving them from memory when they start to question how they are coming across to others.

Some clients may find that video feedback has no impact on their negative self-image, seemingly confirming what they already suspected. This may occur if clients are unable to overcome their information-processing biases when viewing the video. For example, one client admitted watching the video while intoxicated and through a window from a separate room. Clearly this was not an ideal strategy for obtaining an objective impression.

The exercise might also have a limited impact if the video is objectively negative (i.e., they do look anxious or don't perform well). Such an occurrence is uncommon in our experience, and not a reason not to show the client the video. Even if performance is not of a high standard or some symptoms are present, the client's self-image is typically far more negative than the video image. Regardless of the reason for the video feedback task being ineffective in challenging negative self-imagery, therapists should not despair. The following are some options for addressing this problem should it arise:

- "Regardless of whether the image is true, does holding this image help you in your goal of being able to socialize more? What are the consequences of hanging on to this image of yourself? What would be a more helpful image to develop that might be more compatible with your goal of wanting to socialize more?"
- "Regardless of whether the image is true, let's look at the cost. What does it matter if the symptoms of concern are present? You noticed them because you were really attuned to them, which is different from other people noticing and caring. What experiment could we do to find out how much others notice and how much it really matters, even when the symptoms are really obvious?" This paves the way for shame-attacking experiments where symptoms are purposely exaggerated and the consequence of this is observed (see Chapter 6).
- "Is it possible that the symptoms of concern may be more exaggerated in this video task because you are not practiced at public speaking? I am wondering if it would be the same in more general daily social interactions? How could we find

out?" This could lead to experiments aimed at obtaining objective feedback from trusted people in real-world situations (see the earlier section on feedback from others).

- Reframe the video as an opportunity to improve, rather than the only goal being to disprove the negative self-image. "What can you do about it? What specific skills might you need to work on?" (e.g., making more eye contact, speaking in a louder volume). The therapist and client can then begin working on these skills in therapy. In addition, the client might acknowledge that many of the symptoms noticed were actually safety behaviors, which provides a strong rationale for dropping these in future social tasks.

- Given that social anxiety could be thought of as social perfectionism (i.e., demanding that one be socially perfect), could this exercise be used as a good opportunity to tolerate imperfection? "If you could tolerate not being socially perfect, what would that be like for you? What consequences would follow?"

Cautions for Video Feedback

If clients have a current or past eating disorder, body dysmorphia, weight and shape problems, or other body image issues, then you may need to consider whether video feedback is still appropriate. The decision regarding whether to proceed should consider how significant the negative self-image is in maintaining social anxiety, the likelihood of the video task reinforcing or worsening appearance concerns, and whether clients can separate concerns about the observability of their anxiety from other appearance concerns. If clients have been able to successfully take part in mirror retraining, which is recommended in the treatment of BDD (i.e., being able to more objectively describe and view their image when using a mirror), then this is a good sign that they may be able to engage in the video feedback task appropriately.

If the therapist has good evidence based on their observations of the client that the negative self-image is accurate, then the therapist may decide not to proceed with video feedback. However, therapists should make this decision with caution. Therapists might predict that many socially anxious clients would perform poorly or show obvious anxiety during the video task. However, it is often surprising how clients are able to rise to the challenge when the task demands it. We have often been pleasantly surprised by client performances during video feedback, in that most clients look like any person would look when giving an impromptu speech, some nerves but nothing out of the ball park of "normality." In fact, we are frequently very entertained by our clients' humor, knowledge, and warmth when given the opportunity to present. Therapists need to be careful not to get drawn into clients' negative views of themselves, and in turn underestimate clients' capabilities and resilience. Anxiety symptoms are typically far more exaggerated in clients' self-images than in reality. As already mentioned, even if clients' negative images are confirmed, video feedback will help them clearly identify specific behaviors that they can actively work on.

Clinical Case: Modifying Negative Self-Imagery

One client was very preoccupied with the self-image of her jaw and face looking very tense whenever she was anxious. She imagined looking very taut, unnatural, almost statue-like. She believed this was obvious to others, and as a result they would think she was crazy, mentally unstable, and dangerous. In social settings, she would constantly touch her face and move her mouth in an attempt to relax her jaw and would often keep her head down. It was actually these safety behaviors that were more likely to generate negative judgment, rather than her jaw or facial appearance. A speech task was not necessary to elicit her anxiety. Being videotaped in the therapist's office doing nothing was enough to elevate her anxiety sufficiently. The client was videotaped just sitting in the chair, and after a while she was instructed to "amp up" the facial tension that she believed was so obvious. The therapist and client then watched the video together. In true form, there were aspects of her appearance that she didn't like and initially honed in on. However, when the therapist encouraged her to instead focus on assessing how the video image of her jaw matched the predicted self-image of her jaw, she laughed in disbelief, saying "I don't look like a statue, I don't look how I imagined." The client ceased touching her face and the elaborate jaw movements thereafter.

THERAPY SUMMARY GUIDE: Negative Self-Image

Therapy Aim: Identify and modify negative self-images, which typically reflect an overestimation of the observability of anxiety and an underestimation of social performance.

Therapy Agenda Items:

▼ Identify negative self-images:

◢ Worksheet 5, *Thought and Imagery Record,* and general questions for identifying negative social thoughts and images outlined in Chapter 5 may reveal negative self-imagery

◢ Prompt clients to adopt an observer perspective when eliciting negative social images

▼ Provide a rationale for targeting negative self-images:

◢ Have a Socratic discussion about negative self-images promoting self-focused attention, increasing perceived threat, eliciting further negative imagery, and increasing avoidance

◢ The vicious cycle diagram (i.e., Figure 7.1) can accompany this discussion

▼ Modify negative self-images:

◢ Worksheet 6, introduced in Chapter 5 (*Imagery Challenging Record*), can be used, with additional disputation questions specific to challenging self-imagery

◢ Behavioral experiments:

▶ Observer feedback is an option, but may not be ideal if clients cannot establish an objective and believable feedback source.

▶ Video feedback is preferred due to its objectivity. A video-recorded impromptu speech or social interaction can be used to elicit anxiety. Special attention must be given to the way the experiment is set up, using Worksheet 1, the *Speech Form.* to guide this process. Watching and debriefing the video also require careful consideration and planning.

Therapy Materials:

▼ Handouts

◢ Handout 10, *Self-Image: How I Really Appear to Others*

▼ Worksheets

◢ Worksheet 11, *Speech Form*

◢ Worksheet 12, *Speech Rating Form*

CHAPTER 8

Attention Biases

THERAPIST: You mentioned that walking down the street can be really anxiety provoking. Have you ever noticed what you pay most attention to when you are walking down the street?

CLIENT: Not really, I've never thought about it.

THERAPIST: Let's do it now together, if you'd be willing. We will just go outside and walk along the street as you normally would do, but this time just notice what your mind is homing in on . . . [Therapist and Client go out to the surrounding streets and do the exercise, pause, and debrief on the street.] So what did you notice your mind was focused on?

CLIENT: Well, I was looking down most of the time.

THERAPIST: Yeah, I noticed that too. What was the purpose of looking down?

CLIENT: Well, that way I don't have to make eye contact with people, which would be really awkward. They'd be able to tell I'm anxious just from the look on my face.

THERAPIST: So, looking down is one of those safety behaviors we have spoken about, trying to avoid your feared image of others noticing your anxiety if you do make eye contact. I am also curious how looking down might make you more inwardly focused. Did you notice if your mind was getting caught up in things going on inside you?

CLIENT: Yeah, I really noticed how uncomfortable I was feeling, how tight my chest felt, how shaky my hands were, and how self-conscious and awkward I felt doing something as simple as walking. I was really focused on trying to not feel those things, but it wasn't working.

THERAPIST: When your mind focuses in on those symptoms and feelings, and focuses hard on trying to get rid of them, what do you think happens?

155

CLIENT: Well, it probably makes them worse because I am paying so much attention to them, but I can't help it.

THERAPIST: Also, could you tell me anything about any of the sights that we went past? Anything about the cafés or buildings? How many people or cars were out and about on the street? Or how many trees or gardens we passed?

CLIENT: No, I guess I wasn't paying attention to any of those things.

THERAPIST: I am wondering if we could try the exercise again as we walk back to the office, but this time just being aware when your gaze drops to the ground and your mind goes inward, and instead purposely turning your attention to what is going on around you, particularly looking for interesting things around you that you haven't noticed before. Would you be willing to approach the task in this way just to see what it is like?

CLIENT: Because you're here I think I can try it. It would be harder if I was by myself.

THERAPIST: That sounds like an expectation you have, and with more practice we can see if that is really the case . . . [Therapist and Client continue the walking exercise back to the office, the therapist prompting the client to verbalize what enters her awareness and, if necessary, to redirect attention to external stimuli. The debrief commences when back in the therapist's office.] So, what did you notice that time around?

CLIENT: The ground was like a magnet. I kept wanting to look down, I didn't realize how much I did that. When I looked up it was difficult at first, but then I would get drawn to something interesting and when that happened I think I felt less self-conscious for a moment.

THERAPIST: So being less self-focused was difficult, but helpful in managing your anxiety. Anything in particular you noticed out on the street that you hadn't before?

CLIENT: One thing that stood out was that huge pink crane on the construction site across the road. I can't believe I have never noticed that before. Who doesn't notice a pink crane?!

THERAPIST: I wonder what other things you might miss out on, particularly in social situations, when your attention is focused inward?

About This Module: Addressing Attention Biases in SAD

Human beings are hardwired to attend to threat. Attention is the "microscope of the mind," and when we are under genuine threat it is adaptive for this microscope to focus on the threat to the exclusion of all else. All our attentional resources need to focus on aspects of the situation that will increase our chances of survival at that moment. The problem arises when attention is unduly drawn to, and maintained on, perceived rather than real threats.

For socially anxious clients living in a social world, threat is almost everywhere. Perceived threat is not only present in the external environment in the form of judgment from others, but also internally. Anxious feelings and associated physical sensations are perceived as threatening, as clients believe they are observable to others and hence will increase the likelihood of negative evaluation.

Cognitive theory suggests that attention is directed toward information that is congruent with an individual's core beliefs. Attention is therefore biased by what we already believe to be true about ourselves, others, and the world in general. We seek confirmation of our beliefs, not objective information. Our attention gets hijacked by information that fits with our existing knowledge, with any incongruent information that potentially has the power to modify existing knowledge being overlooked. The information we attend to then guides our interpretations and recall, and, in turn, ultimately shapes the thoughts and images that occupy our stream of consciousness in any given situation.

Clients with SAD typically hold negative core beliefs about themselves as being socially inept, inadequate, and unlikable. They also hold negative core beliefs about others being generally critical, judgmental, hostile, and superior. Attention is guided by these beliefs, and thus clients will tend to focus on internal and external evidence (ambiguous or otherwise) of ineptitude, inadequacy, unlikability, criticism, judgment, hostility, and inferiority. One client described this as a "GPS of the mind, which scans and locks on to anything that alerts you to potential social danger." Little attention is paid to the social task at hand, which can adversely impact social performance. Excessive self-focus makes it exceedingly difficult to keep up with the topic of conversations, let alone actively contribute to the dialogue. Neutral and positive social feedback that has the potential to undermine unhelpful core beliefs is largely ignored.

An important task of therapy is to assist clients with SAD to (1) recognize when their attention is not deployed to the present social task but is instead focused on the self or environment in unhelpful ways, and (2) rectify this attentional bias by purposely redirecting attention back to the present social task. This module covers the practicalities of effectively engaging clients in retraining their unhelpful attention biases, with the aim of facilitating greater task-focused attention when socializing. Doing this can not only result in a reduction in perceived social threat and therefore reduced social anxiety but can also enhance and enrich the social experience, and, dare we say, facilitate enjoyment of that which was once feared.

Introducing Attention Biases

Introducing clients to the notion of self-, environment- and task-focused attention can simply be done by asking clients, "Where do you notice your attention is focused when you are in social situations?" If this question is too general, then experientially or imaginally engage clients in a social situation and encourage them to notice where their attention is focused. This self-reflection can then lead into a discussion of the concepts of self-, environment- and task-focused attention.

Self-Focused Attention

Self-focused attention refers to attention being deployed inwardly. The types of internal experiences that might capture one's attention when socially anxious can vary. Self-focused attention may relate to purely being caught up with negative internal experiences, or strategizing how to stop negative internal or external experiences. Clients may be focused on one particular internal experience or a myriad of internal experiences at once, creating a sense of internal chaos. Attention might be captured by the emotional experience itself (i.e., fear, anxiety, panic, self-consciousness, embarrassment), physical sensations that accompany anxious feelings (e.g., sweating, shaking, blushing, heart racing), or negative thoughts and images regarding one's appearance, performance, or negative evaluation from others. Attention could also be focused on intentionally monitoring one's own performance, particularly what one is saying before, during or after it has been said. People with SAD may also be acutely aware of the fact that they are using safety behaviors and may be self-critical or expect criticism from others as a consequence.

Environment-Focused Attention

The little attention that is left over is often focused on environmental threat, in the form of scanning for signs of negative evaluation from others that confirm the clients' negative social images. Ambiguous social cues such as frowns, yawning, a glance at a watch, pauses in conversation, and laughter tend to lure the attention of the socially anxious client. These ambiguous social cues are generally interpreted as signs of negative evaluation, and hence provide fodder for further self-focused attention as a means of trying to reduce the perceived negative feedback.

Task-Focused Attention

Our attentional capacity is finite, and so with self and environmental threats stealing the show, attention to the "task at hand" suffers. During social interactions, the task at hand will likely involve absorbing oneself in the moment, such as concentrating on the topic of conversation, noticing common interests, allowing natural curiosity about what the other person is saying to take over, and making links to one's own experience that can then be followed up in conversation. In observational situations (e.g., walking, eating, writing, working in front of others) and performance situations (e.g., public speaking, music or dance performances), the task at hand involves focusing on what is required to complete and immerse oneself in the activity, including the sensory aspects. During behavioral experiments, the task at hand will also involve directing attention to evidence that may confirm or disconfirm negative thoughts and images.

The Competition for Attention: Self, Environment, and Task

Handout 11, *Self-, Environment- and Task-Focused Attention,* provides useful psychoeducation regarding the competition between these three potential attentional foci. These concepts can also be visually illustrated to clients by collaboratively drawing and talking through an attentional biases diagram similar to Figure 8.1.

Figure 8.1 shows that attention is mostly self-focused on noticing internal emotional experiences or monitoring safety behaviors, adopting an observer perspective of the self and hence getting caught in negative self-imagery, or being distracted by imagery of others' negative reactions. Any attention that can escape this rather enclosed self-focused system then moves to scanning the environment for social threat, either from the current social companion or from further afield in the environment (e.g., other onlookers). Very little attention is left over to focus on the task at hand of conversing with the current social companion.

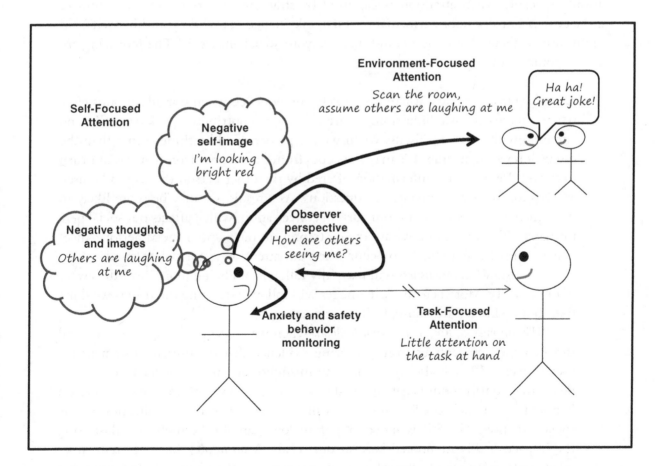

FIGURE 8.1. Illustration of attentional biases: self-, environment-, and task-focused attention.

Impact of Attention Biases

Clients with SAD are usually readily able to recognize that when feeling socially anxious they are not focused on the present task at hand (i.e., the conversation, walking, writing, eating). It is important to normalize this attention bias:

"From an evolutionary perspective we are hardwired to pay attention to threat. In cave-man times if there was a saber-toothed tiger about to eat us, and we were paying attention to something else, then humans wouldn't have lasted very long as a species. Fast-forward to now and the threat isn't a saber-toothed tiger but instead a social situation; however, our attentional instincts are still the same: if we perceive something is threatening, then of course we pay attention to it."

After normalizing this cognitive process as useful in genuinely threatening situations, clients must then be encouraged to recognize the detrimental impact of this attentional bias when it comes to the maintenance of their social anxiety. Some clients will readily recognize this, while others may at first believe that certain aspects of self- and environment-focused attention are helpful in reducing the likelihood of negative evaluation, especially when attention is captured by strategizing about how to minimize anxiety sensations or poor performance. First, ask clients, "How do you think self- and environment-focused attention could increase your social anxiety?" The following are useful points to discuss:

"*Distraction* from the task at hand is a likely consequence when our attention is elsewhere. In the case of a discussion, we are less able to contribute, speak naturally, and come up with topics to discuss when we are preoccupied by things other than the discussion we are having. We may miss cues from the other person that it is our turn to speak. We may miss information offered by the other person that could be used as leads for further comments and questions. As a result, we may be more likely to draw mental blanks when it is our turn in conversation, which affects our social performance. The very thing we are trying to prevent (i.e., a poor social performance) may actually be more likely to occur when our attention is not task focused.

"*Increased self-consciousness* will naturally follow from being more inwardly aware of our anxiety. More negative self-images will follow, reflecting the things we don't like about what we are doing, feeling, and saying.

"*We can miss positive and neutral feedback* when we are so preoccupied with social threat, which prevents us from gathering evidence that disconfirms our negative social images. We are also more likely to misinterpret ambiguous feedback as evidence that confirms our negative social images (e.g., a yawn means the other person is bored rather than tired). This results in an overall negative recollection of the social situation. The following computer analogy can also be useful in illustrating the impact of this attentional bias on our recall: A computer can only remember what we type into the keyboard. Our attention is like the keyboard. Anything that isn't attended to isn't typed into our memory so it can be recalled later. So if we are focusing on threatening information to the exclusion of positive feedback, then our memory of social experiences will be biased toward remembering only the negative aspects of the social situation."

All of these side effects of self- and environment-focused attention generate an increased perception of social threat and therefore more anxiety.

Self- versus Task-Focused Attention Experiment

While a verbal discussion of the negative consequences of not being task focused during social interactions is useful, a more experiential method of illustrating these negative consequences may be more powerful. Clients need to be satisfied that self- and environment-focused attention is unhelpful when it comes to their social anxiety before they are likely to abandon this as a protective strategy.

To experientially illustrate the helpfulness of task-focused attention during social interactions (or the unhelpfulness of self-focused attention), it can be useful to do an experiment that is very similar to the safety behaviors experiment described in Chapter 6. The experiment involves the client manipulating attention during a social task to contrast the impacts of self- versus task-focused attention. In group therapy, as with the safety behaviors experiment, the social task we use is a 5-minute conversation with another group member, contrasting being self-focused in the first conversation versus task focused in the second conversation. In individual treatment, the conversation could be with the therapist or the therapists' colleagues. An alternative social task could be used, as long as it can be completed twice to contrast the two attention conditions, and ideally it can be done in the presence of the therapist rather than as a homework exercise. We find that a conversational task is quite effective, as it usually becomes very clear that self-focused attention hinders social performance, and performance is very much valued by the client.

Worksheet 13, the *Self- versus Task-Focused Attention Experiment,* can guide therapists and clients through the steps of the experiment. Once the social task has been set, typically a conversation on a topic of the client's choosing with a designated person (e.g., fellow group member, therapist, therapist's colleague), clients are then given the instruction to be *self-focused*. For example:

> "During the first conversation, I would like you to focus as much attention as possible on yourself. Notice how you are feeling, what thoughts or images are going through your mind, body sensations you are experiencing, monitor carefully what you are saying or doing. Devote as much attention as possible to yourself."

Ask clients to list on the worksheet the types of things they will focus on so it is very clear where they will place their attention during this first conversation. Allow 5 minutes for the conversation to take place, and once this is completed clients then rate their anxiety, self-consciousness, observability of their anxiety, and social performance during the conversation.

Prior to the second conversation, clients are given the instruction to be *task focused*. For example:

"Now I would like you to engage in a second conversation with the same person, but this time I would like you to focus as much attention as possible on the task at hand. Focus on the topic of the conversation . . . what is being said, how it might relate to your experience, sharing your experience. Really try to get to know the person. Immerse yourself in the other person's story and contribute as much as you can to the topic. If your attention wanders, as best you can shift it back on to the topic of the conversation and try and get yourself lost in the topic."

Again, ask clients to list on the worksheet the types of things they will focus on.

As this condition of the experiment is more foreign to clients, imaginal rehearsal is completed to prepare them to deploy their attention in this unfamiliar manner:

"Before starting this conversation, just close your eyes and imagine yourself being able to focus almost all of your attention on the topic of the conversation. Imaging yourself, from your own perspective, looking at the other person and devoting all your attention to what they are saying. Also, notice that your own contributions to the conversation are coming fairly naturally. You are able to focus your attention on the topic, and this is freeing you up to contribute more to the conversation. If your attention gets sidetracked momentarily, within the image just experience bringing your attention back to the conversation, getting absorbed again in what is being said. Notice what your posture is like as you are engaging in this conversation in a comfortable and relaxed way. How does the other person look as they are appreciating the attention that you are devoting to them and the interest you are showing in the conversation?"

Again, allow 5 minutes for the second conversation to take place, and once this is completed clients again rate their anxiety, self-consciousness, observability of their anxiety, and social performance during the conversation.

The final step is to debrief any discrepancies in ratings across the two conditions, and from these observations draw some conclusions about what clients have learned about the impact of self- versus task-focused attention. Typically, they acknowledge that they felt more anxious and self-conscious, perceived their anxiety to be more observable, and perceived themselves to have performed more poorly when they were self-focused. If this does not occur, question what it was about being self-focused that was more helpful. Hypothesize that the finding may have been an artifact of the task-focused condition being unfamiliar to the client, and hence a more challenging way to interact. Encourage curiosity about whether this finding would hold with more practice or repetition of being task focused. For clients who recognize that task-focused attention was more helpful, therapists can suggest that even though they now know that being task focused is a better way to approach social situations, they may still default to being self-focused because it is so automatic, involuntary, and habitual. This leads nicely into the rationale for attention retraining as a means of assisting clients to acquire the skill of being task focused more often.

Attention Retraining

Based on the previous groundwork, clients should now acknowledge that being task focused is more beneficial for their social anxiety and social performance. They should also be primed to understand that to get the most out of behavioral experiments they need to approach social situations with an open mind, be present in the social task, and be unbiased in the information they attend to. We hope they now realize that this is hard to do when they are anxious and the default attentional bias to threat kicks in. Thus, they need to adjust their default attention setting. We frame this as "attention retraining," which is essentially a specifically focused form of mindfulness practice. Handout 12, *Attention Retraining and Focusing,* can provide useful psychoeducation about these skills.

Rationale for Attention Retraining

The following discussion can be useful to orient clients to attention retraining:

"Before we can focus our attention on the task at hand in social situations, we need to increase our general *awareness* of what our attention is focused on at any given time, and our ability to *flexibly* redirect our attention. We are often oblivious to where our attention is, and it can often be a very automatic, involuntary, unconscious process. It also may not occur to us that we can become more deliberate about where we deploy our attention.

"The strategy we use to increase our attentional awareness and flexibility, making it more deliberate, voluntary and conscious, is called attention retraining. This process involves paying attention to the present moment and 'coming to our senses.' This means focusing on what we can see, hear, feel, touch, and taste in the 'here and now,' using our senses as 'anchors' to the present. We start by doing this with nonsocial activities that are not anxiety provoking (e.g., doing the dishes, hanging the laundry, eating, showering, sitting, walking, breathing), so that eventually we can apply the skill in social situations, helping us to be more task focused when socializing.

"You can think of it this way: before an athlete can use a muscle for its intended purpose (e.g., a big race), the muscle needs to be strengthened (e.g., training in the gym). We use this as a metaphor for attention retraining. Your attention keeps getting locked on social threat, so your attentional muscle needs to be strengthened generally (i.e., with nonsocial activities), which will enable you to use it the way you want (i.e., to be task focused in social situations)."

Clients are then guided through some attention retraining exercises within the therapy session to get a more practical understanding of attention retraining. In session, we typically use short exercises involving attention to breath (see Box 8.1) and sitting (see Box 8.2). We then encourage clients to adopt this same "coming to their senses" approach multiple times daily in all manner of nonsocial tasks as a homework exercise, encouraging them to use Worksheet 14, *Attention Retraining Record,* to monitor their practice. We are not necessarily wedded to a particular mindfulness exercise, as long as

---

BOX 8.1. Attention Retraining Exercise: Breath

"If you feel comfortable doing so, I would like you to close your eyes and sit comfortably in your chair, with your hands resting on your lap or on the arms of the chair. Sitting up in a dignified way with your head comfortably balanced and feet resting on the floor. [pause] Now I would like you to begin by directing your attention to your breath. Just noticing the sensations associated with inhaling and exhaling, without trying to alter your breath. [pause] Observe the entry point of the air into your nose. How does it feel to be drawing air into your body through your nostrils? Does it tickle? Is it numb? Can you start to become aware of the sensations within your nasal cavity that are meeting the new air as it arrives? [pause] Start to follow the path your breath makes all the way down into your windpipe and into the bottom of your lungs . . . and then follow the path of the air from the bottom of your lungs out through your trachea, nasal cavity, and back into the environment . . . allow yourself to follow the path of your breath. [pause] Now becoming aware of the sensations of the muscles in your stomach and chest expanding as you breathe in to the point where they choose to start expelling the air, and contracting and relaxing as they let the air go. [pause] Notice how your whole body feels as you continue to inhale and exhale . . .

"Should your mind wander, that's OK. That's what minds do. Just congratulate yourself for noticing . . . perhaps make a mental note . . . "mind wandering" . . . and then shift your attention back to your breath. [pause] It doesn't matter how many times your mind wanders away from your breath, it is the noticing that is important, and you can just shift your attention back to the sensations of breathing whenever you need to. [pause] If you start to notice any uncomfortable sensations, emotions, thoughts, or images that are distracting you, as best you can, try and make space for them, allow them to be there alongside your breath . . . can you allow them to be as they are for a little while without trying to change them? Allow these experiences to be there, and then when you are ready, without any urgency, guide your attention back to the sensations of the breath. [pause 1 minute] OK, as we end our attention retraining on the breath, when you are ready, open your eyes, bringing your focus back to the room."

Debrief: "What did you experience during the exercise? What did you notice or learn about your attention? How much of your attention was on the task at hand (i.e., the breath)? Were you able to catch your mind wandering? How did you know it was wandering? Where did it wander to? What did you do when you noticed this? What impact did that have? When you were focusing on the present moment, how much attention was left over for thinking about other things?"

Make sure that clients do not see the purpose of the exercise as having to maintain 100% focus on their breath. Frustration is a sure sign that this is their aim. Remind them that the point is to be aware of where their attention is, including when it wanders.

> ## BOX 8.2. Attention Retraining Exercise: Sitting
>
> "We are going to do another attention retraining exercise to demonstrate that we can apply the skill to different activities. I would now like you again to close your eyes if you feel comfortable to do so, and again sit comfortably in your chair. I would like you to direct your attention to the sensations of the chair pushing against your body. Starting with the back of the chair. Noticing the portions of your back that are in contact with the chair and the portions that are not. How does it feel on your back? Is it hard, soft, supportive, uncomfortable . . . just notice these sensations. [pause] Now focus on the part of the chair pushing up against your bottom. How does this feel? What sensations are you noticing? [pause] Now shift your attention down to the parts of your feet that are making contact with the ground. How does the ground pushing up against you feel on the soles of your feet? [pause] OK, we are going to end the attention retraining exercise here, so at your leisure, feel free to come back to the room and open your eyes."
>
> Debrief in a similar manner to the breathing exercise.

the aim of the exercise is the same. That is, developing an awareness of where attention is, choosing to shift attention to present-moment experience, noticing when the mind has inevitably wandered away, and gently and nonjudgmentally redirecting it back to the intended focus. We frequently use the phrase "catch and bring it back" when orienting clients to this aim. We emphasize that the goal is not to be 100% focused on the present moment, but instead to catch where our attention is and bring it back to the task at hand, no matter how many times redirection is required.

Many treatments use various mindfulness-based practices. Most will introduce mindfulness in their own manner with their own rationale and aim, which may well be different from the rationale and aim used in this treatment. The emphasis when using mindfulness exercises in this treatment is on general attentional awareness (i.e., attention as conscious) and choice regarding attentional deployment (i.e., attention as deliberate). Above all, the aim in this case is not to achieve general relaxation or a generally present-focused mindset, but to ultimately help clients to be able to focus their attention away from social threat and onto the social task at hand.

Attention Retraining: A Caution

Attention retraining is not to be used as a safety behavior. Be aware of the potential for some clients to misuse attention retraining as a means of focusing attention away from perceived threat, as a form of distraction or cognitive avoidance of social situations. They may be physically in the social interaction but may use attention retraining exercises to mentally be elsewhere. An example of this is clients doing attention retraining on their breath during social interactions. Using attention retraining in this manner will inhibit clients from challenging their negative social images, as they will miss the opportunity to gather contrary evidence that might be available in the situation because their attention is mostly directed internally (i.e., on their breath). Instead, attention retraining is a means of strengthening attentional awareness, so that when clients are in social situations they can pay attention to more helpful aspects of the situation (e.g., neutral and positive aspects), rather than only focusing on threatening or negative aspects of the situation. As a guideline, clients should always be seeking to deploy their attention on the task at hand. The conversation, rather than the client's breath, would be the task at hand when socializing. It may be helpful to focus on the breath before and after a social situation as a way of tolerating anxiety and settling back to baseline, but not as a form of avoidance. Attention retraining exercises should therefore typically only be completed on nonsocial tasks when the client is not feeling anxious.

Attention Focusing

Once clients have begun to understand and practice their attention retraining exercises, this skill can be extended by introducing the idea of "attention focusing." Clients do not need to be experts in attention retraining before moving to attention focusing. In fact, these skills can often be introduced back to back in one session or across two sessions, providing the client understands the value of regular attention retraining practice in facilitating attention focusing.

Rationale for Attention Focusing

Picking up the athlete metaphor again can be a helpful way of introducing attention focusing:

> "So, initially we focused on strengthening your attention muscle generally using nonsocial activities (i.e., becoming aware of attention and being able to move it). With attention focusing, you then use your attention muscle for a specific purpose (i.e., being task focused during social interactions). To extend the athlete metaphor, we have done the training in the gym and now it is time to use those muscles in the big race for which all that hard training was intended."

Attention focusing is essentially encouraging clients to deliberately practice shifting attention to the task at hand during social encounters. This can be phrased as "getting lost in the conversation" or "getting out of your head and into the situation." Clients are encouraged to develop a new habit when socializing. As soon as they become aware that their attention is focused on themselves or the environment in an unhelpful way, or they recognize that their attention is not on the present social task, this is a cue to reorient their attention back to the task at hand. In social interaction situations, it is clear that the task at hand is the topic of conversation.

What Is the Task at Hand in Observation Situations?

The task at hand is a little less clear in situations when the person might be observed rather than engaged in a social interaction (e.g., eating in public, shopping, walking in a public place). In line with the attention-retraining exercises, it might be tempting for clients to focus solely on the sensory aspects of eating, shopping, or walking. However, deploying their attention in this way could deprive them of the opportunity to gather positive or neutral information about other people's behavior. For example, if clients are focused on the feeling of pressure in their feet as they walk down the street, they may miss out on observing that the other people walking by are generally too preoccupied with themselves to be paying any attention to what they are doing.

When trying to work out with a client what the task at hand is, and hence where attention needs to be focused, behavioral experiments should be prioritized. Behavioral experiments will require attention to be deployed in the service of collecting evidence for and against negative thoughts and images, rather than being tuned to self or environmental threat. During a behavioral experiment, the task at hand is objective evidence gathering, and clients need to use their attention "muscle" to do this. So for the client who finds walking down the street challenging, the task is to do this activity and pay attention in an objective way to whether other people's *actual* reactions match the client's *predicted* negative image. Once the negative thoughts and images have been adequately modified (e.g., <5% belief), clients often report doing these social activities "without thinking," which is a great sign that the anxiety has reduced and new approach behaviors are becoming automatic. At this stage, it might then be appropriate to apply attention retraining exercises to fully immerse oneself in the sensory experience of walking down the street. However, until then, objective evidence gathering must take precedence. Worksheet 7, The *Behavioral Experiment Record,* has a prompt in the "Evidence to Observe" column for clarifying where attention needs to be focused during behavioral experiments.

Attention-Focusing Exercises

To facilitate attention focusing, when this is first introduced clients are asked to choose a specific social interaction that they will participate in as a homework task, and to purposely approach the interaction with the explicit intention of being task focused. To encourage this deliberate attentional focus, clients are aware that following the interaction (as soon as is practicable) they will be required to write as much content as they can remember from the social interaction on Worksheet 15, the *Task-Focused Attention Exercise.* This exercise encourages clients to prioritize focusing as much of their attention as possible on the content of the conversation, to the exclusion of self- and environment-focused attention.

Attention focusing can also be practiced in role plays between client and therapist. The client and therapist could have a conversation with the explicit intention of the client noticing when self-focused attention is occurring and redirecting attention back to the conversation as quickly as possible. Clients can signal with their fingers the number of times they need to redirect attention back to the conversation, so as not to disrupt the conversational flow. Another option is that the therapist could hold two cards, one with the words "self-focused attention" and the other with "task-focused attention." The therapist can hold up each card in turn to signal to the client to switch attention as demanded. This may give clients practice with attention redirection.

All the attention exercises are designed to increase client perception that attention is something that can be deliberately manipulated to either the benefit or detriment of their social anxiety. While being more task focused can reduce social anxiety, likewise clients find that as their social anxiety diminishes they usually observe that their attention is naturally more flexible and that the "threat-seeking GPS" is no longer switched on in social situations.

Clinical Case: Attention Retraining

One client was obviously highly anxious while conducting one of the group behavioral experiments, which involved walking down a main street in single file and performing silly tasks (e.g., pretending to be airplanes, skipping). Her head was down and her eyes fixed on the ground throughout the whole experiment. While other group members progressively became braver with their actions, as they discovered just how hard it was to capture anyone's attention, this client's affect did not shift. During the debrief she reported feeling highly anxious and embarrassed about what the group had just done. The other group members gently challenged her beliefs that other people had noticed or cared what the group had done based on what they had observed. However, the client appeared unable to accommodate this information on an emotional level and the experiment was sadly unsuccessful for her. This example highlights self-focused attention as a critical maintainer of social anxiety. This client's negative thoughts and images could not be effectively challenged while her safety behavior of looking down was in operation. This in turn promoted strong self-focused attention, which negatively biased her processing of the event. In group situations, it is not always possible to titrate exposures to everyone's needs, and fortunately this is rarely a problem. In this instance, having noticed the client's inability to drop her safety behaviors and broaden her attention, the therapist had the option of interrupting the experiment and completing another experiment with this client. Observation of the group completing the task may also have allowed for vicarious learning, without her own anxiety overwhelming her ability to be task focused. In individual therapy, the therapist may have spent more time developing the client's attention retraining and focusing skills prior to conducting behavioral experiments.

THERAPY SUMMARY GUIDE: Attention Biases

Therapy Aim: Increase awareness of attention biases to self and environmental threat, and develop the capacity to be task focused in social situations.

Therapy Agenda Items:

▼ Introduce attention biases:

   ◢ Encourage clients to self-reflect on their attentional focus in social situations generally, or prompt clients to be more aware of their attention deployment during specific *in vivo* or imaginal social situations

   ◢ Discuss self-, environment-, and task-focused attention, and use Figure 8.1 to illustrate the competition between these biases

   ◢ Normalize attentional bias to threat

   ◢ Socratic discussion of the negative impacts of self- and environment- focused attention in SAD, including distraction, self-consciousness, and missing feedback

   ◢ Conduct the self- versus task-focused attention experiment

▼ Attention Retraining:

   ◢ Introduce attention retraining exercises using nonsocial tasks

   ◢ Complete attention retraining exercises in session, such as the breathing and sitting exercises

   ◢ Use Worksheet 14, *Attention Retraining Record,* to self-monitor daily practice

▼ Attention Focusing:

   ◢ Encourage clients to be task focused in all social tasks, clarifying what this means for interaction versus observation situations

   ◢ Worksheet 7, the *Behavioral Experiment Record,* prompts for explicit consideration of attentional focus during behavioral experiments

   ◢ Worksheet 15, *Task-Focused Attention Exercise,* can be used initially to encourage task-focused attention in social interactions

Therapy Materials:

▼ Handouts

   ◢ Handout 11, *Self-, Environment-, and Task-Focused Attention*

   ◢ Handout 12, *Attention Retraining and Focusing*

▼ Worksheets

   ◢ Worksheet 13, *Self- versus Task-Focused Attention Experiment*

   ◢ Worksheet 14, *Attention Retraining Record*

   ◢ Worksheet 15, *Task-Focused Attention Exercise*

CHAPTER 9

Negative Core Beliefs

CLIENT: I picture all eyes are on me. People are sneering, frowning, judging.

THERAPIST: Judging you how?

CLIENT: That I'm . . . not good enough.

THERAPIST: In what way "not good enough"?

CLIENT: In every way . . . looks, intelligence, personality, social skills, money, you name it.

THERAPIST: That idea of not being "good enough," is that something you experience just in this situation, or does it pop up in other situations too?

CLIENT: I always feel like I'm not good enough.

THERAPIST: It might sound like a funny question, but for you what is bad about "not being good enough," what will "not being good enough" lead to?

CLIENT: Well, if you aren't good enough people aren't going to want to know you, and people will sense that you are inferior and find ways to expose and humiliate you.

THERAPIST: Do you believe all people will do these things all the time?

CLIENT: I know that sounds a bit over the top, but I still feel like most people are like that, aside from my closest family. Everyone just seems better than me, more together than me.

THERAPIST: It sounds like you have two types of what we call "negative core beliefs" at play that drive all your specific negative social images that arise in specific social situations. One core belief relates to how you generally see yourself as a person, and this is captured by that idea "I am not good enough." The other belief relates to how you generally see most other people, and this is captured by the idea "Others are better than me, and will reject me or expose and humiliate me." These two beliefs kind of play off one another. Not being good enough leads to the expectation that others will be negative toward you, and the expectation that others will be negative toward you just confirms the idea of not being good enough.

CLIENT: But "not being good enough" is such a part of me, I don't think it is something that will ever change.

THERAPIST: Many of us have these sorts of negative core beliefs, so I hope you don't think you are alone in this. These beliefs usually develop from how we have made sense of certain experiences we had during our life. What can happen with core beliefs is once an idea is established, which often happens when we are quite young—so like a child's understanding of the world—our mind then keeps focusing on things that seem consistent with the belief and our mind ignores things that don't match the belief. So, over time the belief grows very strong.

CLIENT: So how do you change a belief that is that strong and feels so true?

THERAPIST: Rather than try to tackle the belief head on, our best strategy is to start with your behavior. What I mean is putting yourself in the position to have new social experiences that don't fit your beliefs of "not being good enough" or others being "rejecting and unkind," and of course paying close attention to these experiences. It would be interesting to see if over time by doing this you start to see these beliefs as outdated and then feel ready to update them. Think of the beliefs as having initially started out the size of a mouse. But they have been fed over the years by your mind paying so much attention to every possible negative social experience or every minute flaw within you, so these beliefs are now the size of some huge beast. Maybe what we can do is not try to fight or tackle the beast because that probably wouldn't work, but instead we could just stop feeding it for now. Perhaps we could start feeding an alternative more helpful belief, and over time this could grow. If we do this, over time the old belief might start to diminish in strength until it is just in the background, whereas the new, more helpful and fair belief will increase in strength and become the new lens through which you see yourself and others.

About This Module: Addressing Negative Core Beliefs in SAD

Negative core beliefs are negatively valenced, global, overgeneralized, fundamental, central, pervasive, long-standing "truths" of how we see ourselves, others, and the world. Negative core beliefs are generally framed as simple, inflexible absolute facts, such as "I am unlikable," "others are critical," or "the world is dangerous." Core beliefs generally lead to the development of certain rigid rules for how to live one's life and assumptions of what one can expect in life, given the "truth" of the core beliefs. For example, if I hold core beliefs that "I am unlikable" and "others are critical," then I might understandably develop the rule that "I must not get close to other people" and the assumption that "if I get close to others, they won't like what they see and will reject me." These rules and assumptions therefore help me negotiate life and protect me in the context of my core beliefs. In this treatment, we focus most explicitly on negative core beliefs, given that they underpin subsequent rules and assumptions. However, explicitly eliciting and addressing rules and assumptions is still a valid treatment pursuit, particularly for clients with chronic low self-esteem and personality pathology such as avoidant personality disorder.

Negative core beliefs are generally formed by the processing of early or later life experiences (e.g., parenting received, parent modeling, bullying, abuse, criticism, humiliation, ostracism, limited achievements, relationship breakdown), which is influenced by genetic and temperamental factors. As already discussed in Chapter 8 ("Attention Biases"), our attention and interpretive processes are guided by our core beliefs, so that core beliefs become self-perpetuating. That is, our core beliefs guide what we pay attention to and how we interpret sensory input, such that we attend to and interpret the world in a manner that mostly confirms our core beliefs. This leaves our core beliefs firmly in place to then bias the processing of subsequent sensory inputs.

The most prominent negative core beliefs in SAD center on themes of the self as defective and others as rejecting, hostile, or superior. Table 9.1 provides some common examples of negative core beliefs prominent in SAD, most of which are overgeneralized conclusions about the self or others. Some clients will also hold problematic core beliefs that relate to societal conventions and intolerance of anxiety, which can also maintain SAD.

This module first reviews more traditional cognitive-behavioral approaches to eliciting and modifying negative core beliefs. These approaches are still valid and useful. However, the greater focus of this module, and indeed this treatment, is on imagery-based methods for eliciting and modifying negative core beliefs. The practicalities of

TABLE 9.1. Typical Core Beliefs in SAD

Domain	Core belief examples
Self: *I am* . . .	worthless; inadequate; incompetent; unlikable; not good enough; inferior; boring; weak; socially inept; different; weird; not like others; not normal; a loser; stupid; a failure
Others: *Others are* . . .	critical; judgmental; scrutinizing; rejecting; ostracizing; mean; hostile; aggressive; bullies; superior; better; confident; calm; strong
World: *Society* . . .	has strict social rules; demands social perfection; requires good social skills to be successful in life; dictates that there is a right and wrong thing to say and do in social situations; does not tolerate people being different
Emotions: *Anxiety is* . . .	bad; a sign of weakness; unbearable; abnormal; something to be hidden; a sign of being weird or mentally unstable

engaging clients with and effectively applying imagery rescripting and positive imagery are a particular focus. Behavioral action planning to consolidate core belief changes accomplished via these imagery-based strategies is also outlined.

Traditional Approaches to Addressing Negative Core Beliefs

How Do We Change Negative Core Beliefs?

Negative core beliefs can be changed by genuinely and actively attending to, interpreting, encoding, and recalling experiences that are inconsistent with them. An accumulation of disconfirming experiences over time will eventually require accommodation of the new information, leading to the development of new balanced core beliefs that better reflect reality in the here and now.

To gather these new experiences, clients need to do two things:

1. Approach (instead of avoid) situations that provide opportunities to gather disconfirmatory evidence, and
2. Be open, realistic, and balanced in their thinking and imagery about the situation.

Do these two requirements for core belief change sound familiar? Essentially this is what we have already been doing so far in treatment (i.e., behavioral experiments, imagery challenging, and task-focused attention). Accumulating these new positive and neutral experiences, as well as learning how to manage negative experiences in a balanced way, will "chip away at" and undermine negative core beliefs over time, leaving room for more balanced core beliefs. This gradual and cumulative pathway to core belief change necessitates that it is the last factor addressed in treatment. By the time treatment begins to explicitly target core beliefs, clients should already have accumulated a range of experiences that contradict and compete with their negative core beliefs.

While acquiring new experiences is crucial for core belief change, reframing past experiences upon which negative core beliefs are based can also be therapeutic. This process will generally involve assisting clients to understand that past negative experiences, or a lack of positive experiences, were not necessarily their fault or reflective of personal defects. It is also important for clients to understand that these past experiences are relatively isolated to particular people, places, or times, rather than reflecting how all people are likely to behave toward them now. This reunderstanding of the past can be very useful in weakening the foundation upon which negative core beliefs rest.

A Word of Caution

Explicitly highlighting and working with negative core beliefs can be confronting for some clients, as having greater awareness of the negative ways in which they perceive themselves at their very core can be distressing and leave them feeling vulnerable. While explicitly addressing negative core beliefs late in treatment makes strategic sense for the reasons previously outlined, it also places clients in a better position to cope with any distress that is elicited. Later in treatment the therapeutic alliance should be strong. Clients will likely trust their therapist, have experienced success with previous strategies that were also challenging, and therefore be ready to undertake this next challenge. The work they have done will hopefully have already weakened their negative core beliefs, perhaps reducing the intensity of conviction with which they are held. Clients will likely also have acquired meta-learning (e.g., thoughts/images are not facts), that will stand them in good stead to approach their core beliefs with a more detached and curious attitude. Clients will also have acquired emotion regulation skills via strategies already developed in treatment (e.g., imagery challenging, coping imagery, attention training). If high distress is elicited from core belief work, normalize this and encourage the application of these previously learned strategies, as well as the addition of self-soothing behavioral strategies.

Identifying Negative Core Beliefs

Traditional CBT methods of eliciting and adjusting negative core beliefs often start with the "downward arrow technique." CBT therapists will be familiar with this questioning method of starting with negative automatic thoughts or images available in client thought records and then exploring the deeper meanings and implications of these by asking "If this [thought/image] were true, what would this say or mean about you?" This continued chain of questioning elicits the meaning implications of a situation-specific cognition to the deeper core character of the person. An example of how to elicit core beliefs about self and others is provided below.

> THERAPIST: So, when you were in the lunchroom at work, what was going through your mind?
>
> CLIENT: Jason must be regretting the decision to have lunch right now because now he's stuck with me!
>
> THERAPIST: OK, I wonder if this thought is related to any core beliefs about yourself or others. Shall we see if we can find out?
>
> CLIENT: Sure. How do we do that?
>
> THERAPIST: We can use the downward arrow technique. This involves starting with a specific negative thought or image you have in a specific social situation you find anxiety provoking, and then asking the same question until we uncover a broad negative belief about yourself or others. Let's start with core beliefs about yourself. The question we ask is "If it is true that Jason is regretting being stuck with you, what would it say or mean about you?"
>
> CLIENT: Well, that I'm boring.

THERAPIST: OK, so one core belief might be that you are boring. Let's see if we can go any further. If it is true that you are boring, what would that say or mean about you?

CLIENT: That I'm a loser.

THERAPIST: Ok, if it is true that you are a loser, what might this say or mean about you?

CLIENT: That I'll always be alone.

THERAPIST: OK, so the thought that Jason is regretting being in the lunchroom with you might stem from the core beliefs that you are boring, a loser, and will always be alone. If you believed you were no more boring than most other people and that you weren't a loser, would you still think Jason doesn't want to have lunch with you?

CLIENT: No, I don't think so.

THERAPIST: OK, so the negative thought about Jason does seem to stem from these core beliefs about yourself. Now, let's see if there are also any core beliefs about other people at play here. To uncover core beliefs about other people we just change the question slightly to "If this were true, what would this say or mean about other people?" So if it were true that Jason regretted being with you, what would this say or mean about other people?

CLIENT: Well, I don't think it is very nice to be that judgmental. But I don't think that is just about Jason. I think everyone is like that.

THERAPIST: OK, so one of your core beliefs about other people is that they are judgmental. If you hold this core belief about others, then it makes sense that you would expect Jason to be sitting there having negative thoughts about you. If, on the other hand, you believed that most people are usually kind and accepting, you would probably be unlikely to expect negative evaluation from others and you might feel more comfortable. Does that make sense?

Once a core belief has been uncovered via this method, its validity can be questioned. The broad impact of the negative core belief across a variety of domains in the client's life is then considered (e.g., family, friendships, relationships, work, leisure, health/self-care). The aim is to assist clients to recognize the unhelpfulness of the core belief (i.e., it is getting in the way of the life they want) and prepare them for what needs to be done to address it.

Evidence against Negative Core Beliefs

The next step is to develop alternative conclusions that are more helpful in contextualizing and depersonalizing the experiences that have informed negative core beliefs. The therapist assists clients to specifically look for evidence against core beliefs. The aim is to alter clients' attentional biases by setting the task of purposely collecting evidence or experiences that show their core belief is not 100% true all the time. This involves recording historical "evidence against"' their core belief, such as positive treatment by others, positive social experiences, personal achievements, and positive personal qualities. Clients are also encouraged to become more attuned to present "evidence against" their core beliefs daily. For instance, they might be encouraged to record one small thing they do or experience each day that contradicts their core belief, such as positive behavioral experiment outcomes, positive feedback from others, completing a task on time, doing something considerate for others, and attending to daily responsibilities.

Formulating New Core Beliefs

The next step is to formulate a new balanced core belief that better fits the accumulated evidence. CBT has traditionally made a strong case for promoting balanced, believable, and realistic thinking, rather than positive thinking. With this in mind, the therapist might be tempted to guide clients to very modest, moderate core belief statements (e.g., "I am unlikable" might become "Some people will like me some of the time and some people won't, but that is OK and probably says more about them than me"). Christine Padesky's writing in this area gives the therapist some food for thought when considering new core beliefs. Padesky (1994) writes that negative core beliefs tend to be short, basic absolute statements (e.g., I am unacceptable, worthless, unlikable), and as such they tend to pack quite a punch. Padesky advocates that new core beliefs should be positive versions of the same absolute statements (e.g., I am acceptable, worthwhile, likable). But does this approach still fit with the CBT stance of realistic rather than positive thinking?

Padesky (and we) would say yes! Padesky (1994) writes that negative absolutes are usually more extreme as they imply total absence (e.g., if I am unlikable, then there is absolutely nothing likable about me), whereas positive absolutes are less extreme by nature as they imply that a quality is present but not necessarily perfect (e.g., if I am likable, then I am able to be liked by others, but not necessarily everyone will like me). Therefore, when assisting clients to develop new balanced core beliefs, we would recommend that therapists don't shy away from positive statements. The guiding principles to keep in mind are that new core beliefs need to be:

1. Potentially believable to clients. We say "potentially" because they are unlikely to be believable at first, before experiences generated by behavior change have accumulated sufficiently to strengthen them;
2. Reasonable reflections of reality. That is, new core beliefs should not overstate the positive in an unrealistic way (e.g., "I am inferior" to "I am superior"); and
3. Framed in clients' own words, so they can eventually take ownership of these new beliefs.

It may be useful for therapists to keep in mind that longer, more moderate core belief statements may lack emotional "punch."

Putting New Core Beliefs into Action

Once new balanced core beliefs have been developed, the final step is to put them into action across various life domains. This involves assisting clients to find specific ways of "acting as if" their new core beliefs were true. Useful questions include:

- "If you believed you were [insert the new core belief, e.g., likable], what would you be doing differently when it comes to family?"
- "What about your friendships?"
- "What would you be doing differently in terms of your romantic relationships?"
- "What about your work, career, or studies?"
- "How would you be spending your leisure time?"
- "What might you be doing to take care of your health and well-being?"

These questions help clients to understand that the new, more helpful core beliefs will be optimally strengthened and consolidated if comprehensive changes are made across all valued aspects of their lives. The actions identified need to be very concrete and specific, and may need to be graded. The rationale for this approach, which some people describe as "fake it till you make it," rests on the idea that behaving in this new manner places clients in a better position to have new positive and neutral life experiences that will strength the new balanced core beliefs over time.

We all know life is not always smooth sailing and at times certain people can be judgmental or mean. At these times clients are then encouraged to make sense of the experience in a helpful way that doesn't undermine new core beliefs. For example, the negative experience could be seen as the exception rather than the rule, and factors other than core personal defectiveness or an overgeneralized view of others being critical can be considered.

Essentially the end point of working on core belief change is to engage clients in ongoing, unlimited behavioral experiments that are about testing the validity of their new balanced core beliefs. As such this can be framed as a "work in progress" that continues even when formal therapy sessions have finished. This final stage of therapy is about helping clients to modify the way they live their lives so they accumulate experiences that support their new balanced core beliefs and chip away at their old negative core beliefs over time. Core belief modification is not a quick fix. Core beliefs are strongly entrenched, so it will take time and plenty of new experiences to strengthen new, more helpful and adaptive ones.

Difficulties with Traditional CBT Approaches

The approaches just mentioned are useful for many clients, but a common complaint when working in this manner is the disconnect between logic and emotion (e.g., "Logically I can see that when I was bullied at school it wasn't about me personally, that kids can be cruel if they sense anyone is a bit different. But I still feel like it was my fault, that there was/is something wrong with me"). Imagery-based strategies may be particularly valuable in these instances due to the emotional bridge they can facilitate. In this treatment, we favor using imagery to address negative core beliefs, and we do this in two specific ways:

1. *Imagery rescripting* involves using imagery to reexperience, in new ways, past negative events that significantly contributed to the development of negative core beliefs. Imaginally reexperiencing these events and attaching benign or positive meanings to them serves to undermine negative core beliefs.

2. *Positive imagery* involves clients imagining how they would like to be in certain situations and using this ideal image to assist in the identification of new balanced core beliefs. Positive imagery then provides direction for the specific actions required to strengthen these new beliefs.

Imagery Rescripting to Undermine Negative Core Beliefs

What Is Imagery Rescripting?

Imagery rescripting can be used as a broad term that refers to rewriting or transforming problematic images. It can be applied to memories of events or other images that are not based on actual experiences (e.g., intrusive images, nightmares). In this treatment for SAD, imagery rescripting is applied to memories that are consistent with clients' negative core beliefs, and as such support them (Hackmann et al., 2011). In other words, the strategy is applied to address images of past events that have significantly contributed to how clients see themselves, others, and the world now.

Slightly different methods can be used to facilitate imagery rescripting. The method used in this treatment is informed by the work of Arnoud Arntz (Arntz, 2011; Arntz & Weertman, 1999), whose method of imagery rescripting was first developed for working with personality disorders and complex trauma, and has more recently been applied to posttraumatic stress disorder, depression, eating disorders, and SAD (Stopa, 2011). In SAD, researchers have applied imagery rescripting alone (Reimer & Moscovitch, 2015; Wild, Hackmann, & Clark, 2007, 2008) or as part of a treatment package (Clark et al., 2003; McEvoy & Saulsman, 2014; McEvoy et al., 2015), with positive outcomes. Readers interested in using imagery rescripting with clients are encouraged to read further in this area, particularly Hackmann and colleagues (2011) and the special issue of *Cognitive and Behavioral Practice* (2011, Volume 18, Issue 4).

The aim of imagery rescripting is important to remember because at first glance it can seem fanciful or like "playing pretend." The purpose of imagery rescripting is the generation of a *new competing image* of a recalled negative event, with the new image representing *more functional meanings and affect* than the initial memory image. With this in mind, the content of the new image that emerges from the rescripting process does not really matter. It is fine for the new image to seem fanciful or unrealistic when viewing it from a literal perspective. What matters is that the new image represents a new more helpful perspective about the event in terms of its implications about the self or other people, and hence more positive feelings are attached to the image. We must remember that memories are constructions that have been extensively filtered through personal biases and then edited and manipulated through similar biases over time. Therefore, whether they are an exact replication of some "external truth" is not especially important. What is important is the meaning that memories have for clients and the extent to which clients believe them or "feel" them to be true and relevant to now.

The theoretical framework for imagery rescripting is Brewin's (2006) "retrieval competition theory" as already mentioned in previous chapters. During imagery rescripting we are creating a new image representation of a past event that needs to effectively compete with the old negative image of the event, and hopefully win the retrieval competition. From this perspective, fanciful images may be effective because they are likely to be quite distinctive and memorable, hence increasing their chances of retrieval supremacy. During imagery rescripting we are not removing the original memory. Instead we are creating a new image, which is an alternative elaboration of the old memory. The new image considers the wider context of time, place, person, or circumstance and introduces a more helpful perspective regarding the past event. Think back to the logic versus emotion disconnect that some clients complain about during thought challenging. The new image developed via imagery rescripting should capture the logical meaning that clients may concede is true during verbally based discussions of the event with the therapist. However, because by its very nature the image is more emotionally evocative, it may be better able to bridge the gap between logic and emotion, creating a synchrony between the two. Consequently, imagery-based reframes of past experiences that support negative core beliefs should have a greater emotional impact for clients.

Introducing Imagery Rescripting

The Rationale

The most common question asked by therapists new to rescripting is "How do I explain this to clients?" Clinicians can be concerned that it will seem to clients like we are trying to pretend that a bad thing didn't happen. Clinicians may even have firsthand experience of clients discounting the strategy because "that isn't how it happened in reality" or "that couldn't happen in reality so what is the point?" The rationale presented to clients is crucial so that they are on board with the true purpose, which will be lost if we just launch into using imagery rescripting without adequate preparation. Below are the types of concepts we have found useful in orienting clients to effective engagement with imagery rescripting, and they have been reiterated in Handout 13, *Past Imagery Rescripting,* as psychoeducation for clients:

> "So far we have been working on negative images of the present or future (i.e., pictures of ourselves or others' reactions in a current or upcoming social situation). We

are now going to move on to the final bubble in the model—core beliefs (i.e., how we generally see ourselves, others, the world), which tend to be influenced by negative social images from the past (or memories).

"It is common for people with social anxiety to report memories of early negative social experiences that impact what they expect in social situations now. When we have had some negative social experiences in our past we can get 'stuck' in our memories, so that they can recur as echoes of the past, haunting us, and shaping the negative social images we have in the here and now.

"Memories we may have of other events tend to feel like they are firmly in the past and probably rarely rear their head. In social anxiety, negative social memories we may intellectually know are in the past may still feel emotionally relevant to today.

"Now, we can't change that these negative experiences happened. It is awful that you had to go through them in the first place. What is also awful is that these experiences keep affecting your life, coloring and tainting what you expect in social situations now.

"Using a technique we call imagery rescripting, we have the opportunity to go back in our imagination to experience the past event from a new perspective. We can do things we couldn't do at the time, but that in an ideal world we would have liked to have done with no limitations. Doing this seems to have the effect of reprocessing the event in a way that can be helpful for changing its meaning and putting the memory back in its place—as a bad thing that happened in the past with little relevance to the here and now. As we work on these past images, we can learn that these memories don't reflect on ourselves, others, and the world today as we previously thought, that the memory is outdated (specific to a past time, place, or person), and doesn't need to dictate what we expect and how we live our lives now."

PHOTO METAPHOR

"These memories are like a bad photo we have been carrying around in our front pocket and looking at all the time. We can't rip up the photo, but processing these memories can help us to put them in a photo album on the shelf as mementos from the past, rather than carrying them with us now. This can change the way we feel about these past events and their impact on how we see ourselves, others and the world now.

"Working on the past memory image can be upsetting in the short term, though worthwhile in the long run. This idea of short-term pain for long-term gain has been a theme that runs through everything that you have done in treatment so far."

The Three Phases of Imagery Rescripting

After the rationale has been presented, it is important to give clients clear expectations about what will take place during the imagery exercise, so they are prepared to fully engage in the process. You don't want clients to be distracted by wondering what will come next or how long it will take while doing the imagery exercise. Inform them that there are three phases to the imagery exercise, and the time for each will depend on how involved the situation is that they are imagining and how long it takes them to run through the situation in their mind's eye. The three phases are as follows and should be briefly described to clients:

- *Phase 1:* Imaginally reexperiencing the event at the age it occurred as if it were occurring right now.
- *Phase 2:* Imaginally reexperiencing the event at their current age, watching their younger self going through the experience and intervening in any way they wish to protect and care for the younger self.
- *Phase 3:* Imaginally reexperiencing the event at the age it occurred, but this time experiencing their older self intervening and asking the older self for anything else they need.

Spend time discussing the idea of the older self being intervening within the image. Remind clients that they will be manipulating a past image, and so it is essentially creating a fantasy. The technique will involve imaging aspects of the situation that didn't and/ or couldn't have happened in reality, but that they might have liked to have happened. Again, be clear that we are not pretending this awful thing did not happen. We can't change the event, but we can change the meaning of the event. Changing the meaning can, in turn, change associated feelings and reduce the relevance of the past event to life in the here and now. It can be very useful to give examples of how the intervention doesn't have to conform to reality, so clients realize there are no limits on what they can do (e.g., shrinking the bully to the size of a mouse; getting on a dragon and flying away to a village of people who are kind and caring).

Prepare for Distress Tolerance

Therapists should also explain that as they work on the image the therapist will try to remain in the background, simply asking prompting questions, and will not offer comfort unless distress becomes extreme and overwhelming. Therapists should reassure clients by saying, "I don't anticipate this will happen, I just like to cover all bases. If this happens you can just open your eyes, and then we can use your coping image or attention retraining exercises to deal with those feelings." It can be useful to predetermine the client's preferred distress tolerance strategy. This is particularly important if applying imagery rescripting in a group context. To our knowledge, we are the first to have used imagery rescripting in a group therapy setting. Prior to commencing imagery rescripting in group therapy, we ask each group member to nominate their preferred distress tolerance strategy, such as focusing on their breathing, connecting with their five senses in the present moment, or engaging with the specific content of their coping image. Therapists write down each client's preferred strategy so it can be easily referred to should a client's distress need to be contained within a group environment. So far in our experience no client has needed assistance to use a distress tolerance strategy. It may be that the process of nominating a strategy is enough to create a sense of safety in the group so that clients are more willing and able to endure the emotions activated by the technique.

Imagery Rescripting Preparation

Select a Memory to Rescript

Clients with SAD will often easily be able to identify key negative social memories from the past that relate to their social anxiety today. Bullying, embarrassment, criticism, and humiliation, often in their school years, are the most common memories that emerge as significant in SAD. If clients can't readily identify a relevant memory, then ask them to imagine being in a situation where they feel socially anxious, connecting with socially anxious thoughts, images, feelings, and urges. Once they are connected with this experience then ask, "When in your life do you first remember feeling this same way?"

This emotional bridge technique can be very useful for identifying memories of relevance (Hackmann et al., 2011). Once a memory has been selected it is recorded in Worksheet 16, *Past Imagery Rescripting,* which assists with working through the remainder of the imagery rescripting process.

Elicit the Meaning of the Memory

Once a memory is selected, the meaning of the memory to the client must be identified. There are two ways to do this. The first approach is via verbal discussion prior to completing the imagery rescripting exercise. Therapists can simply ask clients what the experience meant to them.

- "From the experience, what did you conclude about yourself as a person?"
- "What did you conclude about what other people are generally like?"
- "What did you conclude about what the world is generally like?"

When eliciting meanings, the therapist can also question the significance or importance of the image per se to identify any metacognitive beliefs relevant to the memory:

- "Does this image seem important in some way, rather than just being a picture of the past?"
- "Does the image seem powerful or scary in any way?"
- "Does it seem like an important image to hold on to for some reason?"
- "Does it help you in some way to hold the image close, rather than lose it to the recesses of your mind like other memories from long ago have been lost?"

Some clients may see the memory as helpful if they believe that remembering the event keeps them vigilant and hence safe from it reoccurring or prepares them for the worst. Some clients might fear bringing the memory to mind, as they perceive it as being too powerful at eliciting emotion or undermining coping (e.g., "the memory is too overwhelming, I won't be able to cope or function if I think about it, I'll have a breakdown").

If verbal discussion of the meaning of the memory is not fruitful, then you could save the sorts of questions above and ask them at the end of Phase 1 within the imagery exercise when they have relived the experience. While they still have their eyes closed and before moving to Phase 2, their emotions related to the event should still be active, which indicates that core beliefs are likely to be activated and more accessible. Phrasing the questions in the following way may be more relevant:

- "How are you seeing yourself?" or "What is this image/event saying about you?"
- "How are you seeing others?" or "What is this image/event saying about others?"
- "How are you seeing the world?" or "What is this image/event saying about the world?"
- "Does the image itself seem important in some way, either in a bad way or in a helpful way? Is there something bad about holding on to it? Is there something helpful about holding on to it?"

Whichever method is used to elicit the meaning of the past event, this should then be recorded in Worksheet 16, *Past Imagery Rescripting*. The strength of belief in each core belief can also be rated (i.e., "Belief before rescripting").

Identify the "Older You" Perspective

Before engaging in imagery rescripting, clients are encouraged to think about what they know about the situation now that they may not have known at the time, and record this "older you" perspective on Worksheet 16. Therapists may say something like:

"The older, more compassionate 'adult you' may know things now that you didn't know then. These things you've learned since the event may have been useful for you to have been aware of at the time of the upsetting event. Although the event may still be emotionally painful to think about, you may be able to understand the situation differently now.

"For instance, if I had been bullied at school I might now have a different perspective compared to when it happened. At the time, I might have assumed this occurred because I was unlikable and a loser. Although I still feel sad about it, I can now see logically that although there were differences between me and the bully, his bullying behavior had less to do with me and more to do with his personality or insecurities. I simply did not deserve this treatment and no child deserves this treatment. Any child who bullies another child is behaving badly, and it need not reflect on the bullied child's character, likability, or worth. In fact, in hindsight we may be able to see that there were aspects of ourselves that were very likable at that time. We might be able to see these things as an adult, but we didn't know them as a child."

If clients have difficulty generating a more helpful perspective on the situation, ideally one that depersonalizes the negative event, the following questions may be helpful.

- "If a friend had been through a similar experience, what advice would you give them?"
- "If you were observing a child go through that same experience right now, what would you think about the situation and the child?"

It can also be useful to brainstorm ideas for ways the older self can intervene before the imagery rescripting exercise is undertaken. This will reduce the likelihood of clients getting stuck when they get to the most distressing point in the image and not knowing what to do. This process also provides the therapist with an opportunity to assess whether clients have the internal resources to intervene in the rescript, or whether the therapist will need to be more active and make suggestions. It can also serve as another reminder to clients that there are no limits on what they can do with the image. This doesn't mean that they must use the ideas generated in verbal discussion during the imagery exercise, but it may help them to be both creative and determined when taking care of the younger self within the image. A key ingredient in the intervention is that the younger self experiences what was emotionally needed at the time of the event in the third phase. The intervention should facilitate a sense of mastery and safety first (e.g., stopping the bullying or bad treatment, power being removed from the perpetrator, increasing one's own power), followed by experiencing soothing and compassion (e.g., experiencing kindness, warmth, and comfort from another). Ideally the rescript should end with the younger self engaging in some form of happy play or comforting activity with a sense of moving past the event.

Imagery Rescripting Guide

The scripts outlined in Box 9.1 provide an example of how imagery rescripting is conducted. These scripts were designed for a group treatment setting specifically and are used verbatim in this context. In an individual treatment setting they are only intended as a guide.

Imagery Rescripting in Individual versus Group Treatment

There are some key differences in conducting imagery rescripting in individual compared to group treatment. In group treatment clients select the memory to be rescripted and discuss the "older you" perspective and ways of intervening in pairs. Therapists can circulate and observe these discussions to ensure that the memories being worked on are

BOX 9.1. Imagery Rescripting Guide

Phase 1: Imagining the event from the perspective of the "younger you"

"Closing your eyes now, sitting comfortably, I would like you to imagine being back in the past situation you have identified, being the age you were when it occurred, and imagine it as vividly as you can from beginning to end, as if you are there experiencing it firsthand right now. Looking through the younger you's eyes . . . What is happening? Who is there? What can you see (hear, smell, taste, feel)? . . . How are you feeling emotionally? How does your body feel—what sensations do you notice? What are you thinking? What is this event meaning to you? What happens next? Take your time to run the image to its conclusion. When you have finished briefly raise your hand and then wait in silence. [Allow up to 10 minutes, although most clients will complete the task within 5 minutes.]"

Note: The Phase 1 script is only applicable if the event is not highly traumatic. If this were the case, the whole event does not need to be imagined. With traumatic memories, the image only needs to be taken to the point the client knows the traumatic event is going to happen and emotion is activated. At this point the image would switch to the therapist intervening (see the chapter section on trauma memories for more information).

Phase 2: Imagining the event from the perspective of the "compassionate older you" offering support to the "younger you"

"Now, go back to the start of the memory. Run through the image again from start to finish, but this time from the perspective of the 'older, compassionate you' at the age you are now, watching the 'younger you' going through the experience. As you look through the older you's eyes and observe the 'younger you' going through the situation, what are you feeling? What are you thinking? What do you want to do to help them? What needs to be done? What does the younger you need? . . . Now do it, intervene and do those things . . . What are you saying and doing? [pause] Make eye contact with the younger you and move closer. What else do you want to do? What else does the younger you need? Keep intervening until you feel satisfied you've done all that is needed. I will now give you some time to do this. Briefly raise your hand when done and wait quietly with eyes closed."

Phase 3: Imagining the event from the perspective of the "younger you" but with the "compassionate older you" intervening and offering all the support needed

"Now, again let's rewind going back to the start of the image. Now run through the image again from start to finish, but this time from the perspective of the 'younger you' receiving the support of the 'older, compassionate you.' Looking through the younger you's eyes, pay close attention to how you feel as the 'older, compassionate you' is intervening. What are they doing and how does that make you feel? [pause] Make eye contact with the 'older you' as you receive their support. [pause] Once you have received all their support, pay attention to what else you need from the older you and ask for it. Continue asking the older you for what you need until you feel safe and comfortable. I will now give you some time to do this. Briefly raise your hand when done and wait quietly with eyes closed.

"As you keep this image in mind, notice what the event means to you now . . .
"What is this image saying about you?
"What is this image saying about others?
"What is this image saying about the world?
"How important does the original image seem now?
"Just note how you are feeling as you think about the event now. Notice how you feel and where you feel it in your body. When you are ready you can open your eyes."

not too traumatic to rescript within the group context and to assess each client's capacity to intervene. The three scripts are read verbatim, and aside from the therapist talking, the exercise is done in silence. As each phase will take different durations for each person, the script gives the instruction that when clients are finished with each phase they can briefly raise their hand to let the therapist know they have finished and then wait in silence until everyone has completed the phase. After each phase clients open their eyes and make the relevant emotion and body ratings on Worksheet 16, *Past Imagery Rescripting,* before closing their eyes again to participate in the next phase. After Phase 3 they record any new conclusions regarding the self, others, world, or the image itself, the strength of belief they have in each of these new conclusions (0 = completely untrue, 10 = completely true), and how they generally feel about the past event now. This is also when they rerate their strength of belief in their initial core beliefs (i.e., "Belief after rescripting"). As a group we then debrief participants' experiences, reflecting particularly on quantitative and qualitative shifts in emotion and meaning across the phases, and their new conclusions about the event and its meaning.

The exercise is more interactive and flexible in individual treatment because clients can verbally respond to the therapist's prompt questions and therapists can adjust the process to account for individual needs. Thus, the scripts are only a guide for individual therapy. The circular questioning guide in Table 9.2 can be useful to assist therapists through the process of imagery rescripting in a more flexible way in individual treatment. Once the scene has been set regarding the specific rescripting phase (i.e., whether the client is taking the perspective of the younger or older self), the therapist can then use questions flexibly to first elicit a description of the situation, followed by emotional and body experiences, cognitions, and then behavioral actions. Behavioral actions in Phase 1 refer to those that actually occurred in the event, either enacted by the client or others involved in the situation. Behavioral actions in Phases 2 and 3 refer to those desired by the older and younger self respectively. The questioning then circles back to the start again, with an update on the situation, and so on.

TABLE 9.2. Imagery Rescripting Circular Questioning Guide

Focus	Phase 1	Phase 2	Phase 3
Situation		What is happening?	
Emotion/body		How are you feeling? Where do you feel it?	
Cognition		What are you thinking?	
Behavior/action	What are you doing? What are others doing?	What do you want to do? Do it	What do you need? Ask for it
	Repeat questions—what's happening now?		

Note. Based on Arntz (2011).

In individual treatment, rather than having clients open their eyes at the end of each phase to make relevant emotion and body ratings on Worksheet 16, the therapist is already eliciting this information during the circular questioning process and can record it on the client's behalf. In this way, there is no need for breaks between the three phases, unless in the therapist's clinical judgment this would be worthwhile, for example if each phase is lengthy and the client is losing focus. As with group treatment, at the end of the process it is important to debrief the client's experience and reflect on the emotion and meaning shifts that have occurred. Reflect on whether clients' feelings are now more consistent with their logical understanding of the situation and assess any shift in the current relevance of the image. This should be followed up over subsequent weeks by asking clients to periodically reflect on how they feel about the event now. Particularly focus on the correction of meaning distortions that are relevant to clients' negative core beliefs, such as coming to understand that the negative event wasn't their fault, wasn't about their personal worth, and was the exception, not the rule of how other people and the world operate. By working through this process, clients can also make metacognitive shifts regarding the broader importance of distressing memories, such as these insights from previous clients following imagery rescripting: "the meaning of memories is malleable," "you can change your perspective on anything," and "I don't need to be scared of my memories."

The process of imagery rescripting can be challenging and exhausting for clients. Ideally a comprehensive debrief will occur immediately afterward to consolidate the new learning. However, sometimes clients feel somewhat dazed and tired after the exercise and find it difficult to elaborate on their learning immediately afterward. On these occasions, it can sometimes be fruitful to keep the debrief relatively short and revisit their experience and shifts in meaning in more detail at the next session. The therapist needs to ensure that the client is emotionally contained and safe before completing the session, which may require some grounding exercises or casual conversation before the client is sufficiently settled. The therapist might encourage clients to bring their new image (i.e., the Phase 3 image) to mind several times over the intervening week between sessions, or if helpful meaning and emotion shifts have not been achieved during the initial exercise, then the exercise may need to be repeated in the next session, with the client imagining a different rewrite of the memory that may be more effective. However, in our experience, if a satisfactory rescript has occurred in session, rescripting the same event is not typically necessary for meaning and emotion shifts to be consolidated.

Other Imagery Rescripting Tips

Multiple Memories

If there are multiple memories, allow clients to choose one they wish to start on. Grading the memories in terms of distress is not essential, unless clients wish to adopt this approach. If there are multiple memories that are similar in meaning, working effectively on one or two memories will often generalize to seeing other significant memories in a different light.

Trauma Memories

In group therapy we encourage clients to work with a past negative *social* experience to rescript. Should clients attribute their social anxiety to a highly traumatic experience (e.g., sexual abuse, physical violence, torture), we would recommend that rescripting of this nature be undertaken in individual and not group therapy. With highly traumatic experiences, clients may be at risk of dissociating or may need more assistance from the therapist with the rescripting process. For example, if clients find it difficult to adopt a more compassionate perspective, the therapist may need to take a far more active role in intervening in the image rather than relying on the client's older self being the interven-ing figure. These issues obviously cannot be accommodated within a group setting. It is important to note that with highly traumatic experiences clients do not need to relive horrific trauma in Phase 1 for rescripting to be effective. In these circumstances, clients only need to imaginally reexperience the event up to the point where they know the traumatic incident is about to occur, and hence the associated emotion is activated. At that point the therapist would step into the image and be the intervening figure, protect-ing the client, and actively providing the safety and comfort required. Again, readers are encouraged to read Hackman and colleagues (2011) and Arntz (2011) for further infor-mation on rescripting under these circumstances.

What about Aggressive or Violent Imagery?

Clients will sometimes want to include violence in their imagery, for example, envis-aging the bully being bullied or clients seeing themselves enacting violent revenge. Therapists sometimes feel uneasy about facilitating vengeful and violent impulses in their clients in case they are encouraged to act them out in real life. Arntz (2012) suggests that the desire for revenge can be common and natural, and that articulating, accept-ing, and learning to tolerate this desire during rescripting may reduce the likelihood of acting it out. Studies investigating the impact of violent imagery have found that safe-place imagery (leaving the situation and entering a positive and safe situation) has a more positive impact on reducing angry emotions and increasing positive emotions compared to imagery rescripting with or without revenge (Seebauer, Froß, Dubaschny, Schönberger, & Jacob, 2014). Interestingly, rescripting with revenge did not help or hin-der the rescripting process compared to rescripting without revenge. Other studies have also found that revenge imagery has not increased the risk of aggressive actions (Arntz, Tiesema, & Kindt, 2007). It is important to note that there have been very few studies of violent imagery in clinical samples. Caution may also be required in forensic settings or with clients who have a history of violence or aggression. Needless to say, people with SAD do not typically fit this profile. If revenge is enacted in fantasy during imagery rescripting, Arntz (2011) suggests that therapists then pay close attention to other needs the client has regarding feeling comforted, supported, and safe.

Imagery Rescripting Summary

Consistent with traditional CBT strategies, imagery rescripting is essentially a method of trying to re-understand "evidence for" negative core beliefs in a new way that undermines them. When the older self tells the bully off, or shrinks him, or lassos him, or sends him to jail, and then people come and support the younger self, telling him it is OK, that they aren't to blame, putting their arm around him, hugging him, asking him to come play on the swings or go for an ice cream—what message do these imagined actions convey? "The bully was the problem, not me." "They were in the wrong, not me." "People are on my side." "People are kind." "I am not weak and defective." "I am strong and likable."

Imagery rescripting brings a new perspective to a negative event that can be more emotionally evocative than a purely verbal reinterpretation of the event. For therapists new to this process, who may be unsure if the way the image has been rescripted is "right," remember that it is just an image that can be played with. Remember it is the meaning of the image that is important. If the meaning and feelings attached to the new image seem appropriate and helpful to both the client and therapist, then it is likely to be helpful for emotional processing of the event. Remember, it is an image, so you can always rewind it and try something else if initial attempts fail to yield demonstrable emotional shifts.

Positive Imagery to Construct New Core Beliefs

The use of positive imagery for the construction of new balanced core beliefs comes from Padesky and Mooney's (2005, cited in Hackmann et al., 2011) "Old System/New System" approach, and particularly their method of "New System" construction. This approach was developed for working with personality disorders, with the aim of helping to address the chronic long-standing interpersonal difficulties these clients face. Mooney and Padesky (2000) are strong advocates of constructing new core beliefs, rather than only challenging the old ones. This is a collaborative creative process between therapist and client that involves the exploration of new possibilities of how the client would like to be in life. Imagery is a particularly useful tool for starting to develop "new ways of being" (Hackmann et al., 2011, p. 181), as essentially clients are encouraged to vividly imagine an alternative, more ideal way of operating in the world. Clients' imagery then provides clues as to the new core beliefs that are required to operate in the desired manner. At first it is OK for clients not to believe the alternative self they are envisioning or the new core beliefs their imagery represents. Following Padesky and Mooney's "New System" approach, behavior change becomes the primary means of strengthening new beliefs. Positive imagery is simply recruited in the construction of new core beliefs, and action planning (i.e., behavioral experiments) is used to strengthen new core beliefs.

Introducing Positive Imagery

It is critical that clients be provided with a strong rationale for using positive imagery so that they can fully engage with the process, otherwise it may be interpreted as "pie in the sky wishful thinking." We have found the following concepts useful in socializing clients to this method:

> "The imagery work done so far has been about uncovering negative images (past, present, and future) that maintain social anxiety, and finding ways to manipulate or change these images by testing their validity through various experiments. Our focus has mostly been on chipping away and breaking down these negative images.
>
> "However, it is equally important to construct positive images. We have already seen the power of imagery in terms of its influence on emotions and actions. Just as negative images influence negative emotions and actions, equally, positive images can promote positive emotions and actions. Developing positive images of how you would ideally like things to be in your life can give us clues about new core beliefs you might like to start developing.
>
> "Hopefully the behavioral experiments and past imagery rescripting have shown you that the old negative core beliefs are outdated. For example, experiments as an adult have shown that others and the world generally aren't as critical and hostile as first believed, or that you are more socially adept than you've given yourself credit for. So it is time for a core belief update.
>
> "The positive images we develop can help us construct these new core beliefs. It is OK and normal if you don't initially believe any of the positive images we generate. We will find ways to strengthen your belief in these positive images over time through the way you act and live your life."

Positive Imagery Guide

There are seven steps involved in developing positive imagery to construct new core beliefs, and these can be divided into three aims: identifying new core beliefs, generalizing new core beliefs, and consolidating new core beliefs. Worksheet 17, *Constructing New Core Beliefs,* and the accompanying Handout 14, *Constructing New Core Beliefs,* can assist the therapist and client through the seven steps. When the positive imagery exercises are completed in a group setting, we pause after each of the three sections to take some time to fill in the worksheet and debrief clients' experiences before moving to the next section. In individual treatment, this process can be more flexible and at the discretion of the therapist. The therapist can often fill in the details required on Worksheet 17 from the client's responses during the imagery exercise. However, the therapist will likely choose to pause and have the client open her eyes at certain points, as the imagery exercise would be very lengthy if all seven steps were done without a break. Below we provide a script for working through the seven steps that has been elaborated from the ideas of Padesky and Mooney's "New System" approach (Hackmann et al., 2011, p. 190; Mooney & Padesky, 2000; Padesky, 2011). This script is delivered verbatim in a group setting and is used as a flexible guide in individual treatment.

Identifying New Core Beliefs

STEP 1: ELICIT A DIFFICULT SITUATION

"If you feel comfortable doing so, close your eyes, sitting comfortably . . . bring to mind a situation in which you have typically experienced strong social anxiety . . . (raise your hand when you have a clear situation in mind)."

STEP 2: IMAGINE A NEW WAY OF OPERATING

"Without changing anything about the situation itself, *how would you like to be*? How would you like to handle the situation? Experience being that way now. What are you doing? [pause] What kind of expression do you have on your face? [pause] How are you holding your body posture? [pause] What self-talk is going through your mind? [pause] Experience being this way now . . . [pause] When you are operating in this way how do you feel? How does that feel in your body? Where do you feel it?"

STEP 3: NEW CORE BELIEF IMPLICATIONS

"When operating in this new way, how do you see *yourself*? [pause] How do you see *others*? [pause] How do you see the *world*? [pause]"

The typical experiences this part of the exercise elicits are visions of the self as calm, at ease, interacting and participating socially, contributing to discussions freely, others engaging with the client positively, the client smiling and standing in a relaxed, engaged, and confident posture with head held high and shoulders back. From these actions, clients can typically infer new core beliefs about the self as socially adept, good enough, adequate, worthwhile, competent, interesting, confident, strong, likable, and so on. Others are seen as equals, welcoming, kind, nonjudgmental, and interested. The world is seen as safe, with flexible social conventions.

Generalizing New Core Beliefs

STEP 4: DIFFERENT LIFE DOMAINS

"Let's reestablish the new positive image again. Closing your eyes again, sitting comfortably . . . bring to mind the same situation as before, seeing yourself operating in this new more positive mode, operating from your new core beliefs (raise your hand when you have this in mind). Now imagine bringing this new way of operating into other situations."

- "*Think about your current relationships* . . . bring an image of a friend, partner, or acquaintance to mind . . . if no one is coming to mind, imagine that you are starting to establish a relationship . . . keep in mind your new core beliefs about yourself, others, and the world . . . maintain these new core beliefs as you develop the image in your mind's eye . . . what would you and the other person be doing to reflect these positive core beliefs ? . . . again being aware of your expression, posture, and how it all feels within you . . . [pause] Make a note of how things are different, what you are doing, how you are feeling, where you notice those feelings in your body . . . [pause]"
- "*Now think about your family.* Bring to mind a vivid image of how things would be different if you were operating from your new, more positive core beliefs. [pause]"
- "Now move on to what you would be doing differently with your *work, studies, or daily responsibilities* if you were operating from your new core beliefs. How would you be approaching these situations? [pause]"
- "Now bring to mind an image of your *leisure time or hobbies,* or other ways that you would spend your time if you were operating in this new system of more positive core beliefs. What would you be doing and how does that feel? [pause]"
- "Finally, bring to mind an image of how your lifestyle might be different when it comes to *health and general well-being*? If you were operating from your new core beliefs, what would you be doing to take care of your health, well-being and self-care? [pause]"

The typical experiences this part of the exercise elicits are seeing oneself more engaged, interactive, and participating in all domains of life, rather than avoiding or being disconnected. Clients envision more positive relationships with current friends, relatives, and partners, or the development of a new social network or intimate relationship. They see themselves involved in desired work or study and being able to progress in these areas. They see themselves attending to the responsibilities of daily living independently, taking up new hobbies and interests, and taking care of their physical health. In general, the vision is of a much improved quality of life when operating from their new core beliefs.

STEP 5: "STORMY WEATHER"

"Unfortunately, life doesn't always go according to plan and we can hit 'stormy weather.' It is important to prepare for these times. Continuing with your eyes closed, I would like you to imagine a social situation that doesn't go so well, for example where you thought you offended someone, or you thought someone didn't like you, or you made a mistake (raise your hand when you have this in mind).

"Now remembering your new core beliefs about how you see yourself, other people, and the world . . . if this were to occur, how could you handle this? What would you need to do? Experience yourself doing it. What would you need to say to yourself? Say these things to yourself now, adopting the body posture and facial expression that would go with this. How do you feel within yourself when you react in this manner? What does that feel like in your body?"

This part of the exercise is about building new core beliefs that are strong enough to accommodate and be resilient to setbacks, rather than reverting to enacting the old negative core beliefs at the first sign of trouble. Generally, clients envision themselves staying calm, depersonalizing the experience, letting it go, and moving on.

Consolidate the New Core Belief

STEP 6: EVIDENCE FOR

"Think of a past occasion where you did something that exemplifies your new core belief. This may be the recent past, perhaps as part of this treatment, or further into the past. Now close your eyes again and visualize this past occasion . . . stay with this image, experiencing yourself in the situation as if it were now . . . what's happening . . . how do you feel? How does your body feel? Spend a few moments reexperiencing this event."

This process is equivalent to what is done in traditional CBT, looking for evidence that supports the new core beliefs. However, by having the client imaginally reexperience the evidence and sit with the feelings this generates it aims to make the evidence more emotionally powerful, memorable, and convincing. This step also instills hope that the new core beliefs may not be "pie in the sky" ideals when clients glimpse evidence of having operated in this way before. Given all the work they have done earlier in treatment, clients may be closer than they think to transitioning to a set of new core beliefs. They may not be building something from scratch, but instead gradually increasing the amount of time or circumstances within which they operate in this new way.

STEP 7: ICONS

"When you imagine operating in this way, what 'icons' come to mind? [you can give a brief personal example] Are there particular songs, images, movies, characters, fairy tales, stories, people, animals, or scenes from nature that represent this way of operating for you? For you, is there something that captures the spirit of your new, more positive core beliefs? If nothing immediately comes to mind that's OK, just give yourself some time for an image to emerge [pause].

"If you have an icon in mind, spend a moment noticing how you feel in your body when you bring this icon to mind. [pause] Consider for a moment how this icon could be used to help you stay in this new way of operating. [pause]

"You can now start broadening your attention back to the room and, when you are ready, open your eyes."

Clients have used icons such as Superman, Wonder Woman, Yoda, a sunset, and a wild horse to represent the spirit of their new core beliefs. Clients are only limited by their creativity. The main aim is to see if clients can develop a shorthand way of stimulating the same mindset and feelings that are linked with their new core beliefs. The icon can then be used as a means of kick-starting the new core belief system when they need some assistance. Clients can then elaborate or strengthen their icons by mentally rehearsing the icon image or finding other mediums that reinforce the icon (i.e., painting, drawing, photos, pictures, songs, objects, pendants). The idea is to make the icon easily accessible and effective in stimulating the new core belief system and emotions, particularly when faced with challenging situations where clients may be tempted to revert to cognitive, emotional, and behavioral cycles reflecting their old negative core beliefs.

For example, one client walked into a party with the theme music of *Star Wars* playing in his mind's ear. This served the purpose of activating the new core belief system (by representing the system and elicit feelings linked to the system), giving him the boost he needed to hold his head high, shoulders back, smile, and approach someone to have a conversation. Doing this meant he was operating consistently with his new core beliefs that "I am competent and others are kind." Other clients might choose to use their new "core belief song" as a ring tone, which will serve as a regular reminder to approach phone conversations in a manner consistent with their new core beliefs.

Action Planning to Strengthen New Core Beliefs

During the positive imagery exercise, and particularly in Step 4 when generalizing new core beliefs to different life domains, clients will have envisioned some specific activities they would be doing differently if they were operating consistently with their new, more balanced core beliefs (e.g., enjoying family gatherings, spending time with new friends, attending a course of study, going to the gym to exercise). These visions of an alternative life offer ideas about what actions clients will need to engage in over the long term to reinforce and strengthen the newly constructed core beliefs. The actions clients need to take across various aspects of their lives may be similar to what they have already been doing in treatment with their behavioral experiments. In practice, strengthening new core beliefs may therefore mean doing more of the same. However, the intention will be not only to challenge their negative social images, but also to test the validity of their new balanced core beliefs.

It is useful to socialize clients to the need to act consistently with their new core beliefs as a means by which to gradually strengthen their conviction in the new core beliefs.

"We know that the best way to build conviction in your new core beliefs is to live your life 'as if' they were true. Some call it 'fake it till you make it,' and what we know is that changing our behavior is the most powerful way to change our beliefs. Behavioral experiments are a prime example of that. So if you start operating, acting, behaving in a way that is consistent with your system of new balanced core beliefs, usually your confidence in the new beliefs will catch up."

Worksheet 18, the *New Core Belief Action Plan,* is then used for collaboratively planning the specifics of operating within clients' new core belief system. This involves identifying a target for change in each life domain, such as participating in family events, starting a course of study, being assertive at work, making new friends, starting an art class, and so on. A specific plan of action is then devised for how to meet this target, and a time frame is placed on when specific actions will be taken to increase the likelihood that the plan will become a reality. A target for change may require more than one action to achieve change, and the actions required are likely to be ongoing over time. This means that clients don't just operate from their new core beliefs in isolated cases but must ensure they are consistently operating from their new core beliefs over time. For example, if the target for change is being more assertive at work, there may be several action steps such as saying no to unreasonable requests, delegating tasks to others, making requests of others, providing constructive feedback where necessary, and raising problems with the boss. Each of these tasks will need to be done multiple times as the opportunity arises. As clients become more familiar with completing their action plans, the structured planning of these behavioral changes may not need to be so formal. Targets for change should be thought of as something that is typically never "achieved" per se, but something one is always working toward.

The idea is for clients to treat each planned action as a behavioral experiment. However, by this point in therapy the experiments generally won't have to be planned as rigorously, using Worksheet 7, the *Behavioral Experiment Record,* as was required for behavior changes early on in therapy. Over time with an accumulation of many behavioral experiments over many life domains, clients' new core beliefs will mostly be supported. The action plan is a road map that guides clients to live their lives in a manner that provides them with many opportunities to strengthen their new set of balanced core beliefs. With time, these new core beliefs will more consistently govern clients' social expectations and how they operate in the world, hence facilitating recovery from SAD.

Clinical Case: Modifying Negative Core Beliefs

During imagery rescripting one client reexperienced being back in early primary school. There was no one specific memory for this person—the image was a conglomeration of the bullying and rejection she received from her peers at the time. It featured being laughed at, being left out of games, being called "weirdo" when she tried to join in on group activities in the playground, and a lot of time spent on the swings alone. As an adult, and when in "safe" company, this client was quite brash and had a great sense of humor. She was generally really fun to work with in therapy. It appeared in her imaginal recount of primary school that her sophisticated sense of humor was present from a young age. She reexperienced the teachers laughing at her jokes, but her peers sitting dumbfounded. These sorts of experiences just reinforced her overall core beliefs that she was "different," "weird," and "didn't belong." During the rescripting process her older self visited her in the school grounds and sat next to her on the swings. The older self gave advice like "who would want to be like those boring jerks, they are all sheep." The older self spoke about how being different was a good thing, something she might even value later in life, seeing her differences as a sign that she was funny, intelligent, creative, unique, and special. The older self gave comfort to the younger self by putting her arm around her and pushing her on the swing. She then brought into the image a person she met later in high school who ended up being a fabulous friend. Imagining that they had met earlier allowed the younger self to experience the sense of belonging and kinship she needed. At the end of the imagery rescripting exercise when the client opened her eyes the first words out of her mouth were an exuberant "I was an awesome kid!" This was an important step in her developing a new core belief about herself, which she phrased as "I am different and that is an awesome thing to be."

THERAPY SUMMARY GUIDE: Negative Core Beliefs

Therapy Aim: Identify and undermine negative core beliefs typically regarding self as defective and others as judgmental, and construct new balanced core beliefs and positive actions to strengthen these new core beliefs.

Therapy Agenda Items:

▼ Traditional CBT methods for identifying and modifying core beliefs can be used; however, this SAD treatment places a strong emphasis on imagery rescripting, positive imagery, and action planning as the main methods for achieving the same aim.

▼ Imagery Rescripting:

- ◢ Introduce clients to imagery rescripting by presenting a rationale, explaining the three phases, and preparing for distress tolerance
- ◢ Use Worksheet 16, *Past Imagery Rescripting,* to guide the entire process:
  - ▶ Prepare for imagery rescripting by selecting a memory, eliciting its meaning, and identifying the "older-you" perspective
  - ▶ Complete imagery rescripting by following the three-phase imagery rescripting guide and/or circular questioning guide
  - ▶ Debrief shifts in meaning and affect regarding the memory

▼ Positive Imagery:

- ◢ Introduce clients to positive imagery by presenting a rationale
- ◢ Use the positive imagery guide and Worksheet 17, *Constructing New Core Beliefs,* to guide the process:
  - ▶ Identify new core beliefs by imagining how clients would like to be in difficult situations and extrapolating new core beliefs
  - ▶ Generalize new core beliefs to different life domains and difficult situations (i.e., "stormy weather")
  - ▶ Consolidate new core beliefs by reexperiencing past confirmatory evidence and developing an icon to activate the new core belief system

▼ Action Planning:

- ◢ Use Worksheet 18, *New Core Belief Action Plan,* to plan specific behavior changes across life domains that will likely strengthen the new core beliefs over time

Therapy Materials:

▼ Handouts

  ◢ Handout 13, *Past Imagery Rescripting*

  ◢ Handout 14, *Constructing New Core Beliefs*

▼ Worksheets

  ◢ Worksheet 16, *Past Imagery Rescripting*

  ◢ Worksheet 17, *Constructing New Core Beliefs*

  ◢ Worksheet 18, *New Core Belief Action Plan*

CHAPTER 10

Maintenance and Relapse Prevention

THERAPIST: Let's review your initial goal that you set for treatment "to be less socially anxious so that I can accept and initiate invitations with friends, join a sporting club, and speak up in work meetings." How much do you feel you have progressed with that goal?

CLIENT: Well, I am doing all of those things. I am going out more with friends, and I have started playing basketball, and I make a point of saying at least one thing in work meetings each week.

THERAPIST: It sounds like you have achieved your goal then?

CLIENT: Yeah, I have.

THERAPIST: That being the case, maybe we should start talking about how we might know we were coming to the end of treatment. I guess one sign would be achieving the goal you had set at the start.

CLIENT: Yes, but I still don't feel confident in all situations, and coming here is good for helping me plan my behavioral experiments for the week. I am not sure how I would go without that.

THERAPIST: It is natural to be a bit cautious about the idea of ending treatment. But let's start to look at other signs that might tell us if you are ready to move to the "winding down" phase of therapy. I wonder what other signs we might look for to make this decision together. I am also wondering about what things we could put in place to help you feel more confident about finishing treatment when the time comes.

About This Module: Completing Treatment

The duration of SAD treatment is going to vary between clients depending on pretreatment symptom severity and speed of skill acquisition. As already discussed, in group therapy the treatment outlined in Chapters 4–9 is completed in 12 weekly 2-hour sessions, with a subsequent 1-month follow-up session. In individual therapy the length of treatment can be flexible depending on client needs. This module covers what to look for in clients to determine when treatment should move into the completion phase. In addition, this module outlines the topics that should be covered and how to address each topic, with the aim of preparing clients to maintain their therapy gains and be resilient to social anxiety setbacks to prevent relapse.

When Are Clients Ready to Complete Treatment?

A sign that treatment can move into the completion phase is when clients are actively and independently engaging in behavioral experiments, and through this process there is a reduction in their perceived social threat. This should mean that while certain situations may still trigger social anxiety, the intensity is reduced, experimentation rather than avoidance now follows, and the threshold for trigger situations is now set higher.

A sure sign that therapy is nearing its end is when sessions become repetitive in nature. For example, sessions may start to focus mainly on setting and debriefing between-session behavioral experiments, the planning may not need to be as meticulous as it was early in treatment (i.e., clients are well aware of how to approach social situations, where to place their attention, and what safety behaviors to drop), and the conclusions from behavioral experiments are becoming repetitive (e.g., "no one is looking," "no one is judging," "the situation went well," "I was able to participate and socialize," "when I screwed up it wasn't a big deal, I was able to move on from that moment rather than getting stuck in it").

Another sure sign that treatment is coming to a natural conclusion is when clients are doing things they want to be doing in life without social anxiety holding them back. For example, they can regularly attend and participate in study or work, can go to a sporting or hobby group they have always wanted to be a part of, they are engaging more with family and friends, and they are establishing some new friendships or relationships. The end point of therapy is not indicated by the absence of anxiety in social settings, but instead the client should be well along the trajectory of living a life that is not dictated by a fear of negative evaluation from others. If clients can do this, then their anxiety will likely continue to diminish over time, and when their anxiety inevitably spikes at times, as it does for all of us, they will be well practiced in knowing how to handle this.

How to Complete Treatment

As treatment starts to wind down, it may be useful to begin spacing sessions further apart, moving from weekly sessions to fortnightly or monthly sessions. Scheduling follow-up sessions at 1-, 3-, or 6-month intervals may also be useful for some clients who lack the confidence that they can maintain or continue their progress without therapist assistance. Follow-up intervals can provide clients with the opportunity to discover for themselves that they can cope independently, and can be framed as behavioral experiments. The therapist might encourage clients by saying:

> "I believe you can do this on your own because it has been you doing the hard work all along. This treatment has been all about training you to become your own therapist. Maybe the follow-up period can be like a behavioral experiment, giving you the opportunity to gather evidence and prove this to yourself, so that you believe it too."

The focus of sessions in the completion phase of therapy should be to review treatment content, review client progress, facilitate maintenance of client gains, plan for preventing relapse, address any therapy termination concerns clients may have, and look forward to the future ahead. This can typically be achieved in two sessions and can be reiterated in follow-up sessions if they have been scheduled.

Reviewing Treatment

When reviewing treatment, therapists might return to Worksheet 1, *My Model of Social Anxiety,* which they completed at the beginning of treatment, and Socratically elicit the main treatment strategies that have been used to address each component of the model. The following treatment components should be reviewed, and clients encouraged to reflect on the components that were most helpful to them. These components can be referred to as their "skills toolbox" and are described in Handout 15, *Skills Toolbox.*

The main treatment components include:

- Imagery monitoring and challenging
- Coping imagery to facilitate engaging in behavioral experiments
- Behavioral experiments to reverse avoidance
- Behavioral experiment hierarchies
- Dropping safety behaviors
- Video feedback to correct a negative self-image
- Attention retraining and focusing to facilitate task-focused attention during behavioral experiments
- Imagery rescripting to change the meaning of past events linked to negative core beliefs
- Positive imagery and action planning to generate new core beliefs

Reviewing Progress

Worksheet 19, *Your Progress,* can be used as a way of focusing discussion on the progress and gains clients have made during treatment. The worksheet encourages clients to consider the following:

- "In what situations are you managing your social anxiety better?"
- "What changes have you made in your life? What things have you done that you had not done before (or not done for a long time)?"
- "What was the most important thing that you learned in treatment that has contributed to reducing your anxiety in social situations?"
- "What new skills learned in treatment are you using regularly?"
- "What skills do you think you would benefit from using more often?"
- "What specific situations do you need to confront to overcome remaining anxieties?"
- "What specific goals can you set to help you address these remaining anxieties?"

Readministration of Worksheet 2, the *Personal Fear and Avoidance List,* and debriefing changes from pre- to posttreatment are also recommended as a method of reviewing progress and determining any future priorities for change. Areas that have changed should be reinforced and those that have not changed can be discussed. Therapist and client can consider together the reasons why change has not occurred (e.g., no behavioral experiments have been conducted in this specific domain, or safety behaviors are still in place and are inhibiting change), and they can specifically target the area by designing relevant behavioral experiment hierarchies and/or action plans. Obviously, readministration of any psychometric pretreatment measures would occur at this time. This will provide an objective indicator of treatment outcome, and appropriate feedback should be provided to the client.

Maintaining Gains

The last four questions of Worksheet 19, *Your Progress,* can also stimulate discussion regarding what clients need to keep doing to maintain and further their progress when formal treatment has finished. Therapists should convey the message that "just because the formal therapy sessions have finished does not mean that the therapy has finished. Therapy and its benefits can be ongoing when you continue to apply the skills you have learned in day-to-day life." Worksheet 18, *New Core Belief Action Plan,* previously completed to strengthen new core beliefs, and any ongoing behavioral experiment hierarchies clients are still working on (see Worksheet 9 and Chapter 6) can facilitate maintenance, giving clients a plan for what specific tasks need to be done to stay on track and progress even further.

The development, maintenance, and treatment of psychological difficulties can be complex. However, in our experience, the main therapy concepts and strategies that will work for clients, and a plan for continuing to apply these in daily life, should be as simple as possible—in fact, simple enough to fit onto a single sheet of paper and/or a 3″ × 5″ flash card. In lieu of ongoing therapy sessions, this brief summary of key lessons from therapy can then serve as a reminder for clients and as a prompt to check in on their progress. If the concepts and strategies learned in therapy are many, vast, complex, and not easily accessible, then the likelihood of sustained application of therapy skills by clients may be compromised.

Preventing Relapse

Recovery from SAD can be a "rocky road." Therapists should explain to clients that the road to recovery is rarely smooth, and there are usually some ups and downs along the way. Sometimes drawing a graph showing the typical peaks and troughs of progress can help to convey this "two steps forward, one step back" message. This message is not intended to be pessimistic, but to normalize setbacks and develop realistic expectations regarding change:

> "Setbacks are normal, the important thing is how we respond to these setbacks. If we think in unhelpful ways like 'I'm back at square one' we will probably start to fall back into old habits of avoiding social situations and reverting back to old safety behaviors. Instead, if we try to learn something from the experience and see it as the ideal opportunity to practice our therapy skills to help overcome the setback, this will build our resilience. Not feeling socially anxious is not the only sign that we have overcome our social anxiety. Feeling socially anxious, coping with those feelings, and not having those feelings stop us from doing what we want to do in life is an equally important sign of social anxiety recovery."

Worksheet 20, *Dealing with Setbacks,* encourages clients to consider potential triggers for setbacks (i.e., When are setbacks in my social anxiety more likely to occur? In what types of circumstances do I tend to have a setback?) and consider early warning signs of setbacks (How do I know when I have had a setback in my social anxiety? Are there any emotional, thinking, behavioral, or physical signals?). With this awareness in mind, clients are then encouraged to consider how they will respond to setbacks by developing a cognitive action plan (i.e., What do I need to focus on and remind myself of when a social anxiety setback occurs?) and behavioral action plan (i.e., What do I need to do when a social anxiety setback occurs?). If follow-up sessions have been scheduled, be sure to prompt clients on whether they have had to use their action plans during the follow-up period, the impact or outcome of this, and whether their action plans require revising.

Addressing Termination Issues

Clients can have mixed feelings about ending therapy. Some may feel ready to move on, some may be glad to move on, and others may find it a loss and be worried about their independent coping abilities. It is important to ensure attention is given to how clients are feeling about completing therapy, so that if they do have fears about therapy termination, you have the opportunity to address them. The spacing of sessions and follow-up sessions can allay some concerns. For those who are concerned, it may be useful to use Worksheet 6, the *Imagery Challenging Record,* to uncover negative images regarding therapy termination, and allow clients to use the skills they have acquired to challenge this image and develop a more helpful image of life beyond therapy.

Looking Forward to the Future

It is within the spirit of the imagery-based approach to end therapy with a final imagery exercise that encourages clients to look to the future with optimism. The following script can be used to facilitate this.

"Closing your eyes, I would like you to consider the question of how you will be heading forward from here. Spend a few minutes imagining yourself at some point in the future, continuing to operate consistently with what you have learned in treatment, operating consistently with your new core beliefs and action plans.

"Where are you? What are you doing? What are you thinking? What is your facial expression and body posture like? How do you feel? Where do you feel this in your body? I will give you a few moments to explore this image looking into the future . . .

"When you are ready you can let go of the image and open your eyes."

In individual therapy, therapists can ask clients to describe what they are imagining during the exercise. In group therapy, the therapist can elicit descriptions afterward. Take some time to debrief the exercise by asking clients about the main features of their future-oriented imagery. Clients will usually envision a life that they desire—participating in study, work, or hobbies, having meaningful friendships, engaging in family events, having a partner, having a family, and so on. They may acknowledge that SAD had previously robbed them of this kind of life. However, through the courage they have demonstrated by participating and persisting with this treatment, this type of life may now be accessible to them, if not immediately, then as a future no longer outside the realms of possibility. As therapist and client end their journey together, both can be satisfied that the short-term pain has been worth the long-term future gain of a life well lived.

Clinical Case: Completing Treatment

For one of our clients, completing university study had always been a struggle due to his social anxiety. Historically, he would begin study and inevitably withdraw at assignment or exam time when he started to miss classes and therefore fall behind in his work. Going back to school had therefore been highly anxiety provoking, with images of past "breakdowns" and "quitting" in his mind. He was very concerned that his social anxiety would get the better of him and history would be repeated yet again. On this occasion, compared to his previous attempts at returning to college, he was undertaking treatment at the same time and hence was well prepared for the challenge. He was now aware of his negative social images and able to challenge these, he saw attendance at classes as continual behavioral experiments, and he was now naturally dropping safety behaviors and being more task focused in these environments. A sign that we were coming to the end of treatment was his ability to continue meeting his university commitments even during times of anxiety "flare-ups." Our sessions were beginning to feel repetitive, and we seemed to have less to cover and would finish the session early. I clearly remember him saying to me, "This time is different from all those previous times I couldn't deal with college, I have different skills now that I didn't have then." It wasn't so much what he said, but the way he said it that struck me. I reminded him that during the imagery challenging we had been doing earlier in therapy to prepare for his return to college, this statement had appeared almost verbatim in his Contrary Evidence column to counter his negative image that "returning to university would be just like all the other times." However, compared to earlier in therapy, I heard a confidence, conviction, and certainty in his voice when he said these words. It was not just the wonderful cognitive and behavioral changes he had made that indicated he was ready to end treatment, but his tone of voice, body language, and attitude when reflecting on those changes gave us both confidence that formal therapy was no longer necessary.

THERAPY SUMMARY GUIDE: Maintenance and Relapse Prevention

Therapy Aim: Complete therapy ensuring clients are: (1) clear and confident regarding what they need to keep doing to maintain and further their gains, and (2) prepared for responding to setbacks to prevent SAD relapse.

Therapy Agenda Items:

▼ Review treatment:

⬥ Map treatment strategies onto clients' previously completed Worksheet 1, *My Model of Social Anxiety*

⬥ Complete handout 15, *Skills Toolbox,* to summarize the treatment components

▼ Review clients' progress:

⬥ Refer to Worksheet 19, *Your Progress*

⬥ Readminister Worksheet 2, *Personal Fear and Avoidance List,* and provide feedback on changes

⬥ Readminister any relevant psychometric measures and provide feedback on changes.

▼ Facilitate maintenance of gains:

⬥ Use relevant questions on Worksheet 19, *Your Progress*

⬥ Ensure that previously completed Worksheet 18, *New Core Belief Action Plan,* and/ or any uncompleted behavioral experiment hierarchies (Worksheet 9) are clear and can serve as guides to continued behavior change over time

⬥ Simplify on one page or a flash card in clients' own words the most helpful concepts and strategies from treatment that they will continue to apply regularly

▼ Prevent relapse:

⬥ Normalize setbacks

⬥ Use Worksheet 20, *Dealing with Setbacks,* to plan a response

▼ Address termination concerns where necessary:

⬥ Schedule follow-up sessions

⬥ Use imagery challenging skills

▼ Close treatment on an optimistic note with the Looking Forward to the Future Imagery Exercise

Therapy Materials:

▼ Handouts
  ◢ Handout 15, *Skills Toolbox*
▼ Worksheets
  ◢ Worksheet 19, *Your Progress*
  ◢ Worksheet 20, *Dealing with Setbacks*

APPENDIX

Reproducible Worksheets and Handouts

WORKSHEETS

HANDOUTS

My Model of Social Anxiety

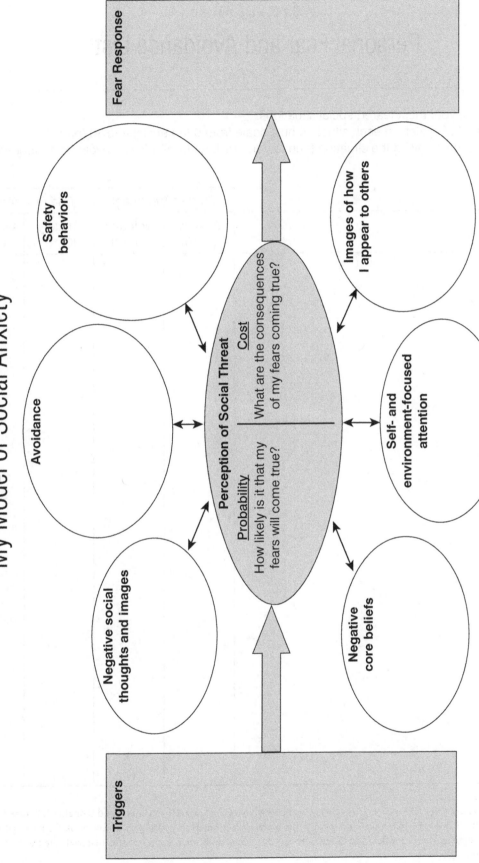

From *Imagery-Enhanced CBT for Social Anxiety Disorder* by Peter M. McEvoy, Lisa M. Saulsman, and Ronald M. Rapee. Copyright © 2018 The Guilford Press. Permission to photocopy this material is granted to purchasers of this book for personal use or use with clients (see copyright page for details). Purchasers can download additional copies of this material (see the box at the end of the table of contents).

Personal Fear and Avoidance List

Name: _____

1. List up to 10 of your most feared social situations.
2. Rate your level of <u>anxiety</u> in each situation on a scale from 0 (no anxiety) to 10 (panic).
3. Rate how much you <u>avoid</u> the situation (due to your anxiety) from 0 (never avoid) to 10 (always avoid).

Situation	Start of Treatment		End of Treatment	
	Anxiety (0–10)	Avoidance (0–10)	Anxiety (0–10)	Avoidance (0–10)

From *Imagery-Enhanced CBT for Social Anxiety Disorder* by Peter M. McEvoy, Lisa M. Saulsman, and Ronald M. Rapee. Copyright © 2018 The Guilford Press. Permission to photocopy this material is granted to purchasers of this book for personal use or use with clients (see copyright page for details). Purchasers can download additional copies of this material (see the box at the end of the table of contents).

Looking Forward

1. Close your eyes and imagine what your life would be like if your social anxiety did not change and you continued along the same path you are currently traveling. What would your life look like in 10 years' time? Write down what life would be like.

2. Now close your eyes and imagine how your life might be in 10 years' time if you make changes in your life and overcome your social anxiety. Write down what life would be like.

3. What kinds of things might get in the way of making the life changes necessary to overcome your social anxiety? What sorts of issues might act as obstacles or roadblocks for you?

4. The positive aspects of changing to a life without social anxiety are pretty obvious, but what about the negative aspects? Is there anything that you stand to lose by changing?

From *Imagery-Enhanced CBT for Social Anxiety Disorder* by Peter M. McEvoy, Lisa M. Saulsman, and Ronald M. Rapee. Copyright © 2018 The Guilford Press. Permission to photocopy this material is granted to purchasers of this book for personal use or use with clients (see copyright page for details). Purchasers can download additional copies of this material (see the box at the end of the table of contents).

Thought/Image–Feeling Connection

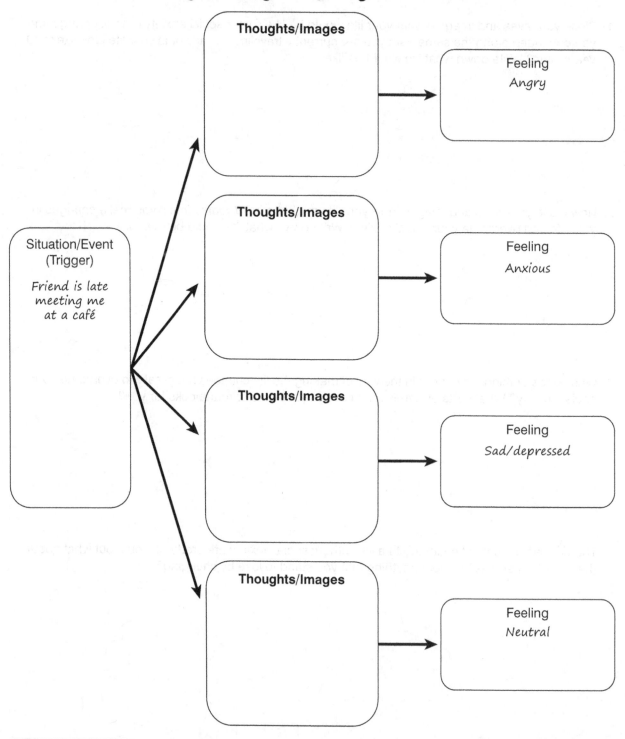

From *Imagery-Enhanced CBT for Social Anxiety Disorder* by Peter M. McEvoy, Lisa M. Saulsman, and Ronald M. Rapee. Copyright © 2018 The Guilford Press. Permission to photocopy this material is granted to purchasers of this book for personal use or use with clients (see copyright page for details). Purchasers can download additional copies of this material (see the box at the end of the table of contents).

Thought and Imagery Record

Trigger/Situation What is happening? Where am I?	Thoughts What thoughts are going through my mind?	Visual Image What specific images arise from these thoughts about the situation?	Sensations What sensations are part of the image (body, taste, smell, sound)?	Emotion How did I feel? SUDS 0–10?

From *Imagery-Enhanced CBT for Social Anxiety Disorder* by Peter M. McEvoy, Lisa M. Saulsman, and Ronald M. Rapee. Copyright © 2018 The Guilford Press. Permission to photocopy this material is granted to purchasers of this book for personal use or use with clients (see copyright page for details). Purchasers can download additional copies of this material (see the box at the end of the table of contents).

Imagery Challenging Record

1. Trigger Situation What was/is happening? Where am I?	2. Negative Image What visual images/thoughts are going through my mind? Body sensations, taste, smell, touch, sound?	3. Emotion How do I feel? How intensely (SUDS 0–10)?	4. Contrary Evidence What evidence do I have that does not support these thoughts/images? Alternative ways to view the situation?	5. Realistic Probability and Consequences How likely is it that my negative thoughts/images are accurate? If something bad happened, then so what? Would it really be that bad? Would I cope?	6. Helpful Image Describe as a picture the most realistic outcome and/or a more helpful image.	8. Rerate Emotion Describe and rate emotions during helpful image (SUDS 0–10).
					7. Visualize the helpful image as if it were actually occurring now.	

From *Imagery-Enhanced CBT for Social Anxiety Disorder* by Peter M. McEvoy, Lisa M. Saulsman, and Ronald M. Rapee. Copyright © 2018 The Guilford Press. Permission to photocopy this material is granted to purchasers of this book for personal use or use with clients (see copyright page for details). Purchasers can download additional copies of this material (see the box at the end of the table of contents).

Behavioral Experiment Record

Negative Image Describe your prediction. Specifically, what do you envision happening?	SUDS (/10) How anxious do you feel?	Experiment Specifically, what could you do to test this image? **Safety behaviors to drop?**	Evidence to Observe Specifically, what do you need to look for to confirm or disconfirm your image? **Where to focus attention?**	Results What happened? What clear evidence did you collect? Stick to unambiguous facts.	Conclusion What conclusion follows from your results?

Close eyes and update image based on results and conclusions.

From *Imagery-Enhanced CBT for Social Anxiety Disorder* by Peter M. McEvoy, Lisa M. Saulsman, and Ronald M. Rapee. Copyright © 2018 The Guilford Press. Permission to photocopy this material is granted to purchasers of this book for personal use or use with clients (see copyright page for details). Purchasers can download additional copies of this material (see the box at the end of the table of contents).

Safety Behaviors Experiment

Situation: _____

Image(s) of the worst possible outcome in this situation (describe in words or pictures):

My safety behaviors in this situation are: _____

_____

_____

_____

With safety behaviors	How anxious did I feel?	How self-conscious did I feel?	How anxious did I appear to others?	How good was my social performance?
Rating (0–10)				

What I will do instead of using safety behaviors: _____

_____

_____

_____

Without safety behaviors	How anxious did I feel?	How self-conscious did I feel?	How anxious did I appear to others?	How good was my social performance?
Rating (0–10)				

Conclusion—What did I learn about safety behaviors? _____

_____

_____

_____

_____

From *Imagery-Enhanced CBT for Social Anxiety Disorder* by Peter M. McEvoy, Lisa M. Saulsman, and Ronald M. Rapee. Copyright © 2018 The Guilford Press. Permission to photocopy this material is granted to purchasers of this book for personal use or use with clients (see copyright page for details). Purchasers can download additional copies of this material (see the box at the end of the table of contents).

Behavioral Experiment Hierarchy

Area for change: _____

Image(s) in these situations (describe in words or pictures):

| |
| |
| |
| |
| |

Goal:	SUDS (/10)

TIP: When thinking about the steps, consider what would make it harder or easier for you to complete the experiment. **What** will you do? **Where** will you do it? **When** will you do it? **Who** is there? By manipulating these variables you can create harder or easier steps.

From *Imagery-Enhanced CBT for Social Anxiety Disorder* by Peter M. McEvoy, Lisa M. Saulsman, and Ronald M. Rapee. Copyright © 2018 The Guilford Press. Permission to photocopy this material is granted to purchasers of this book for personal use or use with clients (see copyright page for details). Purchasers can download additional copies of this material (see the box at the end of the table of contents).

Coping Imagery

Describe in detail (in words or pictures) your coping image.

┌───┐
│   │
│   │
│   │
│   │
│   │
│   │
└───┘

How vivid is this image (circle)?

Not at all vivid				Moderately vivid			Like seeing a movie/photo		
1	2	3	4	5	6	7	8	9	10

How do you feel emotionally when you hold this image?

How do you feel physically when you hold this image?

Meaning of image: What does this image mean about you or your anxiety? What is the image trying to convey to you?

How can you strengthen this image?

How can you use this image to help manage your anxiety in the future?

From *Imagery-Enhanced CBT for Social Anxiety Disorder* by Peter M. McEvoy, Lisa M. Saulsman, and Ronald M. Rapee. Copyright © 2018 The Guilford Press. Permission to photocopy this material is granted to purchasers of this book for personal use or use with clients (see copyright page for details). Purchasers can download additional copies of this material (see the box at the end of the table of contents).

Speech Form

Before the speech:

1. Task: _____

2. Topic of your choosing: _____
   (Note: Make sure the topic will create at least 5/10 anxiety for you.)

3. For 2 minutes create a mental image of how you think you will appear to others as you are giving the speech. Write a brief description or draw a picture of this image.

   ┌───┐
   │   │
   │   │
   │   │
   │   │
   │   │
   │   │
   └───┘

4. How clearly were you able to see yourself in the image (0 = not at all vivid, 10 = extremely vivid)?

   _____

5. Complete the first column of the Speech Rating Form (pre-speech). Rate each item to reflect how you think you will perform on the 5-point scale.

After the speech, but before watching the recording:

6. Now that you have completed the speech task, close your eyes and form a clear image of how you think you came across during the speech. Do your best to construct an "internal video" of how you think you will appear on the recording. Write a brief description or draw a picture of this image.

   ┌───┐
   │   │
   │   │
   │   │
   │   │
   │   │
   └───┘

7. How clearly were you able to see yourself in the image (0 = not at all vivid, 10 = extremely vivid)?

   _____

8. Now predict what you will see in the recording by completing the second column of the Speech Rating Form (post-speech).

Review of the Recording

Before watching the recording we need to be clear about the difference between how you felt while giving the speech (and how you feel watching it) and how you *look*. You need to pay attention to how you look rather than how you felt. Try watching as if you were viewing a friend or someone else you cared about.

   Now watch the recording once.

(continued)

From *Imagery-Enhanced CBT for Social Anxiety Disorder* by Peter M. McEvoy, Lisa M. Saulsman, and Ronald M. Rapee. Copyright © 2018 The Guilford Press. Permission to photocopy this material is granted to purchasers of this book for personal use or use with clients (see copyright page for details). Purchasers can download additional copies of this material (see the box at the end of the table of contents).

After watching the recording once:

9. Rerate yourself using the third column on the Speech Rating Form.
10. Do your best to construct an "internal video" of how you actually look on the recording. Write a brief description or draw a picture of this image.

[blank box]

11. How clearly were you able to see yourself in the image (0 = not at all vivid, 10 = extremely vivid)?

_____

After watching the recording four times:

12. Rerate yourself using the fourth column on the Speech Rating Form.
13. Do your best to construct an "internal video" of how you actually look on the recording. Write a brief description or draw a picture of this image.

[blank box]

14. How clearly were you able to see yourself in the image (0 = not at all vivid, 10 = extremely vivid)?

_____

15. Conclusions: Make a note of what you learned from this task. What do you notice when you compare your ratings? What does this tell you about the accuracy of your initial image? How could this new information help to reduce your "perception of social threat" in the future? Within imagery, take a few moments to see yourself completing upcoming speech tasks or engaging in conversations in a way that is consistent with this new self-image.

[blank box]

Speech Rating Form

Use the "Pre-speech" column to rate how anxious you think you will feel and look while giving the speech. Then list the specific symptoms you believe will be obvious and rate how much you think they will show on the recording. In the remaining columns, rate your anxiety and observable symptoms after giving the speech and then after watching the recording.

Not at all		Mild			Moderate			High		Extreme
0	1	2	3	4	5	6	7	8	9	10

	Pre-speech	Post-speech	After watching recording once	After watching recording four times
How anxious will/did I feel? (0–10)				
How anxious will/did I look? (0–10)				
Below list your anxiety symptoms (e.g., blushing, shaking, mind going blank) and rate how obvious you think they will be/are on the recording. (0–10)				

From *Imagery-Enhanced CBT for Social Anxiety Disorder* by Peter M. McEvoy, Lisa M. Saulsman, and Ronald M. Rapee. Copyright © 2018 The Guilford Press. Permission to photocopy this material is granted to purchasers of this book for personal use or use with clients (see copyright page for details). Purchasers can download additional copies of this material (see the box at the end of the table of contents).

Self- versus Task-Focused Attention Experiment

1. **Experiment situation:** Having a conversation with . . .

2. ***Self*-focused attention:** List what you pay attention to when you are self-focused.

| |
| |
| |

3. **Conversation with self-focused attention**

4. **Rate yourself.**

	How anxious did you feel?	How self-conscious did you feel?	How anxious did you appear to others?	How good was your social performance?
Rating (0–10)				

5. ***Task*-focused attention:** List what you pay attention to when you are task focused.

| |
| |
| |

6. **Imagine yourself being task focused during the conversation.**

7. **Complete the conversation with task-focused attention.**

8. **Rate yourself.**

	How anxious did you feel?	How self-conscious did you feel?	How anxious did you appear to others?	How good was your social performance?
Rating (0–10)				

9. **Conclusions:** What was the impact of self- versus task-focused attention?

| |
| |
| |

From *Imagery-Enhanced CBT for Social Anxiety Disorder* by Peter M. McEvoy, Lisa M. Saulsman, and Ronald M. Rapee. Copyright © 2018 The Guilford Press. Permission to photocopy this material is granted to purchasers of this book for personal use or use with clients (see copyright page for details). Purchasers can download additional copies of this material (see the box at the end of the table of contents).

Attention Retraining Record

Date/ Time	Attentional Task (e.g., breath, walking, eating, sitting)	Duration	Concentration Level (0–10)	Comments

From *Imagery-Enhanced CBT for Social Anxiety Disorder* by Peter M. McEvoy, Lisa M. Saulsman, and Ronald M. Rapee. Copyright © 2018 The Guilford Press. Permission to photocopy this material is granted to purchasers of this book for personal use or use with clients (see copyright page for details). Purchasers can download additional copies of this material (see the box at the end of the table of contents).

Task-Focused Attention Exercise

Practice task-focused attention during at least one social interaction this week. Devote as much of your attention as possible to the task at hand. Below there is space for you to recall the content of the conversation in as much detail as you can. Knowing that you are planning to recall these details may help you to continue reorienting your attention back to the content of the conversation.

Date: _____

Situation/interaction: _____

Anxiety level (0–10): _____

Details of interaction (especially content of conversation)

_____

_____

_____

_____

_____

_____

_____

_____

_____

_____

_____

_____

_____

_____

_____

_____

_____

_____

Self-focused attention: _____%

Environment-focused attention: _____%

Task-focused attention: _____%

From *Imagery-Enhanced CBT for Social Anxiety Disorder* by Peter M. McEvoy, Lisa M. Saulsman, and Ronald M. Rapee. Copyright © 2018 The Guilford Press. Permission to photocopy this material is granted to purchasers of this book for personal use or use with clients (see copyright page for details). Purchasers can download additional copies of this material (see the box at the end of the table of contents).

Past Imagery Rescripting

Past image: Describe a past distressing situation. (What happened? When did it happen? Where did it happen? Who was there?) *Note.* If you can't think of a specific event, describe your earliest memory of feeling the way you do in social situations.

Meaning of the experience and image: What meaning did you take from this experience?	Belief before rescripting 0 = completely untrue, 10 = completely true	Belief after rescripting 0= completely untrue, 10 = completely true
I am . . .		
Others are . . .		
The world is . . .		
The image is . . .		

Perspective of the "older" you: What do you know now that would have been helpful to know at the time of the event? Logically, what do you know now? If a friend experienced the same situation, what perspective might you offer him or her?

After Phase 1: Imagining the event from the perspective of the "younger you"

What emotions are you feeling?	Where in your body are you feeling them?	How strong is the emotion? 0 = none, 10 = strongest ever

After Phase 2: Imagining the event from the perspective of the "compassionate older you" offering support to the "younger you"

What emotions are you feeling?	Where in your body are you feeling them?	How strong is the emotion? 0 = none, 10 = strongest ever

After Phase 3: Imagining the event from the perspective of the "younger you," but with the "compassionate older you" intervening and offering all the support you need

What emotions are you feeling?	Where in your body are you feeling them?	How strong is the emotion? 0 = none, 10 = strongest ever

Conclusions What did you learn from this?	Strength of belief 0 = completely untrue, 10 = completely true
I am . . .	
Others are . . .	
The world is . . .	
The image is . . .	
How do you feel when you think about the event now?	

From *Imagery-Enhanced CBT for Social Anxiety Disorder* by Peter M. McEvoy, Lisa M. Saulsman, and Ronald M. Rapee. Copyright © 2018 The Guilford Press. Permission to photocopy this material is granted to purchasers of this book for personal use or use with clients (see copyright page for details). Purchasers can download additional copies of this material (see the box at the end of the table of contents).

Constructing New Core Beliefs

1. A situation in which I have typically experienced strong social anxiety is . . .

2a. How would I like to be in social situations . . . ?

Actions

Expression on my face

Body posture

Self-talk

2b. How would that feel? (emotionally, physically)

Emotions

Sensations in my body

3. When operating in this new way . . .

I see **myself** as

I see **others** as

I see **the world** as

(continued)

From *Imagery-Enhanced CBT for Social Anxiety Disorder* by Peter M. McEvoy, Lisa M. Saulsman, and Ronald M. Rapee. Copyright © 2018 The Guilford Press. Permission to photocopy this material is granted to purchasers of this book for personal use or use with clients (see copyright page for details). Purchasers can download additional copies of this material (see the box at the end of the table of contents).

4. When I see myself, others, and the world in this way, what do I see myself doing (or not doing) in the following areas of my life? (Be very specific.)

My relationships

My family life

Work/study

Leisure/hobbies

Health/well-being

Other important aspects of my life

5. When I see myself, others, and the world in these more positive and helpful ways, if I were to hit "stormy weather" (e.g., something bad *does* happen), how would I like to respond?

Actions

Self-talk

Body posture

Expression on my face

Emotions

Sensations in my body

For a few minutes imagine myself being this way . . .

(continued)

6. **A past occasion when I did something that exemplifies my new core beliefs was . . .**

Now spend a few minutes visualizing this occasion.

7. **When I imagine operating in this way, what "icons" come to mind?** Are there particular songs, images, movies, characters, fairy tales, stories, people, animals, or scenes from nature that represent this way of operating? Is there something that really captures the spirit of my new, more positive core beliefs?

How do I feel in my body after bringing this icon to mind?

How could this icon be used to inspire or motivate me to continue operating within the new system of more positive core beliefs?

New Core Belief Action Plan

EXAMPLE:

New core beliefs (self, others, world)	Life domain	Target for change	Specific actions	Time frame
Self: likable Others: caring, supportive World: safe	Work	Be more assertive at work	Ask boss for a meeting to say that I need more help	Tomorrow
Self: likable Others: friendly World: safe	Relationships	Initiate more social outings	Invite work colleague for coffee at lunchtime	Ask Thursday if colleague wants to meet for coffee on Friday

My New Core Beliefs
Self:
Others:
World:

Life domain	Target for change	Specific actions	Time frame
My relationships			

(continued)

From *Imagery-Enhanced CBT for Social Anxiety Disorder* by Peter M. McEvoy, Lisa M. Saulsman, and Ronald M. Rapee. Copyright © 2018 The Guilford Press. Permission to photocopy this material is granted to purchasers of this book for personal use or use with clients (see copyright page for details). Purchasers can download additional copies of this material (see the box at the end of the table of contents).

New Core Belief Action Plan *(page 2 of 2)*

Life domain	Target for change	Specific actions	Time frame
My family life			
Work/study/ career			
My leisure/ hobbies			
My health/ well-being			
Other important areas of my life			

Your Progress

1. In what situations are you managing your social anxiety better?

2. What changes have you made in your life? What things have you done that you had not done before (or not done for a long time)?

3. What was the most important thing that you learned in treatment that contributed to reducing your anxiety in social situations?

4. What new skills are you using regularly?
   - ☐ Imagery monitoring
   - ☐ Imagery challenging
   - ☐ Coping imagery
   - ☐ Behavioral experiments
   - ☐ A structured behavioral experiment hierarchy
   - ☐ Dropping safety behaviors
   - ☐ Recalling an accurate self-image (even when anxious)
   - ☐ Attention retraining
   - ☐ Attention focusing
   - ☐ Rescripting past images
   - ☐ Action planning to strengthen your new core beliefs

5. What skills do you think you would benefit from using more often?

6. What specific situations do you need to confront to overcome remaining anxieties?

7. What specific goals can you set to help you combat these remaining anxieties?

From *Imagery-Enhanced CBT for Social Anxiety Disorder* by Peter M. McEvoy, Lisa M. Saulsman, and Ronald M. Rapee. Copyright © 2018 The Guilford Press. Permission to photocopy this material is granted to purchasers of this book for personal use or use with clients (see copyright page for details). Purchasers can download additional copies of this material (see the box at the end of the table of contents).

Dealing with Setbacks

Setbacks are normal; it is how I respond to setbacks that is most important.

My Triggers (When are setbacks in my social anxiety more likely to occur? In what types of circumstances do I tend to have a setback?)

My Warning Signs (How do I know when I have had a setback in my social anxiety? Are there any emotional, thinking, behavioral, or physical signals?)

ACTION PLAN:	
What do I need to focus on and remind myself when a social anxiety setback occurs?	What do I need to do when a social anxiety setback occurs?

From *Imagery-Enhanced CBT for Social Anxiety Disorder* by Peter M. McEvoy, Lisa M. Saulsman, and Ronald M. Rapee. Copyright © 2018 The Guilford Press. Permission to photocopy this material is granted to purchasers of this book for personal use or use with clients (see copyright page for details). Purchasers can download additional copies of this material (see the box at the end of the table of contents).

What Is Social Anxiety Disorder?

Everyone experiences anxiety from time to time, but when anxiety debilitates someone in important ways (e.g., work, social life, relationships), then he or she may be experiencing an anxiety disorder. Although you might feel alone in your struggle with anxiety, the reality is that anxiety disorders are very common. In fact, **around 1 in 5 people will experience an anxiety disorder in the course of a lifetime.**

Anxiety disorders do not discriminate, and they can affect any kind of person at any stage in of life. People can suffer from anxiety disorders regardless of their circumstances, youthful or elderly, male or female, wealthy or poor. So remember, you are not alone. In fact, you're not even very unusual!

"Social anxiety" is used to describe anxiety that occurs in response to social situations. The anxiety may occur before, during, or after the social situations, and quite often at all three time points. Of course, most people feel anxious about some social situations, such as public speaking and job interviews. Worrying about whether the speech or interview will go well, or what other people will think, is quite common. Most people will also feel relieved when it is over. For some people, however, the anxiety may be so distressing that they avoid the situation at all costs.

In clinical practice, the term "social anxiety disorder" or "social phobia" is used to describe intense, long-standing, and debilitating fear of social situations. Often people with social anxiety disorder (or SAD) will avoid social situations if they can. They worry that they will be embarrassed or humiliated in some way and that they will be evaluated negatively or criticized by other people. SAD is one of the most common anxiety disorders. Although the prevalence differs in different countries, around 8–16% of people are likely to meet criteria for the disorder in their lifetimes.

Half of all people who experience SAD will develop the disorder by the age of 13 years. Many people report always being shy or socially anxious. Unfortunately, SAD is often a chronic disorder that does not disappear without treatment and people usually suffer for many years before seeking help. **The good news is that treatment can be very effective at helping people to better manage their anxiety.**

People with SAD may fear most social situations or one or two specific situations. Therefore, just as with any other problem, people with SAD can vary in the range and severity of their difficulties.

WHAT CAUSES SAD?

There is no single or simple answer to the question of what causes SAD. Contributing factors are many, and they can vary for different individuals. However, some important factors have been identified that can increase someone's chance of developing SAD. These factors can be divided into biological and psychological causes.

Biological factors such as a family history of anxiety disorders or depression increase your

(continued)

From *Imagery-Enhanced CBT for Social Anxiety Disorder* by Peter M. McEvoy, Lisa M. Saulsman, and Ronald M. Rapee. Copyright © 2018 The Guilford Press. Permission to photocopy this material is granted to purchasers of this book for personal use or use with clients (see copyright page for details). Purchasers can download additional copies of this material (see the box at the end of the table of contents).

chances of having an anxiety disorder. The more family members you have who suffer with anxiety or depression, and the closer they are to you genetically, the more likely you are to develop an anxiety disorder. We are also born with our own temperaments, which may be inherited to some degree. Many people with SAD report that they were shy or inhibited as very young children. While most children will grow out of early shyness, if they are shyer and more timid than their peers, this also increases their chances of developing SAD later in life.

Having a biological vulnerability does not necessarily mean that someone will develop an anxiety disorder. It also may depend on the lifestyle of the person, the types of life stressors they have encountered, and their early learning. Many people with SAD report experiencing bullying or abuse during their childhood or adolescence. Some report having one or two particularly distressing social experiences that have stuck in their minds, while others report experiencing regular criticism early in life. Some report that their families did not socialize much during their childhood, so they did not have the opportunity to develop confidence in their ability to develop relationships with others.

Ultimately it probably takes a combination of biological, temperamental, and social factors for someone to develop SAD. The good news is that regardless of the causes of your SAD, effective treatment is available.

WHAT KEEPS SAD GOING?

The diagram on the last page of this handout (based on Worksheet 1) illustrates the model of SAD that will be used to guide your treatment. On the left there is a shaded box labeled triggers, which includes a range of social situations that can trigger a perception of social threat. Our perception of social threat is basically how strongly we believe that a "social catastrophe" will occur. This perception is divided into two parts: probability and cost. The probability refers to how likely our fears are to happen. If we believe our fears are highly likely to come true, then our fear response is more likely to be triggered. The cost refers to how bad we believe it will be if our fears do come true. For example, if you believe it is very likely that you will appear nervous and make a mistake when delivering a presentation (high probability), and that if this does happen you will be criticized or humiliated by others (high cost), then you are likely to feel very anxious about the presentation.

Once the perception of social threat is triggered (i.e., perceived social danger is high) you will experience a strong fear response. This usually results in physical symptoms such as:

- Trembling or shaking
- Blushing
- Pounding heart
- Mind going blank
- Nausea
- Sweating
- Overbreathing or hyperventilation
- Difficulty concentrating
- Urge to escape

(continued)

These symptoms are part of the fight-or-flight response, the body's protective mechanism. If we are under real threat (e.g., a robber) our body must ready itself to fight or flee from the threat. As a result, we get a surge of adrenaline and our respiration rate increases (to get more oxygen to the body), we sweat (to cool the body), our muscles tense (to prepare for fighting or fleeing), our heart rate increases (to pump more blood around the body), our attention narrows and focuses on the threat (so that we aren't distracted from dealing with the threat), and so on. As you can see, all these changes are designed to help us deal with the threat.

In most social situations we can't simply fight or run away at top speed, so we aren't able to use all the extra resources (e.g., adrenaline, oxygen) in our body. As a consequence, we subjectively experience these bodily changes as intense anxiety. Some people may also experience a "freeze" fear response, which is again part of our survival instinct and designed to provide another means of protecting ourselves when we can't fight or flee.

So the shaded areas of the model explain the link between the triggers, the perception of social danger (probability and cost), and the fear response. The question is, what maintains the perception of social danger? This is where the bubbles around the model come in.

NEGATIVE SOCIAL THOUGHTS AND IMAGES

Most people, when they are upset, have upsetting things going through their minds. Sometimes they are in the form of thoughts or words, and sometimes in the form of pictures or feelings in the body. These images may initially be vague or fuzzy, or they might be as clear as if you were watching a movie. They may be about past, present, or future social situations.

Images may involve multiple senses. We may *see* a visual image as if it is a film. We may *hear* sounds or verbalizations. We may associate *touch*, *taste*, or other physical or behavioral reactions with the image, as if we were in the actual situation.

Let's demonstrate. Close your eyes and imagine biting into a lemon and sucking out as much juice as you can. What reactions do you notice? Can you see the lemon wedge as you put it to your mouth? Can you imagine how it feels in your hand? Can you taste the lemon? How does your mouth respond to the taste? Do you notice an urge to take another bite, or an urge to screw up your mouth and spit it out?

People can have images before, during, and after social events. Just like the lemon, these images may have a powerful impact on multiple senses and ultimately on our emotions. Common social anxiety images may include:

- Saying something stupid and others laughing
- Other people talking about me behind my back
- Seeing myself trembling, shaking, and looking as bright red as a beet
- Seeing myself sitting away from the crowd, or not contributing
- Imagining other people looking at me as if I am very odd

(continued)

Although negative thoughts are very common, we will be focusing more on negative social images in this treatment. If you notice negative thoughts, you will be encouraged to try and transform the thoughts into images. The main reasons for this are that images (1) are more specific, (2) are more strongly linked to emotion, and (3) become less scary when we don't avoid them.

Images are often more specific than thoughts.

Many of the negative thoughts people have when they are socially anxious are catastrophic, abstract, and overgeneralized. By abstract and overgeneralized, we mean that they tend to refer to something bad happening in general or to some general negative label. For example, if you are asked about what you think will happen in a particular social situation, an overgeneralized thought might be "I will look like an idiot" or "they will think I am an idiot." The problem is that when we make such a general statement, it is unclear exactly what we mean. Specifically, what does looking like an "idiot" actually mean? Our fears remain quite vague, which makes it difficult to find ways to challenge, test, and change our fears.

Imagery forces you to be really specific about what you fear socially, which is important for effective treatment. So if instead you were asked to close your eyes and describe what you see happening in the same social situation, you might say, "I see myself shaking, stuttering, bright red, having nothing to say" (which is more specific than "looking like an idiot") or "I see others laughing at me, criticizing me, turning away and avoiding speaking to me" (which is more specific than "they will think I am an idiot").

The more specific and detailed you are about what concerns you the most socially, the better position you are in to be able to target your concerns. We now have testable fears we can work with (i.e., did you actually shake, stutter, go bright red, have nothing to say, did others actually laugh, criticize, turn away and avoid you).

Images are more strongly linked to emotion.

Research has shown that images have a very strong association with the parts of the brain that generate emotions, including anxiety. In fact, imagining something either positive or negative generates much more emotion within us than merely thinking about that same thing. So thinking in images can have a more powerful impact on our emotions (in either a negative or positive direction) than merely thinking in words. Given that we are trying to overcome the emotion of anxiety in social settings, we need to work in the "mode" most likely to impact that emotion (i.e., imagery rather than words).

The reason images are more strongly linked to our emotions is that images can be as powerful as the real thing. Research has also shown that many of the same brain pathways are involved in imagining something and actually doing it. So imagining something can have the same impact on our brain and body as if the thing we imagined were real and actually happening to us. For social anxiety, an image of being rejected prior to socializing can elicit the same feelings as actual rejection and hence stop you from socializing. Conversely, an image of being socially competent can elicit the same feelings as actual social competence and make you more inclined to socialize.

(continued)

Running images on past their worst point can make them less scary.

It is likely that when you have a negative social image pop into your head, you dwell on the worst part of it for a little bit, then when it becomes too distressing you suppress it, trying to push the image out of your mind. However, research shows that thought suppression often backfires, making you think even more about the thing you don't want to think about. So you kind of get stuck in the worst part of the image as you think about it, then suppress it, think about it, then suppress it, and so on. Overall this keeps your anxiety and concerns about the situation very high. The alternative is to think about the negative social image fully from beginning to end, rather than suppressing it. By doing this you won't get stuck at the worst point. Instead you can run it on past this point and see what you discover about yourself and other people. It is likely that when you take this approach, your anxiety and concerns will be more like a wave, subsiding when you allow yourself to move past the worst point.

AVOIDANCE

In order to stop feeling anxious, most people with social anxiety try to avoid social situations, including:

- Interacting in groups/going to parties
- Initiating and maintaining conversations
- Meeting new people/dating
- Public speaking
- Being watched while writing, eating, or drinking
- Being assertive with others
- Using public toilets

People with social anxiety might also try to avoid the negative imagery. They may use cognitive and/or behavioral avoidance strategies.

Cognitive avoidance may include:
- Distracting yourself from the images
- Suppressing the images (actively trying to push them out of your mind)
- Criticizing yourself for having the thoughts in the first place
- Worrying or ruminating about the situation (research shows that repetitively thinking about the situation in *words* helps us to *avoid* having as many distressing negative *images*)
- Thinking about ways of escaping the situation or image

Behavioral avoidance may include:
- Escaping from the situation, or avoiding it in the first place, to avoid the negative images
- Using subtle avoidance behaviors to try and prevent our images from coming true (e.g., avoiding eye contact, not contributing to conversations, only speaking with "safe" people). These are called "safety behaviors" (see below for more detail).

(continued)

Avoidance makes sense in the short term because it may provide some relief from the anxiety. However, the relief is only temporary because the underlying perception of social threat is never directly tested, challenged, and modified. As a consequence, the social fear maintains indefinitely. In fact, avoidance usually results in increasing anxiety in more and more situations as people learn that they cannot cope with social situations. Avoidance also causes a lot of practical problems and interference in people's lives.

SAFETY BEHAVIORS

Sometimes it is not possible to completely avoid social situations. In these cases, socially anxious people often use "safety" behaviors to help them feel more comfortable. Safety behaviors are any things you do within social situations to try and prevent your fears from coming true. Common safety behaviors include:

- Using alcohol or drugs
- Not making eye contact
- Not contributing to discussions/meetings
- Wearing inconspicuous clothes
- Asking a lot of questions so you don't need to disclose personal information
- Making excuses to leave early
- Covering up your anxiety symptoms in some way (e.g., using makeup to cover blushing)
- Perfectionistic behaviors such as overpreparation for presentations/meetings
- Carrying or taking antianxiety medications "when needed"
- Only talking to specific "safe" people

We might feel like these "tricks of the trade" are helping to reduce our anxiety and prevent social catastrophes, but in fact they just stop us from learning that our fears are less likely to happen than we think (probability) and less catastrophic when they do happen (cost). If a social situation goes well it doesn't seem to make a difference to our social anxiety because we attribute the success to our safety behavior, rather than learning that the situation itself is safe and we can cope socially. Safety behaviors can actually make things worse because they can cause us to become more self-focused and appear less engaged in the social situation.

IMAGE OF HOW I APPEAR TO OTHERS

Close your eyes and see if you can create a mental image of how you think you appear to other people when you are feeling socially anxious. Most people with social anxiety imagine that they are performing very badly and that this is blatantly obvious to other people. In our "mind's eye" we may see ourselves blushing bright red, shaking, trembling, looking away, sweating, and stumbling over our words. However, we know that many people who feel anxious in social situations do not have accurate views about how they appear to others. It is very likely that although you

(continued)

may feel anxious, others cannot see this. In fact, most people with social anxiety come across far better than they think they do. Inaccurate and overly negative images of your social performance can therefore mislead you and increase your perception of social threat.

SELF- AND ENVIRONMENT-FOCUSED ATTENTION

People with social anxiety focus their attention in ways that increase their anxiety in social situations. In particular, socially anxious people focus most of their attention on themselves, including their physical symptoms of social anxiety and their negative thoughts and images (self-focused attention). They may also look around their environment for any evidence that they are in fact being negatively evaluated (e.g., people laughing in another part of the room, anyone looking in my direction; environment-focused attention). When most of our attention is directed toward ourselves and/or looking for threats in our environment, very little attention is left over to focus on the "task at hand" (task-focused attention). The effects of this are to increase self-consciousness and anxiety, and it interferes with social performance because you are not focusing on what you are trying to do (e.g., maintain a conversation).

CORE BELIEFS

The final "bubble" in the model refers to core beliefs. Many people with SAD recall early life events (childhood, adolescence, early adulthood) that were associated with significant social anxiety. There may be one or two situations, or many early experiences, that you identify as substantially contributing to your social anxiety. These early experiences may be associated with important meanings about ourselves, others, and the world in general (i.e., core beliefs), which then manifest as negative images in the here and now. For example, if I was bullied I may have formed core beliefs such as "I am unlikable" or "I am inferior." I might also have come to believe that "others are hostile or critical." As a consequence, when I think about entering a social situation now, I envision my "inferiority" as being obvious and I expect to be criticized by others. Core beliefs are not necessarily conscious thoughts, but are more like unwritten rules or assumptions through which people interpret what is happening around them. They can act like filters that guide our images and expectations in the here and now.

All of the bubbles in this model work together to cause you to feel anxious and uncomfortable in social situations. So you can see that social anxiety has a mix of factors maintaining the problem. The good news is that the components of this model can also work for us because making a change in any one of the bubbles can flow through to the others.

The treatment you are undertaking will help you to make changes in each bubble within the model of social anxiety.

(continued)

MODEL OF SOCIAL ANXIETY

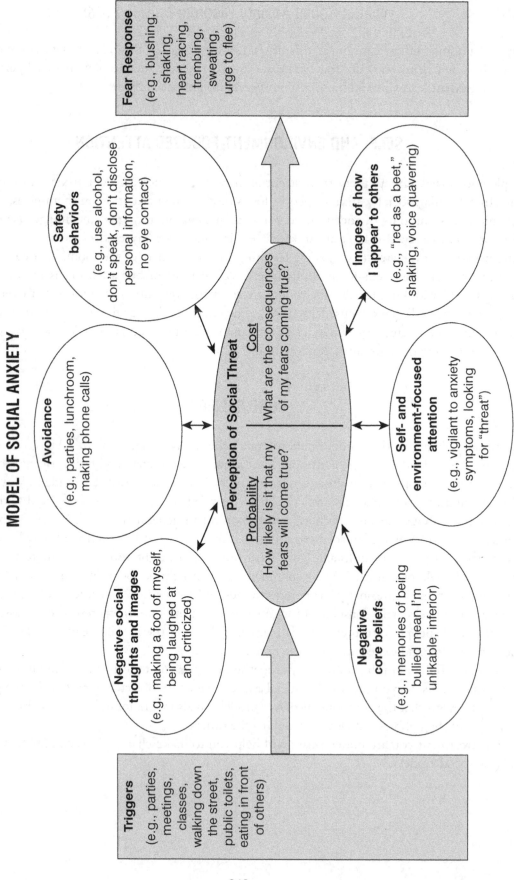

Triggers

(e.g., parties, meetings, classes, walking down the street, public toilets, eating in front of others)

Negative social thoughts and images

(e.g., making a fool of myself, being laughed at and criticized)

Avoidance

(e.g., parties, lunchroom, making phone calls)

Safety behaviors

(e.g., use alcohol, don't speak, don't disclose personal information, no eye contact)

Perception of Social Threat

<u>Probability</u>
How likely is it that my fears will come true?

<u>Cost</u>
What are the consequences of my fears coming true?

Negative core beliefs

(e.g., memories of being bullied mean I'm unlikable, inferior)

Self- and environment-focused attention

(e.g., vigilant to anxiety symptoms, looking for "threat")

Images of how I appear to others

(e.g., "red as a beet," shaking, voice quavering)

Fear Response

(e.g., blushing, shaking, heart racing, trembling, sweating, urge to flee)

Recording Thoughts and Images

Most people have thoughts and/or "pictures" or images going through their minds before, during, and after anxiety-provoking social situations. Some people also hear the sounds of people's voices; experience the body in various ways, like feeling small and fragile or feeling stuck in a box; or experience imaginary tastes or smells. These images may initially be vague or fuzzy and may not seem to make sense, but they may still turn out to be the worth tuning in to.

You may be very aware of such thoughts and imagery, or you may not. During this treatment you will be encouraged to start "tuning in" to thoughts and images going through your mind when you feel anxious. These thoughts and images may be of past experiences or about what is happening during a social interaction, or they may reflect future expectations.

You are encouraged to increase your awareness of various elements of your thoughts and images, which are outlined in the *Thought and Imagery Record* (Worksheet 5). Use this form to keep track of your imagery.

If you are having difficulty noticing your thoughts and imagery during the week, practice closing your eyes and thinking back to a past *social* situation in which you felt anxious. Don't start with the most anxiety-provoking social experience. The Subjective Units of Distress Scale (SUDS) can help you to monitor the intensity of your anxiety, with a SUDS of 10 being the most severe social anxiety you've ever experienced, 7–8 being high, 5 being moderate, 2–3 being mild, and 0 being no anxiety at all (see the scale below). A good place to start is by recalling a past situation with a SUDS rating of around 5/10. Imagine the *social* situation as vividly as possible and complete a *Thought and Imagery Record* for this situation. An example is provided on the next page.

SUDS = SUBJECTIVE UNITS OF DISTRESS SCALE

No anxiety		Mild			Moderate		High		Extreme anxiety	
0	1	2	3	4	5	6	7	8	9	10

(continued)

From *Imagery-Enhanced CBT for Social Anxiety Disorder* by Peter M. McEvoy, Lisa M. Saulsman, and Ronald M. Rapee. Copyright © 2018 The Guilford Press. Permission to photocopy this material is granted to purchasers of this book for personal use or use with clients (see copyright page for details). Purchasers can download additional copies of this material (see the box at the end of the table of contents).

Recording Thoughts and Images *(page 2 of 2)*

THOUGHT AND IMAGERY RECORD—EXAMPLE

Trigger/Situation What is happening? Where am I?	Thoughts What thoughts are going through my mind?	Visual Image What specific images arise from these thoughts about the situation?	Sensations What sensations are part of the image (body, taste, smell, sound)?	Emotion How did I feel? SUDS 0–10?
I'm about to go into the lunchroom at work.	I hate being the center of attention, my colleagues will think I'm a loser and that I'm really boring.	Everyone stares at me as I walk in. I sit down, they are all interacting loudly with each other I'm not saying anything. They deliberately ignore me.	I get this sensation of being in the heat of a bright spotlight. My body feels really jittery and small. I can hear the other people talking and laughing loudly. I can almost smell the coffee and toast in the lunchroom.	Anxious and embarrassed 8/10

Challenging Negative Thoughts and Images

So far you have been "tuning in" to your negative thoughts and images when you feel socially anxious. It is now time to start scrutinizing these negative thoughts and images. Effective challenging of anxious thoughts and images involves eight steps. The *Imagery Challenging Record* (Worksheet 6) can help to guide you through this process. An example is provided on the next page.

Step 1: Trigger Situation: What is the situation? Where am I? Briefly describe what was (past event) or is (present event) happening and who is there.

Step 2: Negative Image: Describe the negative visual images going through your mind. Also describe other senses in the image (i.e., sounds, body/touch sensations, tastes, smells). If thoughts in the form of words are the most prominent thing on your mind, close your eyes and see what picture represents those thoughts.

Step 3: Emotion: Describe the emotions you are feeling and indicate their intensity using SUDS ratings.

Step 4: Contrary Evidence: Look for contrary evidence and consider alternative images and thoughts.

It is easy to fall into the trap of only recognizing or remembering experiences that confirm our fears, while ignoring contrary experiences. The best way to counteract this bias or "filter" is to think about evidence that does not support your negative images. The types of questions you can ask yourself are:

- *Have I had any experiences that show that this image is not completely true all of the time?*
- *Are there any small things that contradict my image that I might be ignoring?*
- *Have I been in this type of situation before? What happened? Is there anything different between this situation and previous ones? What have I learned from prior experiences that could help me now?*
- *Is my image based on facts, or am I "mind reading"? What evidence do I really have?*
- *Am I jumping to conclusions that are not completely justified by the evidence?*
- *If someone who loves me knew I was having this image, what would they say to me? What evidence would they point out that would suggest that my image was not 100% true?*
- *Are there other ways of looking at this situation?*
- *What are all the possible explanations in this situation? Are there any alternatives to mine?*
- *What's the best that could happen?*
- *What's the worst that could happen? What's so bad about that? Could I cope with this? Would life go on? What could I do that would help?*
- *Will this still bother me in 1 week/month/year?*
- *If the roles were reversed, how might I judge the situation/other person?*
- *Regardless of whether the image is true, is it helpful to think this way? What are the negative consequences of thinking this way? What would be a more helpful way to think or a more helpful image to hold?*

Step 5: Realistic Probability and Consequences: Given the contrary evidence and alternative perspectives, now consider the most realistic probability and consequences. What is the most likely outcome? What are the most likely consequences?

Step 6 Helpful Image: Describe the most realistic outcome and/or a more helpful image.

Step 7: Now spend a few moments visualizing this helpful image.

Step 8: Describe and rate the strength of your emotions as you visualized the new helpful image.

(continued)

From *Imagery-Enhanced CBT for Social Anxiety Disorder* by Peter M. McEvoy, Lisa M. Saulsman, and Ronald M. Rapee. Copyright © 2018 The Guilford Press. Permission to photocopy this material is granted to purchasers of this book for personal use or use with clients (see copyright page for details). Purchasers can download additional copies of this material (see the box at the end of the table of contents).

Challenging Negative Thoughts and Images *(page 2 of 2)*

IMAGERY CHALLENGING RECORD—EXAMPLE

1. Trigger Situation What was/is happening? Where am I?	2. Negative Image What visual images/thoughts are going through my mind? Body sensations, taste, smell, touch, sound?	3. Emotion How do I feel? How intensely (SUDS 0–10)?	4. Contrary Evidence What evidence do I have that does not support these thoughts/images? Alternative ways to view the situation?	5. Realistic Probability and Consequences How likely is it that my negative thoughts/images are accurate? If something bad happened, then so what? Would it really be that bad? Would I cope?	6. Helpful Image Describe as a picture the most realistic outcome and/or a more helpful image.	8. Rerate Emotion Describe and rate emotions during helpful image (SUDS 0–10).
I'm about to go into the lunchroom at work.	Everyone will stare at me as I walk in.	Anxious and embarrassed 8/10	People don't always look up whenever I enter a room.	It is likely (50%) that some people will look at me, but not everyone. It is unlikely they will actually stare (i.e., look longer than 3 seconds)	A couple of people glance as I walk in the room and then go back to their conversation.	Still a bit anxious (5/10), but not embarrassed (2/10)
	They will all interact with each other, but I won't say anything.		I am often quiet and don't say anything unless someone asks me a question, but not always.	It is very likely (90%) that I will be quiet and not say anything unless I'm spoken to.	I sit at the table and a couple of people say hi. I listen to the conversation.	
	They will deliberately ignore me.		Sometimes people do make small talk with me.		One person asks me a question.	
	Bright spotlight.		It would be pretty rude to just stare at someone who had just walked in.	It is possible (30%) that someone will try to speak with me.	I focus on eating my lunch, and making the effort to talk and ask them a question back.	
	I feel jittery, small.		If they don't include me it might be because they are caught up in the conversation they are already having.	If some people do look at me I will feel uncomfortable, but then they will probably just go back to what they are doing.	My colleagues are mostly friendly and are just interested in whatever conversation is going on.	
	I hear their loud voices.			If no-one speaks to me then I will just read my magazine.	The times I am silent are OK by everyone.	
	I can smell the lunchroom.			My colleagues are unlikely to ignore me in a rude or critical way.		

7. Visualize the helpful image as if it were actually occurring now.

The Cycle of Avoidance and Anxiety

People with social anxiety often rely on avoidance as a way to minimize their anxiety. On the one hand, avoidance seems like a very sensible strategy. Anyone who had very negative expectations about social situations would want to avoid them. This makes perfect sense. On the other hand, avoidance is one of the main reasons that social anxiety persists. In fact, social anxiety is likely to persist indefinitely until social fears are directly tested.

WHAT'S THE PROBLEM WITH AVOIDANCE?

Although in the short term avoidance may help us to feel safer and less anxious, in the longer term avoidance keeps us anxious for a number of reasons.

1. *We never get to test our negative images.* When we avoid a social situation we are assuming that our negative images are accurate reflections of reality. However, avoidance never gives us an opportunity to directly test our fears. If we did, we might discover that our images are actually inaccurate. We might learn that in fact our fears rarely come true and instead that things often turn out pretty well. We might also find that even if social experiences don't go according to plan sometimes, we can cope with this as well. So avoidance prevents us from getting an accurate impression of the true probability and cost of our fears coming true.

2. *We never get opportunities for positive experiences.* As long as we avoid social situations, we have no chance of having positive social experiences that would motivate us to engage more socially over time.

3. *Loss of self-esteem.* Because people with social anxiety aren't doing what they would really like to do (i.e., have more satisfying relationships) they tend to be very self-critical and can have low self-esteem. They may ruminate a lot about aspects of life that are passing them by, which leaves them more vulnerable to further anxiety and depressed mood. In fact, people with social anxiety can often use their avoidance as just another reason to criticize themselves.

4. *Avoidance and anxiety can generalize.* As we avoid and lose confidence in one area of our lives (e.g., relationships with peers), our anxiety can start to generalize to more and more domains of life (e.g., work, family relationships).

(continued)

From *Imagery-Enhanced CBT for Social Anxiety Disorder* by Peter M. McEvoy, Lisa M. Saulsman, and Ronald M. Rapee. Copyright © 2018 The Guilford Press. Permission to photocopy this material is granted to purchasers of this book for personal use or use with clients (see copyright page for details). Purchasers can download additional copies of this material (see the box at the end of the table of contents).

For all these reasons, it is crucial that the cycle of avoidance and increasing anxiety is broken. Behavioral experiments are a very effective way of achieving this.

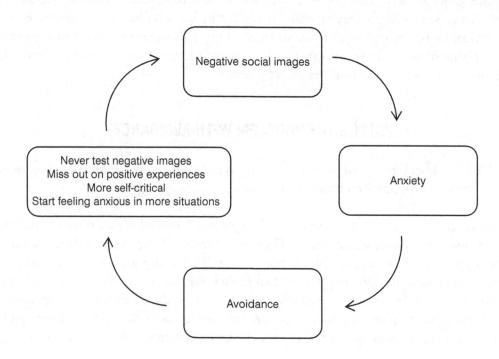

Safety Behaviors

It is very difficult to completely avoid all social situations. However, when people with social anxiety can't avoid social situations they often rely on more subtle forms of avoidance called **safety behaviors**. Safety behaviors are used in an attempt to prevent feared predictions from coming true and to feel more comfortable in social situations. Examples of common safety behaviors include:

Safety Behavior	Function: Why Use It?
No/limited eye contact	To avoid drawing attention to myself To avoid seeing negative reactions from others
Alcohol/drugs	I don't believe I can interact with other people without it I think my anxiety will overwhelm me without it
Don't contribute to conversations	I believe I'll say something stupid and be criticized Something bad will happen if I'm the focus of attention
Rehearse/plan what I'm about to say	To make sure it isn't stupid To make sure I don't stumble over my words
Wear inconspicuous clothes	To avoid drawing attention to myself
Wear makeup	To cover blushing

List some of your safety behaviors.

_____

_____

_____

_____

_____

_____

_____

_____

_____

_____

_____

_____

(continued)

From *Imagery-Enhanced CBT for Social Anxiety Disorder* by Peter M. McEvoy, Lisa M. Saulsman, and Ronald M. Rapee. Copyright © 2018 The Guilford Press. Permission to photocopy this material is granted to purchasers of this book for personal use or use with clients (see copyright page for details). Purchasers can download additional copies of this material (see the box at the end of the table of contents).

SO WHAT IS THE PROBLEM WITH SAFETY BEHAVIORS?

While safety behaviors may help people to feel safer in the short term, unfortunately they serve to maintain social anxiety in the longer term because . . .

1. *Safety behaviors stop us from directly testing our fears.* Although we haven't avoided the situation completely, by using our safety behaviors we are not directly testing our fears. For instance, if I attend a work meeting but don't contribute, I never get to test my image of "saying something stupid and other people laughing or looking confused at my answers." When the next meeting comes along the same image will come to mind and again I will be gripped by fear. If I directly tested my fear by making a comment in the meeting I would have an opportunity to discover that my negative image was inaccurate. After I test the image numerous times and find that it does not come true then the negative image can be seen for what it is—just an image that does not reflect reality. It will have less emotional impact, and it will no longer need to dictate what I do.

2. *Safety behaviors can become "self-fulfilling prophecies."* Safety behaviors can actually cause the outcomes we are trying to prevent by using them. For instance, if I use alcohol because otherwise I don't believe that I could interact with people, I might find myself overindulging at times and acting in ways that result in negative evaluation from others (e.g., drunken behavior). So the "safety behavior" has *increased* the chances of negative evaluation rather than reduced it. Similarly, my boss might get more frustrated with me for not contributing to meetings than if I did contribute from time to time.

3. *If our fears don't come true we mistakenly "thank" the safety behavior.* If we use our safety behaviors and our fears don't come true, we might believe that the safety behaviors "prevented" this from happening. As a result we can become very dependent upon our safety behaviors and start to feel even more anxious if they can't be used (e.g., no alcohol available, not given time to overprepare for meetings). The truth may be that our fears wouldn't have come true even without the safety behavior, but we never discover this as long as we continue relying on them.

4. *Safety behaviors increase our self-focused attention.* Safety behaviors often involve people scrutinizing themselves (what they are doing, how they are doing it, monitoring their thoughts), which can be very distracting. Self-focused attention hijacks attention from the task at hand (e.g., the conversation), which can make it even more difficult to keep up with conversations and contribute.

So, as you can see, safety behaviors may not in fact help to reduce our anxiety in the longer term. If your anxiety remains high after repeatedly confronting a social situation, chances are you are using safety behaviors that are preventing you from directly testing your fears.

Behavioral Experiments

Just like a scientist using an experiment to test a prediction, behavioral experiments are designed to test our negative images or beliefs about social situations. Behavioral experiments provide a structured way of systematically and directly testing our fears once and for all.

There are a number of steps to conducting a behavioral experiment that enable us to learn as much as possible from social experiences. Use the *Behavioral Experiment Record* (Worksheet 7) to help you with the process of planning your experiment and collecting the results. An example is provided on the next page.

Step 1: Negative Image: Identify a social situation that triggers anxiety for you and bring to mind an image of what you think will happen in this situation. Write a description (in words or pictures) of this image. What are you seeing happen? What are other people doing? How are they responding to you? How will they respond to you in the future as a consequence? What are you doing? How does the image start and end?

Step 2: SUDS: Rate the intensity of your anxiety about this situation (0 = no anxiety, 10 = maximum anxiety).

Step 3: Experiment: Plan your experiment. What could you do to find out how accurate this image is? How could you create a situation that would enable you to test the accuracy of this image?

Step 4: Evidence to Observe: What evidence would you need to look for to confirm or disconfirm the accuracy of your image? This evidence must be unambiguous (i.e., clear, observable, objective evidence). Would the evidence hold up in a court of law, or would the judge "throw it out of court" because it was subjective/speculative?

Step 5: Do the Experiment.

Step 6: Results: Note the results. Specifically, what evidence (for and against your negative image) did you observe?

Step 7: Conclusion: Develop some conclusions. What do the results tell you about your initial negative image?

Step 8: Update Imagery. Close your eyes and spend a few minutes now re-creating the image in your mind, but this time incorporating what you learned from your experiment. How is your experience of this image different from your initial negative image? How does this new image make you feel?

(continued)

From *Imagery-Enhanced CBT for Social Anxiety Disorder* by Peter M. McEvoy, Lisa M. Saulsman, and Ronald M. Rapee. Copyright © 2018 The Guilford Press. Permission to photocopy this material is granted to purchasers of this book for personal use or use with clients (see copyright page for details). Purchasers can download additional copies of this material (see the box at the end of the table of contents).

Behavioral Experiments *(page 2 of 2)*

BEHAVIORAL EXPERIMENT RECORD—EXAMPLE

Negative Image Describe your prediction. Specifically, what do you envision happening?	SUDS (/10) How anxious do you feel?	Experiment Specifically, what could you do to test this image? **Safety behaviors to drop?**	Evidence to Observe Specifically, what do you need to look for to confirm or disconfirm your image? **Where to focus attention?**	Results What happened? What clear evidence did you collect? Stick to unambiguous facts.	Conclusion What conclusion follows from your results?
I walk into the lunchroom and my colleagues ask me a question that I can't answer. I hesitate, stumble over my words, and feel an adrenaline rush. I can't finish my sentence, my colleagues look very confused, and I get up and leave abruptly.	9/10	Go into the lunchroom when two colleagues are there. Instead of not speaking and looking down pretending I am reading, look up and make a contribution to their conversation.	Can I finish a sentence without stumbling? Do my colleagues listen? Do they stop and look confused or does the conversation just continue?	I made one comment and they agreed. I couldn't see any sign of confusion. I felt anxious but was able to finish my sentence. There was no evidence that they didn't understand my point or that they were being critical.	My image wasn't accurate this time. I need to keep testing it. My negative image was telling me that my work colleagues were going to act like bullies, but that wasn't the case.

Close eyes and update image based on results and conclusions.

252

Behavioral Experiment Menu

Many behavioral experiments are designed to test the likelihood/probability of our fears occurring, and by now you might be recognizing that your fears are much less likely to come true than you initially thought. But how about the cost/consequences, should they come true?

We are now going to test, once and for all, the true cost of drawing attention to ourselves. How much does it really *need* to matter?

The activities from the list below can be completed as behavioral experiments. Select a task that you find anxiety provoking and complete the first four steps of a *Behavioral Experiment Record* (Worksheet 7). Complete the rest of the record after doing the experiments.

1. Devise three questions you could ask people about their anxiety in social situations. Then approach shoppers and ask them to participate in a brief survey about social anxiety.
2. Look upward and point to the sky for 5 minutes.
3. Pretend to be a street performer and sing a song on a busy street corner.
4. Walk around with a sign on your back proclaiming your support for a sports team.
5. Sit down in a busy café or fast-food outlet and sing happy birthday to yourself . . . then repeat.
6. Walk around with a party hat and a whistle.
7. Skip down the street.
8. Yell "hey" at people and wave.
9. Dance down the street with the most humorous moves you can think of.
10. Take a piece of fruit or other item "for a walk" on a piece of string.
11. Walk down the street with your sweater or shirt on back to front and inside out.
12. Walk down the street with toilet paper hanging out of the back of your pants.
13. Approach strangers and give them a compliment
14. Approach strangers and ask them for the time, preferably while wearing a watch.
15. Go to a shop and buy something, then immediately ask to return it.
16. Ask a salesperson in a shop for help and deliberately look nervous.
17. Deliberately spill a drink while by yourself in a restaurant.
18. Go to a bookshop and ask an employee to help you find a book about social anxiety.
19. Go to a small clothing boutique and try on some expensive clothes that you have no intention of buying.
20. Go into a drug store or supermarket and ask a clerk for a packet of colored condoms.
21. At the supermarket ask an employee where an item is when you're right in front of it.
22. Deliberately drop an item while waiting in line at the supermarket.
23. Without giving a reason, ask people in front of you in a line if you can go ahead of them.
24. Strike up a conversation with people at the checkout and tell them something personal about yourself.
25. Do something in public and simulate the anxiety symptoms you are concerned about (e.g., shaking, blushing, sweating, trembling, stumbling over words).

From *Imagery-Enhanced CBT for Social Anxiety Disorder* by Peter M. McEvoy, Lisa M. Saulsman, and Ronald M. Rapee. Copyright © 2018 The Guilford Press. Permission to photocopy this material is granted to purchasers of this book for personal use or use with clients (see copyright page for details). Purchasers can download additional copies of this material (see the box at the end of the table of contents).

Behavioral Experiment Hierarchies

A behavioral experiment hierarchy is a tool for planning behavioral experiments in increasing order of difficulty. Experiments that generate mild anxiety (say, around 3–4 out of 10) will be at the bottom of the hierarchy, those that generate moderate anxiety (5–7 out of 10) will be in the middle, and those that generate high anxiety (8–10 out of 10) will be at the top. The basic process is to:

1. *Identify an area for change.* What would you like to be different? Or in what area of your life are you having difficulties that you would most like to change?
2. *Identify your negative image* of what you predict will happen in this situation or area of your life. What are you worried may happen? What image do you have of this situation?
3. *Design as many experiments as possible* that will help you test this predicted image.
4. *Place these experiments in order of difficulty* using the *Behavioral Experiment Hierarchy* (Worksheet 9).

HOW TO COME UP WITH DIFFERENT STEPS ON YOUR HIERARCHY

Try and think about what makes social situations more or less difficult for you. Ask yourself the following questions:

- **What** am I doing?
- **Where** am I doing it? How familiar/unfamiliar is the place?
- **When** am I doing it?
- **Who** is there? How many people are there? How familiar/unfamiliar are the people?

As you consider these questions, you may be able to manipulate these variables to make a task more or less challenging. For instance, I might feel more anxious if there are more people around. So walking down the street at quieter times of the day might be ranked around the bottom of my hierarchy and walking down the street at busier times of day might be closer to the top.

Write down what variables make you feel more or less anxious (e.g., number of people, gender of other person, formal or informal situations):

_____

_____

_____

Now use these variables to design your behavioral experiment hierarchy (see Worksheet 9). Some examples to get you thinking are on the following pages.

(continued)

From *Imagery-Enhanced CBT for Social Anxiety Disorder* by Peter M. McEvoy, Lisa M. Saulsman, and Ronald M. Rapee. Copyright © 2018 The Guilford Press. Permission to photocopy this material is granted to purchasers of this book for personal use or use with clients (see copyright page for details). Purchasers can download additional copies of this material (see the box at the end of the table of contents).

BEHAVIORAL EXPERIMENT HIERARCHY—EXAMPLE 1

Area for change: *Increase my social network*

Image(s) in these situations (describe in words or pictures):

I have nothing to say. I am stumbling over my words or not saying anything. People are criticizing me for being boring or they are laughing at me. They don't want to speak to me any further.

	SUDS (/10)
Goal: *Join a sports team*	
Go to a social function with teammates.	10
Sign up to join the team. Attend training and speak to a couple of my teammates.	9
Attend one training session, just to watch. Introduce myself to the coach.	8
Phone the local soccer club and find out information about the team. Ask at least three questions.	7
Initiate a conversation with someone before a class. Ask two questions and say one thing about myself. Speak to the same person briefly after the class.	6
Sit next to the person again in the next class and ask her a question.	5
Say one thing to the person I sit next to in class.	4
Initiate a conversation with my neighbor (1–2 minutes).	3

(continued)

BEHAVIORAL EXPERIMENT HIERARCHY—EXAMPLE 2

Area for change: *Be more assertive*

Image(s) in these situations (describe in words or pictures):

> *Others are getting hostile toward me for saying no or expressing my own opinion. They are being critical, dismissive, and rude. They turn away from me, not wanting anything to do with me. I can't handle the feeling of others not liking me.*

Goal: *Express my own opinion/be able to disagree*	**SUDS (/10)**
Ask my boss for a raise.	*10*
Tell my colleague that I cannot help her with her project until next week.	*9*
Complain to a waiter about the food at a restaurant.	*8/9*
When someone makes a suggestion (e.g., restaurant/activity), provide an alternative suggestion.	*8*
Suggest a particular restaurant for dinner with friends/family.	*7*
Buy something at a large chain store, then take it back and ask for a refund right away.	*6*
Catch the bus and pay the driver with a $50 bill.	*5*
Try something on in a large chain clothing store and don't buy it.	*4*
Walk past a salesperson at the store and say "No, thanks" immediately without stopping.	*3*

(continued)

BEHAVIORAL EXPERIMENT HIERARCHY—EXAMPLE 3

Area for change: *Feel more comfortable being the center of attention*

Image(s) in these situations (describe in words or pictures):

I am blushing, stumbling over my words, and my mind is blank. I don't make any sense. People can see how anxious I am. They are smirking and whispering among themselves about me.

	SUDS (/10)
Goal: *Make a speech at my sister's wedding*	
Give a presentation at the main work meeting with all colleagues.	*10*
Make a brief presentation at a small work meeting.	*9*
Practice my speech in front of my partner and sister.	*8*
Make at least one contribution to a work meeting.	*8*
Meet with my boss alone to make a suggestion for change.	*7*
Intentionally be the last one to enter the room for a meeting.	*6*
Wear a brightly colored shirt to work.	*5*
Walk down the street without sunglasses on.	*4*
Speak on the phone within earshot of a colleague.	*3*

(continued)

257

BEHAVIORAL EXPERIMENT HIERARCHY—EXAMPLE 4

Area for change: _Initiate conversations more often_

Image(s) in these situations (describe in words or pictures):

I don't know what to say. I feel awkward. I am silent. I blurt out stupid comments that don't make sense to break the silence. The other person is looking at me with a weird expression on his or her face.

	SUDS (/10)
Goal: *Initiate a conversation with someone I'm very physically attracted to*	
Try to maintain a longer (5–10 min) conversation with a friend at college who I am moderately physically attracted to.	*10*
Initiate a short conversation with a friend at college who I am moderately physically attracted to.	*9*
Initiate a short conversation with a friend at college about a controversial topic (e.g., politics, religion).	*8*
Initiate a short conversation with a friend about a sports team he follows, and then say that I root for a different team and why I think they are better.	*8*
Say hi to someone who is sitting next to me on the bus, then ask how her day is going.	*7*
Initiate a short conversation with a friend at college. Disclose one thing about myself (e.g., an opinion on something).	*6*
Speak to my housemate over dinner. Ask at least three questions.	*5*
Tell a checkout clerk one thing about my day.	*4*
Ask a checkout clerk how his day is going.	*3*

Coping (Metaphorical) Imagery

Metaphors are symbols/objects that represent our experiences or feelings (as opposed to being real or literal). We often talk and think in metaphors without realizing it ("being put through the wringer" "like a caged animal," "deer in the headlights," "my back to the wall").

Putting our feelings into words can be hard, and metaphors seem to be a really good way of capturing how we are feeling emotionally. Also, metaphorical images seem to connect to our feelings more strongly than words.

Developing a metaphorical (or coping) image that represents your anxiety can help you to see your anxiety from a different perspective, which can help you persevere through difficult experiences and develop confidence in your ability to pursue your goals.

Some examples of coping images include:

Anxious Image	Coping Image
Anxiety as a giant ocean wave I am drowning in	Surfing the wave in to shore
Anxiety is like hiding in a dark cave	I am stepping out of the cave into the light of a beautiful sunny garden
My anxiety is like being trapped under a cage	A loved one lifting the cage up and freeing me
My anxiety feels like a big rock weighing down on my chest	Pushing the rock off my chest, standing up, and taking a breath

Developing an image that represents your anxiety can give you an opportunity to allow a coping image to arise that symbolizes or represents the feeling of coping. It can take time and it may feel strange, that's OK.

Developing a coping image involves doing the following . . .

Let an image arise in your mind that represents your anxiety. Take some time to pay attention to what it is like (e.g., size, color, lighting, how it looks from different angles, texture, weight, smells, sounds, tastes). Consider what this image means about you or your anxiety. What meaning is the image trying to convey?

Consider what would need to be different in the anxious image for you to feel better or to resolve the problem that is going on in the image. What needs to change in the image? It may involve introducing some new action, or new person, or new object, or seeing the image from a different vantage point that allows other things to enter it. Think about what is needed to change the image for the better.

Now that you know what needs to change, try to see these changes taking place now. Find ways of making these changes happen in the image. It may take a number of tries, but keep persisting until the problem in the image has a satisfactory resolution.

Notice how the new image (which we will call your **coping image**) makes you feel emotionally. What sensations do you notice in your body?

Try to bring this new coping image to mind when you are confronting anxiety-provoking situations. Notice the impact it has on how you feel and your ability to persevere as you confront your anxiety and pursue your goals.

From *Imagery-Enhanced CBT for Social Anxiety Disorder* by Peter M. McEvoy, Lisa M. Saulsman, and Ronald M. Rapee. Copyright © 2018 The Guilford Press. Permission to photocopy this material is granted to purchasers of this book for personal use or use with clients (see copyright page for details). Purchasers can download additional copies of this material (see the box at the end of the table of contents).

Self-Image: How I *Really* Appear to Others

Research has shown that socially anxious people underestimate their social performance relative to others. This is because people who are socially anxious base their judgments on how they are feeling, rather than how they are actually performing. This is called "emotional reasoning," whereby the person has decided that "because I feel anxious I must look anxious."

If the image we have of ourselves is very negative, this will increase our perception of social threat. For instance, if I feel warmth in my cheeks and notice that I am shaking and sweating, I might imagine "in my mind's eye" that my face is as bright as a beet, I am shaking like a leaf, and sweating profusely. The image I have is that these symptoms are highly obvious to everyone around me, which may lead me to expect negative evaluation from others.

But what if our symptoms aren't anywhere near as obvious to others as we think they are? What if we find that in fact many of the symptoms you thought were obvious are actually very mild (or unnoticeable) from other people's perspective (the observer perspective)? What impact would that have on your expectations of negative evaluation?

You can obtain feedback in a number of ways. If you are getting feedback from other people, it is important to choose someone you can trust who will give you honest and balanced feedback (i.e., not overly positive or negative). It will also be helpful if you ask for feedback that directly addresses your specific concerns/fears (e.g., "do I sweat profusely when I socialize?"). You should therefore identify in as clear and detailed a manner as possible the features of your performance you are concerned about beforehand and have a trusted person observe you socially and give feedback on these areas of concern.

As a way of illustrating the power of feedback, and how self-perceptions can sometimes be inaccurate, we can also set up an experiment where you watch and evaluate a video of yourself giving an impromptu speech, which is something that makes most people anxious. We need you to be anxious, so we can then compare what you see on the video to your initial judgments of how obvious you imagine your anxiety symptoms are to others. It is therefore important that you try and make these judgments as objective as possible. It may be helpful to watch the video a number of times first to reduce that initial self-consciousness or "yuk" reaction. You may also want to try and watch it as if it is someone else on the video. Would you be making the same judgments if it were someone else (e.g., someone you cared for or respected) doing exactly the same thing? The idea is to be fair and balanced about your self-evaluations.

It is important to also have reasonable expectations. Perhaps you have avoided giving speeches for many years. Either way, giving an impromptu speech is likely to be challenging for most people. Remember, the aim is not to evaluate your public speaking ability (which is a skill that can be developed), but to see how you really look when you are anxious, and whether your anxiety is as obvious as you have always imagined.

If you do notice something that you would prefer to change, try to think about it as a learning experience. At least you know about it now and you can work on that in the future. Our goal is to have a realistic image of ourselves, not an unrealistically positive or negative one.

From *Imagery-Enhanced CBT for Social Anxiety Disorder* by Peter M. McEvoy, Lisa M. Saulsman, and Ronald M. Rapee. Copyright © 2018 The Guilford Press. Permission to photocopy this material is granted to purchasers of this book for personal use or use with clients (see copyright page for details). Purchasers can download additional copies of this material (see the box at the end of the table of contents).

Self-, Environment-, and Task-Focused Attention

Most people with social anxiety notice that most of their attention is self-focused. They might be focusing on their physical sensations of anxiety, negative thoughts/images, their use of safety behaviors, and/or judgments about what they are saying or doing.

At the same time they might also scrutinize the environment for social threats. For example, you might be looking around for people who are laughing at you or could potentially be criticizing you.

We all have a limited attention span—we simply cannot take in all the information around us, so we must select what we are going to focus on. Our attention is like the keyboard on a computer—the computer can only "attend to" what we are typing. The computer can therefore only encode and remember what is typed into it. Similarly, our brains can only encode and remember what *we* attend to. Now, if most of our attention is focused on ourselves and on potential threats in the environment, then that's what we will remember most from our social experiences (i.e., how awful it felt and any sign of "threat" from the environment). We will miss positive feedback from others—it won't be noticed or remembered.

The problem is that if we are too self-focused and environment focused it doesn't leave much attention left over to focus on the task at hand. The pie chart below illustrates the proportion of our attention that is usually self-focused, environment focused, and task focused when feeling socially anxious.

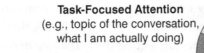

Task-Focused Attention
(e.g., topic of the conversation, what I am actually doing)

Environment-Focused Attention
(looking for signs of "social threat," e.g., people laughing, looking)

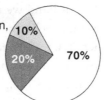

Self-Focused Attention
(physical symptoms, negative thoughts/images, behavior, etc.)

Self- and environment-focused attention maintains social anxiety by . . .

1. *Distracting us from the task at hand:* When we are self- and environment focused we are less able to pay attention to what is being said in conversations and less able to come up with our own contributions. This can have a negative impact on the quality of our conversations.

2. *Increasing the perception of threat:* If we are always looking for threat in the environment, this can increase our sense that something bad will happen.

3. *Missing nonthreatening feedback:* The little bit of attention that is left over to focus on the task at hand may not capture any positive feedback we get from the other person. Instead, our impression is skewed by what we are noticing about ourselves (thoughts, feelings, behavior) and the environment (e.g., what other people in the room are doing). Our memory of the social situation will therefore also be negatively skewed.

4. *Making us more likely to misinterpret ambiguous feedback:* If we are looking for social threat, we may be more likely to misinterpret ambiguous feedback from others. For example, if I start a conversation looking for signs that I am boring, then I am more likely to interpret someone yawning (ambiguous behavior) as proof that the person is bored. I'm unlikely to think that perhaps she is just tired.

The goal then is to become aware of when we are being too self- and environment focused and, as best we can, redirect our attention back to the task at hand.

From *Imagery-Enhanced CBT for Social Anxiety Disorder* by Peter M. McEvoy, Lisa M. Saulsman, and Ronald M. Rapee. Copyright © 2018 The Guilford Press. Permission to photocopy this material is granted to purchasers of this book for personal use or use with clients (see copyright page for details). Purchasers can download additional copies of this material (see the box at the end of the table of contents).

Attention Retraining and Focusing

The pie chart below illustrates the proportion of our attention that we would ideally place on the task at hand (i.e., at least 80%) so that we can immerse ourselves in helpful aspects of the social experience rather than focus on perceived threat.

Self-Focused Attention
(physical symptoms, negative
thoughts/images, behavior, etc.)

Environment-Focused Attention
(looking for signs of "social threat,"
e.g., people laughing, looking)

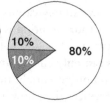

Task-Focused Attention
(e.g., topic of the conversation,
what I am actually doing)

ATTENTION RETRAINING

Before we can direct our attention to the task at hand we need to increase our awareness of where our attention is in the first place. When we are feeling anxious, research has shown that we will search for threat. If you think about it, if there is a real threat it is a good thing that we become very focused on the threat, so that we can do something to protect ourselves. However, when social anxiety is excessive we become too threat focused (i.e., self- and environment focused), which affects our ability to focus on the task at hand.

Attention retraining involves paying attention to the present moment by "coming to our senses." By this we mean deliberately choosing to notice what we can see, hear, smell, taste, and touch right now. We can train our attention at any time of day, regardless of what we are doing. For example, we can attend to:

- The breath
- Sensations while walking
- Taste/smells of food/drink
- Sensations of water on body while swimming

- Sensations of water on body during a shower
- Feel of the water and plates while washing dishes
- Sensations of the chair on your body as you sit
- Sounds while walking in the park

When you try to maintain your attention on the present moment you will notice that your mind will wander—you might start to think about the future, the past, or something else that captures your attention. This is OK. This is what minds do. The task is to notice when your mind wanders and gently escort it back to the task at hand (i.e., whatever it is that you are choosing to focus on).

(continued)

From *Imagery-Enhanced CBT for Social Anxiety Disorder* by Peter M. McEvoy, Lisa M. Saulsman, and Ronald M. Rapee. Copyright © 2018 The Guilford Press. Permission to photocopy this material is granted to purchasers of this book for personal use or use with clients (see copyright page for details). Purchasers can download additional copies of this material (see the box at the end of the table of contents).

Practice attention retraining exercises multiple times throughout the day. Think of it as strengthening a muscle. If you were an athlete, you would train your muscles every day so that they were ready when you really needed them during competition. Attention retraining is like strengthening your ability to (1) be aware of what you are focusing on, (2) notice when your attention wanders, and (3) shift it back to the task at hand. Once you have practiced these skills on nonsocial tasks you will be better equipped to use them within social situations.

One of the advantages of being more present focused is that it is virtually impossible to be present focused and be worrying at the same time.

ATTENTION FOCUSING

Attention focusing involves taking all the skills you have learned from attention retraining and using them to direct your attention more constructively in social situations. The aim is to try to maximize task-focused attention, that is, directed attention toward the behavior required in any specific situation. In social interactions this will mainly involve your attention being focused on really listening to what other people are saying when they are speaking, and then switching focus onto your own message when it is your turn in conversation. This is not easy, and like other skills, it requires regular practice.

Past Imagery Rescripting

So far we have been working on negative images of the present or future (i.e., pictures of ourselves or others' reactions in a current or upcoming social situation). We are now going to move on to the final bubble in the model—core beliefs (i.e., how we generally see ourselves, others, and the world), which tend to be influenced by negative social images from the past (or memories).

It is common for people with social anxiety to report memories of early negative social experiences that impact what they expect in social situations now. When we have had some negative social experiences in our past we can get "stuck" in our memories, so that they can recur as echoes of the past, haunting us and shaping the negative social images we have in the here and now.

Memories we may have of other events tend to feel like they are firmly in the past, and probably rarely rear their heads. In social anxiety, negative social memories we may intellectually know are in the past may still feel very relevant to today emotionally.

Now, we can't change the fact that these negative experiences happened. It is awful that you had to go through them in the first place. What is also awful is that these experiences keep affecting your life, coloring and tainting what you expect in social situations now.

Using a technique we call *imagery rescripting*, we have the opportunity to go back in our imagination to experience the past event from a new perspective. We can do things we couldn't do at the time but that in an ideal world with no limitations we would have liked to have done. While initially this may seem a bit like "make-believe" or just a "fantasy," doing this seems to have the effect of reprocessing the event in a way that can be helpful for *changing its meaning and putting the memory back in its place—as a bad thing that happened in the past with little relevance to the here and now.* As we work on these past images, we can learn that these memories don't reflect on ourselves, others, and the world today, as we previously thought, that they are outdated (specific to a past time, place, or person), and that they don't need to dictate what we expect and how we live our lives now.

Think of these memories as being like a bad photo we have been carrying around in our front pocket and looking at all the time. We can't rip up the photo, but processing these memories can help us to put them in a photo album on the shelf as mementos from the past, rather than carrying them with us now. This can change the way we feel about these past events and their impact on how we see ourselves, others, and the world now.

IDENTIFYING PAST IMAGERY

The first step to working on past imagery is to try and recall an early social experience that you believe may have shaped some of the images you now have when feeling socially anxious. For some people it may be instances of bullying or of being criticized, embarrassed, or humiliated.

If no clear examples are coming to mind, that's OK. Think back to when in your life you first remember having the same sorts of thoughts, feelings, and sensory experiences that are present when you feel socially anxious.

(continued)

From *Imagery-Enhanced CBT for Social Anxiety Disorder* by Peter M. McEvoy, Lisa M. Saulsman, and Ronald M. Rapee. Copyright © 2018 The Guilford Press. Permission to photocopy this material is granted to purchasers of this book for personal use or use with clients (see copyright page for details). Purchasers can download additional copies of this material (see the box at the end of the table of contents).

If you are aware of multiple images, then choose one that is meaningful to you. You might decide to choose the most distressing one first, or you might choose a less distressing one to start with. The choice is yours.

PERSPECTIVE OF THE "OLDER, COMPASSIONATE YOU"

Once you have an image from the past, think about what you know about the situation now that you may not have known at the time it happened. The older, more compassionate "adult you" may know things that you didn't know then. These things you've learned since may have been useful for you to have been aware of at the time of the upsetting event. Although the event may still be emotionally painful to think about, you may be able to understand the situation differently now.

For example, if I was bullied at school I might have initially assumed it was because I was unlikable and worthless. However, as a compassionate adult I can see that the bullying had less to do with me and more to do with the bully's insecurity. I simply did not deserve the bullying, no child deserves it. Any child who bullies another child is behaving poorly, and it does not reflect on the bullied child's character, likability, or worth. In fact, I may be able to see now that I had qualities that were very likable at the time of the bullying.

RESCRIPTING THE PAST IMAGE

Now that we have an image and a new perspective about the image, we can start to rescript or update it. There are three stages to this process, and you can keep track of your experiences in each stage by using Worksheet 16, *Past Imagery Rescripting*. The three phases are:

Phase 1: Imagining the event at the age you were when it occurred as if it were occurring right now.

Phase 2: Rewinding and imagining the event at your current age, watching the younger you going through the experience and intervening in any way you wish in order to protect and care for yourself. You can do anything you like, there are no limits!

Phase 3: Rewind for the last time and imagine the event again at the age you were when it occurred, but this time experiencing the older you intervening and also asking the older you for anything else you need to make you feel safe, secure, calm, and content.

CONCLUSION

The way we have made sense of past negative events has shaped the negative core beliefs we hold today about ourselves, other people, and the world generally. Using imagery rescripting to create a "fantasy" of how we would have liked things to be can help us understand these negative events in a new, more helpful way, changing their meaning for the better. This can then help to undermine our negative core beliefs, paving the way for letting them go and developing new balanced core beliefs.

Constructing New Core Beliefs

The imagery work done so far has been about uncovering negative images that fuel your social anxiety and finding ways to manipulate or modify these images. Chipping away at, modifying, and updating these negative images is very important for changing the way you feel about social situations.

However, it is equally important that you build up more helpful, constructive, positive, and balanced images. We have already seen that images are powerfully linked to our emotional reactions. Just as your negative images are associated with negative emotions and actions, more positive images can promote more positive emotions and actions.

Developing positive images of how we would ideally like things to be in our life can give us clues for what new core beliefs we might want to start developing. Remember, core beliefs are the essence of how we generally see ourselves, other people, and the world around us, and these global views that we hold play a central role in our social anxiety. Hopefully all the behavioral experiments you've done have shown you that your old negative core beliefs might be a little outdated. So, it might be time for a core belief update, and building positive imagery can be a way to start this process. Below we guide you through the sections of Worksheet 17, *Constructing New Core Beliefs*.

Sections 1–3: Generating More Positive Imagery

1. You can start the process of generating more positive imagery by bringing to mind a situation in which you have typically experienced strong social anxiety.
2. Without changing anything about the situation itself, consider how you would like to be within the situation.

What would you be doing? Specifically, what would that look like? What kind of expression would you have on your face? How would you be holding your body? How would you be talking to yourself? Take a few moments to visualize being this way . . .

As you are visualizing being the way you want it to be, how does that feel? How does it feel in your body? Where do you feel it?

3. When you are operating this way, how do you see yourself? Others? The world?

For now you may not fully believe any of these new core beliefs and positive images, but that's OK. We will find ways to strengthen your belief in these positive images over time via your actions.

Section 4: Road-Testing Your New Core Beliefs in Different Life Domains

Our core beliefs can affect our images, behavior, and feelings in many important areas of our lives. Now that you have identified some new, more positive core beliefs, consider how you might "act

(continued)

From *Imagery-Enhanced CBT for Social Anxiety Disorder* by Peter M. McEvoy, Lisa M. Saulsman, and Ronald M. Rapee. Copyright © 2018 The Guilford Press. Permission to photocopy this material is granted to purchasers of this book for personal use or use with clients (see copyright page for details). Purchasers can download additional copies of this material (see the box at the end of the table of contents).

as if" these new core beliefs were true in your life more generally. If you were "acting as if" your new more positive core beliefs were true, what would you be doing (or not doing) in these areas of your life?

- Current relationships (friends, partners)
- Your family (e.g., parents, siblings, children)
- Work, school, career
- Daily responsibilities
- Leisure, hobbies
- Health, well-being, self-care
- Other ways you would be spending your time (or not spending your time)

Your new core beliefs might be associated with doing more of something (e.g., making more phone calls to friends or family) or less of something (relying less on alcohol in social situations). Spend some time imagining yourself operating consistently with your new core beliefs in each of these areas of your life. Write these changes down because they will be used as the basis for your *Action Plans* later.

Section 5: "Stormy Weather"

Sometimes social situations do not go as planned. In fact, we all encounter some very challenging social situations from time to time (e.g., we unintentionally offend someone, someone does not like us for some reason, we make a mistake). Consider what you can do to maintain the new way you would like things to be in difficult times like these. If you were acting in accordance with your new core beliefs, how would you manage these situations? What would you need to do? What would you need to say to yourself? Spend some time imagining yourself responding in these ways to a difficult social situation. See yourself adopting the body posture and facial expression that would go with this. How do you feel within yourself when you react in this manner?

Section 6: Identifying "Evidence For"

Bring to mind a past occasion when you did something that exemplifies your new core beliefs and spend a few moments visualizing this occasion.

Section 7: Identifying an "Icon"

When you imagine operating in this way, what icons come to mind? Are there particular songs, images, movies, characters, fairy tales, stories, people, animals, or scenes from nature that represent this way of operating for you? Is there something that really captures the spirit of your new, more positive core beliefs? If nothing springs to mind, give yourself time for an image to emerge.

Consider for a moment how this icon could be used to help you stay in this new mode of being, which is consistent with your new, more positive, more helpful core beliefs. How could you strengthen the icon and be reminded of it when you need it?

One way you could use your new core belief icon is to prepare for anxiety-provoking situations. Before you approach a social situation, elicit an image of the situation in your mind and

(continued)

bring your icon to mind and see yourself operating from your new core belief. Notice what you are doing and, as best you can, adopt the posture and facial expression that goes with that image. Notice how this feels emotionally. Notice how you feel in your body and where you feel it. Remember your icon and your new core beliefs about yourself, other people, and the world before you enter the situation.

Another time to use your icon might be during or after a challenging anxiety-provoking social situation. Bring your icon to mind and remember your new core beliefs to help you handle the situation and your feelings.

Action Planning

The best way to build conviction in your new core beliefs is to live your life as if they are true. Some call it "faking it till you make it." Changing our behavior is the most powerful way to change our beliefs—behavioral experiments are a prime example of that. So if you start operating, acting, and behaving in a way that is consistent with your system of new balanced core beliefs, your confidence in the new beliefs will catch up.

The positive images you uncovered for different domains of your life in Section 4 of Worksheet 17 can be used to give you some ideas about how to live your life as if you believed your new core beliefs. You can now take these ideas and use them in Worksheet 18, the *New Core Belief Action Plan*, to help you plan a "road map" of specific actions that will lead you to build belief in your new positive core beliefs over time. In many ways it is like continuing to do behavioral experiments in lots of areas of your life, but by this time the experiments may not need to be planned as formally as earlier in treatment, and this time they might be more about strengthening positive images of yourself than discrediting negative ones.

Skills Toolbox

Congratulations on making it to the end of treatment. Change is very challenging, but hopefully you have found the hard work well worth it. We have covered a range of tools you can use, which are summarized below.

Consider how helpful each of these tools has been for you and commit to applying them regularly. If you continue to apply your new skills you will continue to improve.

Tools
Imagery monitoring Starting to become more aware of your negative social images was the first step toward being able to work with this imagery during treatment. You may have been very aware of your imagery at the start of treatment, or you may have had to work hard to generate imagery that reflected your anxious thoughts or feelings. Research has shown that imagery has very powerful links to emotions, so we have focused on working with imagery rather than working only with thoughts.
Imagery challenging You learned that your initial negative social images may just be images rather than facts. You learned how to start looking for contrary evidence that does not fit your images, and we started to consider alternative, more helpful or realistic images.
Coping imagery You learned how to develop coping imagery to help you see your anxiety from a different perspective. We elicited an image that reflects your anxiety and then manipulated it so that it was more benign or positive, or demonstrated coping behavior. Bringing this coping image to mind can help you persevere through difficult experiences and develop confidence in your ability to pursue your goals.
Behavioral experiments You learned that avoiding images and situations that trigger anxiety stops you from directly testing your negative images and therefore keeps your social anxiety going. Behavioral experiments encourage us to be curious about our fears rather than avoid them. Behavioral experiments were used to directly test your negative images. They involved: • Being very specific about your predictions (using imagery) • Planning how you could test the predicted negative image • Carefully considering what evidence you needed to observe to support or disconfirm your predicted image • Doing the experiment • Reflecting on the results • Drawing conclusions based on the results. • Updating your image to better reflect what you had learned from the experiment Developing a behavioral experiment hierarchy helped ensure that your behavioral experiments were working toward a valued goal.

(continued)

From *Imagery-Enhanced CBT for Social Anxiety Disorder* by Peter M. McEvoy, Lisa M. Saulsman, and Ronald M. Rapee. Copyright © 2018 The Guilford Press. Permission to photocopy this material is granted to purchasers of this book for personal use or use with clients (see copyright page for details). Purchasers can download additional copies of this material (see the box at the end of the table of contents).

Behavioral experiments typically show us that our negative images are less likely to come true than we think, and that even when aspects of our negative images do occur we can cope. Shame-attacking experiments in particular show us that even when we do something unusual socially, the consequences are not as catastrophic as we expect. In fact, it can be hard to draw people's attention, and when we do, no costly consequence occurs.

Dropping safety behaviors

We use safety behaviors to prevent our fears from coming true, or so we think! You learned that safety behaviors actually keep anxiety going because they are just more subtle forms of avoidance. They also keep us self-focused, can create negative evaluation rather than prevent it, and ultimately stop us from directly testing our fears. If things go well, we conclude that the safety behavior saved us . . . rather than learning that our fears were just less likely to come true than we thought. You have learned the importance of dropping your safety behaviors generally, and particularly during behavioral experiments.

Video feedback

You recorded yourself giving a speech, an exercise designed to reveal if your self-image was accurate or not. You discovered that even when we are highly anxious our symptoms are not as obvious as we think. You learned that when we are anxious we don't need to be so focused on other people noticing our anxiety.

Attention retraining and focusing

You learned that when your attention is focused on yourself or on looking for threats in the environment you cannot be very focused on the task at hand. Self- and environment-focused attention just distracts us from the task (e.g., conversation), which is then likely to affect our memory of the social situation in three ways. First, we are only likely to remember negative aspects of the situation (e.g., how anxious I was feeling) because that's what we were most focused on. Second, we are likely to miss positive aspects of the situation that would challenge our fears (e.g., positive feedback from others). Third, it is going to be much more difficult to keep up with the task at hand (e.g., topic of the conversation) because we are so distracted with ourselves. You learned how to be more aware and deliberate with your attention generally (attention retraining), and particularly how to shift your attention back to the social task at hand (attention focusing).

Past imagery rescripting

You learned that images from past negative social experiences can contribute to the images and anxiety you are currently experiencing. You learned how to take a more compassionate approach to your early experiences by revisiting those experiences (1) as they originally occurred, (2) with your older and more compassionate self intervening to help and support your younger self, and (3) as your younger self receiving support from your older self. The aim of rescripting past images is to put them in context and to reexamine the meanings we took from the initial events, when we didn't have the same perspective that we do now. Doing this can help chip away at our negative core beliefs, which often arise from these past negative social experiences.

Positive imagery and action planning

You learned how to generate more positive imagery of how you would ideally like to be socially, which reflects more positive core beliefs about yourself that can be applied across various domains of life (e.g., relationships, work, family). You also learned how to turn this positive imagery into action plans so that you could continue to act in accordance with these new core beliefs to build strength in these beliefs over time. We also identified an "icon" that can represent and trigger your new, more positive way of operating within the world.

References

Acarturk, C., Cuijpers, P., van Straten, A., & de Graaf, R. (2009). Psychological treatment of social anxiety disorder: A meta-analysis. *Psychological Medicine, 39,* 241–254.

Aderka, I. M. (2009). Factors affecting treatment efficacy in social phobia: The use of video feedback and individual vs. group formats. *Journal of Anxiety Disorders, 23,* 12–17.

Alden, L. E., & Taylor, C. T. (2004). Interpersonal processes in social phobia. *Clinical Psychology Review, 24,* 857–882.

American Psychiatric Association. (1980). *Diagnostic and statistical manual of mental disorders* (3rd ed.). Washington, DC: Author.

American Psychiatric Association. (1987). *Diagnostic and statistical manual of mental disorders* (3rd ed., rev.). Washington, DC: Author.

American Psychiatric Association. (1994). *Diagnostic and statistical manual of mental disorders* (4th ed.). Washington, DC: Author.

American Psychiatric Association. (2000). *Diagnostic and statistical manual of mental disorders* (4th ed., text rev.). Washington, DC: Author.

American Psychiatric Association. (2013). *Diagnostic and statistical manual of mental disorders* (5th ed.). Arlington, VA: Author.

Amir, N., Najmi, S., & Morrison, A. S. (2012). Image generation in individuals with generalized social phobia. *Cognitive Therapy and Research, 36,* 537–547.

Andersson, G., Cuijpers, P., Carlbring, P., Riper, H., & Hedman, E. (2014). Guided Internet-based vs. face-to-face cognitive behavior therapy for psychiatric and somatic disorders: A systematic review and meta-analysis. *World Psychiatry, 13,* 288–295.

Andrews, G., Cuijpers, P., Craske, M. G., McEvoy, P., & Titov, N. (2010). Computer therapy for the anxiety and depressive disorders is effective, acceptable and practical health care: A meta-analysis. *PLOS ONE, 5,* e13196.

Arnberg, F. K., Linton, S. J., Hultcrantz, M., Heintz, E., & Jonsson, U. (2014). Internet-delivered psychological treatments for mood and anxiety disorders: A systematic review of their efficacy, safety, and cost-effectiveness. *PLOS ONE, 9,* e98118.

Arntz, A. (2011). Imagery rescripting for personality disorders. *Cognitive and Behavioral Practice, 19,* 466–481.

Arntz, A. (2012). Imagery rescripting as a therapeutic technique: Review of clinical trials, basic studies, and research agenda. *Journal of Experimental Psychopathology, 3,* 189–208.

Arntz, A., Tiesema, M., & Kindt, M. (2007). Treatment of PTSD: A comparison of imaginal exposure with and without imagery rescripting. *Journal of Behavior Therapy and Experimental Psychiatry, 38,* 345–370.

Arntz, A., & Weertman, A. (1999). Treatment of childhood memories: Theory and practice. *Behaviour Research and Therapy, 37,* 715–740.

Asher, M., Asnaani, A., & Aderka, I. M. (2017). Gender differences in social anxiety disorder: A review. *Clinical Psychology Review, 56,* 1–12.

Beck, A. T., & Dozois, D. J. (2011). Cognitive therapy: Current status and future directions. *Annual Review of Medicine, 62,* 397–409.

Beck, A. T., Rush, A. J., Shaw, B. F., & Emery, G. (1979). *Cognitive therapy of depression.* New York: Guilford Press.

Beidel, D. C., Alfano, C. A., Kofler, M. J., Rao, P. A., Scharfstein, L., & Sarver, N. W. (2014). The impact of social skills training for social anxiety disorder: A randomized controlled trial. *Journal of Anxiety Disorders, 28,* 908–918.

Beidel, D. C., Turner, S. M., & Morris, T. L. (1999). Psychopathology of childhood social phobia. *Journal of the American Academy of Child and Adolescent Psychiatry, 38,* 643–650.

Bennett-Levy, J., Butler, G., Fennell, M., Hackmann, A., Mueller, M., & Westbrook, D. (2004). *Oxford guide to behavioural experiments in cognitive therapy.* New York: Oxford University Press.

Blanco, C., Heimberg, R. G., Schneier, F. R., Fresco, D. M., Chen, H., Turk, C. L., et al. (2010). A placebo-controlled trial of phenelzine, cognitive behavioral group therapy, and their combination for social anxiety disorder. *Archives of General Psychiatry, 67,* 286–295.

Boden, M. T., John, O. P., Goldin, P. R., Werner, K., Heimberg, R. G., & Gross, J. J. (2012). The role of maladaptive beliefs in cognitive-behavioral therapy: Evidence from social anxiety disorder. *Behaviour Research and Therapy, 50,* 287–291.

Boettcher, J., Carlbring, P., Renneberg, B., & Berger, T. (2013). Internet-based interventions for social anxiety disorder: An overview. *Verhaltenstherapie, 23,* 160–168.

Borkovec, T. D. (1994). The nature, functions, and origins of worry. In G. C. L. Davey & F. Tallis (Eds.), *Worrying: Perspectives on theory, assessment, and treatment* (pp. 5–33). New York: Wiley.

Borkovec, T. D., Alcaine, O., & Behar, E. (2004). Avoidance theory of worry and generalized anxiety disorder. In R. G. Heimberg, C. L. Turk, & D. S. Menin (Eds.), *Generalized anxiety disorder: Advances in research and practice* (pp. 77–108). New York: Guilford Press.

Brewin, C. R. (2006). Understanding cognitive behaviour therapy: A retrieval competition account. *Behaviour Research and Therapy, 44,* 765–784.

Brown, T. A., & Barlow, D. H. (2014). *Anxiety and Related Disorders Interview Schedule for DSM-5 (ADIS-5)—Adult Version.* New York: Oxford University Press.

Burstein, M., He, J.-P., Kattan, G., Albano, A. M., Avenevoli, S., & Merikangas, K. R. (2011). Social phobia and subtypes in the National Comorbidity Survey—Adolescent Supplement: Prevalence, correlates, and comorbidity. *Journal of the American Academy of Child and Adolescent Psychiatry, 50,* 870–880.

Cain, S. (2012). *Quiet: The power of introverts in a world that can't stop talking.* New York: Crown.

Canton, J., Scott, K. M., & Glue, P. (2012). Optimal treatment of social phobia: Systematic review and meta-analysis. *Neuropsychiatric Disease and Treatment, 8,* 203–215.

Carleton, R. N., Collimore, K. C., Asmundson, G. J., McCabe, R. E., Rowa, K., & Antony, M. M. (2009). Refining and validating the Social Interaction Anxiety Scale and the Social Phobia Scale. *Depression and Anxiety, 26,* E71–E81.

Carleton, R. N., Thibodeau, M. A., Weeks, J. W., Teale Sapach, M. J., McEvoy, P. M., Horswill, S. C., et al. (2014). Comparing short forms of the Social Interaction Anxiety Scale and the Social Phobia Scale. *Psychological Assessment, 26,* 1116–1126.

Carroll, J. S. (1978). The effect of imagining an event on expectations for the event: An interpretation in terms of the availability heuristic. *Journal of Experimental Social Psychology, 14,* 88–96.

Carver, C. S., & Scheier, M. F. (1978). The self-focusing effects of dispositional self-consciousness, mirror presence, and audience presence. *Journal of Personality and Social Psychology, 36,* 324–332.

Chiupka, C. A., Moscovitch, D. A., & Bielak, T. (2012). In vivo activation of anticipatory vs. post-event autobiographical images and memories in social anxiety. *Journal of Social and Clinical Psychology, 31,* 783–809.

Clark, D. M. (2001). A cognitive perspective on social phobia. In W. R. Crozier & L. E. Alden (Eds.), *International handbook of social anxiety* (pp. 405–430). Chichester, UK: Wiley.

Clark, D. M., Ehlers, A., Hackmann, A., McManus, F., Fennell, M., Grey, N., et al. (2006). Cognitive therapy versus exposure and applied relaxation in social phobia: A randomized controlled trial. *Journal of Consulting and Clinical Psychology, 74,* 568–578.

Clark, D. M., Ehlers, A., McManus, F., Hackmann, A., Fennell, M., Campbell, H., et al. (2003). Cognitive therapy versus fluoxetine in generalized social phobia: A randomized placebo-controlled trial. *Journal of Consulting and Clinical Psychology, 71,* 1058–1067.

Clark, D. M., & Wells, A. (1995). A cognitive model of social phobia. In R. G. Heimberg, M. R. Liebowitz, D. A. Hope, & F. R. Schneier (Eds.), *Social phobia: Diagnosis, assessment and treatment* (pp. 69–93). New York: Guilford Press.

Clark, G. I., & Egan, S. J. (2015). The Socratic Method in cognitive behavioural therapy: A narrative review. *Cognitive Therapy and Research, 39,* 863–879.

Clauss, J. A., & Blackford, J. U. (2012). Behavioral inhibition and risk for developing social anxiety disorder: A meta-analytic study. *Journal of the American Academy of Child and Adolescent Psychiatry, 51,* 1066–1075.

Coles, M. E., Turk, C. L., Heimberg, R. G., & Fresco, D.

M. (2001). Effects of varying levels of anxiety within social situations: Relationship to memory perspective and attributions in social phobia. *Behaviour Research and Therapy, 39,* 651–665.

Cox, B. J., Turnbull, D. L., Robinson, J. A., Grant, B. F., & Stein, M. B. (2011). The effect of Avoidant Personality Disorder on the persistence of Generalized Social Anxiety Disorder in the general population: Results from a longitudinal, nationally representative mental health survey. *Depression and Anxiety, 28,* 250–255.

Craske, M. G., Treanor, M., Conway, C., Zbozinek, T., & Vervliet, B. (2014). Maximizing exposure therapy: An inhibitory learning approach. *Behaviour Research and Therapy, 58,* 10–23.

Cuming, S., Rapee, R. M., Kemp, N., Abbott, M. J., Peters, L., & Gaston, J. E. (2009). A self-report measure of subtle avoidance and safety behaviors relevant to social anxiety: Development and psychometric properties. *Journal of Anxiety Disorders, 23,* 879–883.

Davidson, J. R., Hughes, D. L., George, L. K., & Blazer, D. G. (1993). The epidemiology of social phobia: Findings from the Duke Epidemiological Catchment Area Study. *Psychological Medicine, 23,* 709–718.

Demyttenaere, K., Bruffaerts, R., Posada-Villa, J., Gasquet, I., Kovess, V., Lepine, J. P., et al. (2004). Prevalence, severity, and unmet need for treatment of mental disorders in the World Health Organization World Mental Health Surveys. *Journal of the American Medical Association, 291,* 2581–2590.

DeWit, D. J., Ogborne, A., Offord, D. R., & MacDonald, K. (1999). Antecedents of the risk of recovery from DSM-III-R social phobia. *Psychological Medicine, 29,* 569–582.

Edwards, D. (2007). Restructuring implicational meaning through memory-based imagery: Some historical notes. *Journal of Behavior Therapy and Experimental Psychiatry, 38,* 306–316.

Fenigstein, A., Seheier, M. E., & Buss, A. H. (1975). Public and private self-consciousness: Assessment and theory. *Journal of Consulting and Clinical Psychology, 43,* 522–527.

Fergus, T. A., Valentiner, D. P., McGrath, P. B., Gier-Lonsway, S. L., & Kim, H. S. (2012). Short forms of the Social Interaction Anxiety Scale and the Social Phobia Scale. *Journal of Personality Assessment, 94,* 310–320.

First, M. B., Williams, J. B. W., Karg, R. S., & Spitzer, R. L. (2016). *Structured Clinical Interview for DSM-5 Disorders—Clinician Version (SCID-5-CV).* Arlington, VA: American Psychiatric Association.

Foa, E. B., Huppert, J. D., & Cahill, S. P. (2006). Emotional processing theory: An update. In B. O. Rothbaum (Ed.), *Pathological anxiety: Emotional processing in etiology and treatment* (pp. 3–24). New York: Guilford Press.

Foa, E. B., & Kozak, M. J. (1986). Emotional processing of fear: Exposure to corrective information. *Psychological Bulletin, 99,* 20–35.

Furmark, T. (2002). Social phobia: Overview of community surveys. *Acta Psychiatrica Scandinavica, 105,* 84–93.

Furmark, T., Tillfors, M., Stattin, H., Ekselius, L., & Fredrikson, M. (2000). Social phobia subtypes in the general population revealed by cluster analysis. *Psychological Medicine, 30,* 1335–1344.

Fyer, A. J., Mannuzza, S., Chapman, T. F., Martin, L. Y., & Klein, D. F. (1995). Specificity in familial aggregation of phobic disorders. *Archives of General Psychiatry, 52,* 564–573.

Gaston, J. E., Abbott, M. J., Rapee, R. M., & Neary, S. A. (2006). Do empirically supported treatments generalize to private practice?: A benchmark study of a cognitive-behavioural group treatment programme for social phobia. *British Journal of Clinical Psychology, 45,* 33–48.

Gilbert, P. (2001). Evolution and social anxiety: The role of attraction, social competition, and social hierarchies. *Psychiatric Clinics of North America, 24,* 723–751.

Gilbert, P. (2009). Introducing compassion-focused therapy. *Advances in Psychiatric Treatment, 15,* 199–208.

Glass, C. R., Merluzzi, T. V., Biever, J. L., & Larsen, K. H. (1982). Cognitive assessment of social anxiety: Development and validation of a self-statement questionnaire. *Cognitive Therapy and Research, 6,* 37–55.

Goldin, P. R., Morrison, A., Jazaieri, H., Brozovich, F., Heimberg, R., & Gross, J. J. (2016). Group CBT versus MBSR for social anxiety disorder: A randomized controlled trial. *Journal of Consulting and Clinical Psychology, 84,* 427–437.

Grant, B. F., Hasin, D. S., Blanco, C., Stinson, F. S., Chou, S. P., Goldstein, R. B., et al. (2005). The epidemiology of social anxiety disorder in the United States: Results from the National Epidemiologic Survey on Alcohol and Related Conditions. *Journal of Clinical Psychiatry, 66,* 1351–1361.

Hackmann, A., Bennett-Levy, J., & Holmes, E. A. (2011). *Oxford guide to imagery in cognitive therapy.* Oxford, UK: Oxford University Press.

Hackmann, A., Clark, D. M., & McManus, F. (2000). Recurrent images and early memories in social phobia. *Behaviour Research and Therapy, 38,* 601–610.

Hackmann, A., Surawy, C., & Clark, D. M. (1998). Seeing yourself through others' eyes: A study of spontaneously occurring images in social phobia. *Behavioural and Cognitive Psychotherapy, 26,* 3–12.

Harvey, A. G., Clark, D. M., Ehlers, A., & Rapee, R. M. (2000). Social anxiety and self-impression: Cognitive preparation enhances the beneficial effects of video feedback following a stressful social task. *Behaviour Research and Therapy, 38,* 1183–1192.

Haug, T. T., Blomhoff, S., Hellstrøm, K., Holme, I., Humble, M., Madsbu, H. P., et al. (2003). Exposure therapy and sertraline in social phobia: 1-year follow-up of a randomised controlled trial. *British Journal of Psychiatry, 182,* 312–318.

Heimberg, R. G., Brozovich, F. A., & Rapee, R. M. (2010). A cognitive-behavioral model of social anxiety disorder. In S. G. Hofmann & P. M. DiBartolo (Eds.), *Social anxiety: Clinical, developmental, and social perspectives* (2nd ed., pp. 395–422). New York: Academic Press.

Heimberg, R. G., Brozovich, F. A., & Rapee, R. M. (2014). A cognitive-behavioral model of social anxiety disorder. In S. G. Hofmann & P. M. DiBartolo (Eds.), *Social anxiety: Clinical, developmental, and social perspectives* (3rd ed., pp. 705–728). Waltham, MA: Academic Press.

Heimberg, R. G., Mueller, G. P., Holt, C. S., Hope, D. A., & Liebowitz, M. R. (1992). Assessment of anxiety in social interaction and being observed by others: The Social Interaction Anxiety Scale and the Social Phobia Scale. *Behavior Therapy, 23,* 53–73.

Hinrichsen, H., & Clark, D. M. (2003). Anticipatory processing in social anxiety: Two pilot studies. *Journal of Behavior Therapy and Experimental Psychiatry, 34,* 205–218.

Hirsch, C. R., Clark, D. M., Mathews, A., & Williams, R. (2003). Self-images play a causal role in social phobia. *Behaviour Research and Therapy, 41,* 909–921.

Hirsch, C. R., Mathews, A., Clark, D. M., Williams, R., & Morrison, J. A. (2006). The causal role of negative imagery in social anxiety: A test in confident public speakers. *Journal of Behavior Therapy and Experimental Psychiatry, 37,* 159–170.

Hirsch, C. R., Meynen, T., & Clark, D. M. (2004). Negative self-imagery in social anxiety contaminates social interactions. *Memory, 12,* 496–506.

Hofmann, S. G., & DiBartolo, P. M. (2000). An instrument to assess self-statements during public speaking: Scale development and preliminary psychometric properties. *Behavior Therapy, 31,* 499–515.

Hofmann, S. G., Newman, M. G., Ehlers, A., & Roth, W. T. (1995). Psychophysiological differences between subgroups of social phobia. *Journal of Abnormal Psychology, 104,* 224–231.

Hofmann, S. G., & Suvak, M. (2006). Treatment attrition during group therapy for social phobia. *Journal of Anxiety Disorders, 20,* 961–972.

Hofmann, S. G., Wu, J. Q., & Boettcher, H. (2014). Effect of cognitive-behavioral therapy for anxiety disorders on quality of life: A meta-analysis. *Journal of Consulting and Clinical Psychology, 82,* 375–391.

Holmes, E. A., Lang, T. J., & Shah, D. M. (2009). Developing interpretation bias modification as a "cognitive vaccine" for depressed mood: Imagining positive events makes you feel better than thinking about them verbally. *Journal of Abnormal Psychology, 118,* 76–88.

Holmes, E. A., & Mathews, A. (2005). Mental imagery and emotion: A special relationship? *Emotion, 5,* 489–497.

Holmes, E. A., & Mathews, A. (2010). Mental imagery in emotion and emotional disorders. *Clinical Psychology Review, 30,* 349–362.

Hook, J. N., & Valentiner, D. P. (2002). Are specific and generalized social phobias qualitatively distinct? *Clinical Psychology: Science and Practice, 9,* 379–395.

Kashdan, T. B. (2007). Social anxiety spectrum and diminished positive experiences: Theoretical synthesis and meta-analysis. *Clinical Psychology Review, 27,* 348–365.

Keller, M. B. (2003). The lifelong course of social anxiety disorder: A clinical perspective. *Acta Psychiatrica Scandinavica, 108*(Suppl. 417), 85–94.

Kendler, K. S., Aggen, S. H., Knudsen, G. P., Røysamb, E., Neale, M. C., & Reichborn-Kjennerud, T. (2011). The structure of genetic and environmental risk factors for syndromal and subsyndromal common DSM-IV axis I and all axis II disorders. *American Journal of Psychiatry, 168,* 29–39.

Kennerley, H. (2007). *Socratic method.* Oxford, UK: Oxford Cognitive Therapy Centre.

Kessler, R. C., Avenevoli, S., Costello, E. J., Georgiades, K., Green, J. G., Gruber, M. J., et al. (2012). Prevalence, persistence, and sociodemographic correlates of DSM-IV disorders in the National Comorbidity Survey Replication Adolescent Supplement. *Archives of General Psychiatry, 69,* 372–380.

Kessler, R. C., Berglund, P., Demler, O., Jin, R., Merikangas, K. R., & Walters, E. E. (2005). Lifetime prevalence and age-of-onset distributions of DSM-IV disorders in the National Comorbidity Survey Replication. *Archives of General Psychiatry, 62,* 593–602.

Kessler, R. C., Petukhova, M., Sampson, N. A., Zaslavsky, A. M., & Wittchen, H. U. (2012). Twelve-month and lifetime prevalence and lifetime morbid risk of anxiety and mood disorders in the United States. *International Journal of Methods in Psychiatric Research, 21,* 169–184.

Kessler, R. C., Stein, M. B., & Berglund, P. (1998). Social phobia subtypes in the National Comorbidity Survey. *American Journal of Psychiatry, 155,* 613–619.

Kosslyn, S. M. (1994). *Image and brain: The resolution of the imagery debate.* Cambridge, MA: MIT Press.

Kosslyn, S. M., Ganis, G., & Thompson, W. L. (2001). Neural foundations of imagery. *Nature Reviews Neuroscience, 2,* 635–642.

Kupper, N., & Denollet, J. (2012). Social anxiety in the general population: Introducing abbreviated versions of SIAS and SPS. *Journal of Affective Disorders, 136,* 90–98.

Lang, P. J. (1979). A bio-informational theory of emotional imagery. *Psychophysiology, 16,* 495–512.

Laposa, J. M., & Rector, N. A. (2011). A prospective examination of predictors of post-event processing following videotaped exposures in group cognitive behavioural therapy for individuals with social phobia. *Journal of Anxiety Disorders, 25,* 568–573.

Laposa, J. M., & Rector, N. A. (2016). Can I really do this?: An examination of anticipatory event processing in social anxiety disorder. *Journal of Cognitive Psychotherapy, 30,* 94–104.

Lecrubier, Y., Sheehan, D. V., Weiller, E., Amorim, P., Bonora, I., Harnett-Sheehan, K., et al. (1997). The Mini International Neuropsychiatric Interview (MINI): A short diagnostic structured interview: Reliability and validity according to the CIDI. *European Psychiatry, 12,* 232–241.

Levine, B., Svoboda, E., Hay, J. F., Winocur, G., & Moscovitch, M. (2002). Aging and autobiographical memory: Dissociating episodic from semantic retrieval. *Psychology and Aging, 17,* 677–689.

Libby, L. K., Shaeffer, E. M., Eibach, R. P., & Slemmer, J. A. (2007). Picture yourself at the polls: Visual perspective in mental imagery affects self-perception and behavior. *Psychological Science, 18,* 199–203.

Lieb, R., Wittchen, H. U., Hofler, M., Fuetsch, M., Stein, M. B., & Merikangas, K. R. (2000). Parental psychopathology, parenting styles, and the risk of social phobia in offspring: A prospective-longitudinal community study. *Archives of General Psychiatry, 57,* 859–866.

Liebowitz, M. R. (1987). Social phobia. *Modern Problems of Pharmacopsychiatry, 22,* 141–173.

Liebowitz, M. R., Heimberg, R. G., Schneier, F. R., Hope, D. A., Davies, S., Holt, C. S., et al. (1999). Cognitive-behavioral group therapy versus phenelzine in social phobia: Long-term outcome. *Depression and Anxiety, 10,* 89–98.

Lincoln, T. M., Rief, W., Hahlweg, K., Frank, M., von Witzlenben, I., Schroeder, B., et al. (2003). Effectiveness of an empirically supported treatment for social phobia in the field. *Behaviour Research and Therapy, 41,* 1251–1269.

Lincoln, T. M., Rief, W., Hahlweg, K., Frank, M., von Witzlenben, I., Schroeder, B., et al. (2005). Who comes, who stays, who profits?: Predicting refusal, dropout, success, and relapse in a short intervention for social phobia. *Psychotherapy Research, 15,* 210–225.

Makkar, S. R., & Grisham, J. R. (2011). Social anxiety and the effects of negative self-imagery on emotion, cognition, and post-event processing. *Behaviour Research and Therapy, 49,* 654–664.

Marks, D. F. (1973). Visual imagery differences in the recall of pictures. *British Journal of Psychology, 64,* 17–24.

Mathers, C., Vos, T., & Stevenson, C. (1999). *Burden of disease and injury in Australia* (Cat. No. PHE 17). Canberra: Australian Institute of Health and Welfare.

Mattick, R. P., & Clarke, J. C. (1998). Development and validation of measures of social phobia scrutiny fear and social interaction anxiety. *Behaviour Research and Therapy, 36,* 455–470.

Mayo-Wilson, E., Dias, S., Mavranezouli, I., Kew, K., Clark, D. M., Ades, A. E., et al. (2014). Psychological and pharmacological interventions for social anxiety disorder in adults: A systematic review and network meta-analysis. *Lancet Psychiatry, 1,* 368–376.

McEvoy, P. M. (2007). Effectiveness of cognitive behavioural group therapy for social phobia in a community clinic: A benchmarking study. *Behaviour Research and Therapy, 45,* 3030–3040.

McEvoy, P. M., Erceg-Hurn, D. M., Saulsman, L. M., & Thibodeau, M. A. (2015). Imagery enhancements increase the effectiveness of cognitive behavioural group therapy for social anxiety disorder: A benchmarking study. *Behaviour Research and Therapy, 65,* 42–51.

McEvoy, P. M., Grove, R., & Slade, T. (2011). Epidemiology of anxiety disorders in the Australian general population: Findings of the 2007 Australian National Survey of Mental Health and Wellbeing. *Australian and New Zealand Journal of Psychiatry, 45,* 957–967.

McEvoy, P. M., Nathan, P., Rapee, R. M., & Campbell, B. N. C. (2012). Cognitive behavioural group therapy for social phobia: Evidence of transportability to community clinics. *Behaviour Research and Therapy, 50,* 258–265.

McEvoy, P. M., & Saulsman, L. M. (2014). Imagery-enhanced cognitive behavioural group therapy for social anxiety disorder: A pilot study. *Behaviour Research and Therapy, 55,* 1–6.

McEvoy, P. M., Thibodeau, M. A., & Asmundson, G. J. (2014). Trait repetitive negative thinking: A brief transdiagnostic assessment. *Journal of Experimental Psychopathology, 5,* 382–398.

McLeod, B. D., Wood, J. J., & Weisz, J. R. (2007).

Examining the association between parenting and childhood anxiety: A meta-analysis. *Clinical Psychology Review, 27,* 155–172.

Mooney, K. A., & Padesky, C. A. (2000). Applying client creativity to recurrent problems: Constructing possibilities and tolerating doubt. *Journal of Cognitive Psychotherapy, 14,* 149–161.

Mörtberg, E., Clark, D. M., Sundin, O., & Åberg Wistedt, A. (2007). Intensive group cognitive treatment and individual cognitive therapy vs. treatment as usual in social phobia: A randomized controlled trial. *Acta Psychiatrica Scandinavica, 115,* 142–154.

Moscovitch, D. A. (2009). What is the core fear in social phobia?: A new model to facilitate individualized case conceptualization and treatment. *Cognitive and Behavioral Practice, 16,* 123–134.

Moscovitch, D. A., Gavric, D. L., Merrifield, C., Bielak, T., & Moscovitch, M. (2011). Retrieval properties of negative vs. positive mental images and autobiographical memories in social anxiety: Outcomes with a new measure. *Behaviour Research and Therapy, 49,* 505–517.

National Institute for Health and Care Excellence. (2013). *Social anxiety disorder: Recognition, assessment and treatment* (Clinical guideline no. CG159). Manchester, UK: Author.

Ng, A. S., Abbott, M. J., & Hunt, C. (2014). The effect of self-imagery on symptoms and processes in social anxiety: A systematic review. *Clinical Psychology Review, 34,* 620–633.

Norton, A. R., Abbott, M. J., Norberg, M. M., & Hunt, C. (2015). A systematic review of mindfulness and acceptance-based treatments for social anxiety disorder. *Journal of Clinical Psychology, 71,* 283–301.

Öst, L. G. (2014). The efficacy of Acceptance and Commitment Therapy: An updated systematic review and meta-analysis. *Behaviour Research and Therapy, 61,* 105–121.

Padesky, C. A. (1993, September). *Socratic questioning: Changing minds or guiding discovery?* Paper presented at the European Congress of Behavioural and Cognitive Therapies, London.

Padesky, C. A. (1994). Schema change processes in cognitive therapy. *Clinical Psychology and Psychotherapy, 1,* 267–278.

Padesky, C. A. (2011, October). *Simplifying personality disorder treatment: A new paradigm for CBT.* Workshop presented at the 34th Australian Association for Cognitive Behaviour Therapy (AACBT) National Conference, Sydney, Australia.

Padesky, C. A., & Mooney, K. A. (2005, May). *Cognitive therapy for personality disorders: Constructing a new personality.* Paper presented at the 5th International Congress of Cognitive Psychotherapy, Gotenburg, Sweden.

Peters, L. (2000). Discriminant validity of the Social Phobia and Anxiety Inventory (SPAI), the Social Phobia Scale (SPS) and the Social Interaction Anxiety Scale (SIAS). *Behaviour Research and Therapy, 38,* 943–950.

Peters, L., Sunderland, M., Andrews, G., Rapee, R. M., & Mattick, R. P. (2012). Development of a short form Social Interaction Anxiety (SIAS) and Social Phobia Scale (SPS) using nonparametric item response theory: The SIAS-6 and the SPS-6. *Psychological Assessment, 24,* 66–76.

Pictet, A. (2014). Looking on the bright side in social anxiety: The potential benefit of promoting positive mental imagery. *Frontiers in Human Neuroscience, 8,* 43.

Pictet, A., Coughtrey, A. E., Mathews, A., & Holmes, E. A. (2011). Fishing for happiness: The effects of positive imagery on interpretation bias and a behavioral task. *Behaviour Research and Therapy, 49,* 885–891.

Powers, M. B., Sigmarsson, S. R., & Emmelkamp, P. M. G. (2008). A meta-analytic review of psychological treatments for social anxiety disorder. *International Journal of Cognitive Therapy, 2,* 94–113.

Rachman, S., Grüter-Andrew, J., & Shafran, R. (2000). Post-event processing in social anxiety. *Behaviour Research and Therapy, 38,* 611–617.

Rapee, R. (1995). Descriptive psychopathology of social phobia. In R. G. Heimberg, M. R. Leibowitz, D. A. Hope, & F. R. Schneier (Eds.), *Social phobia: Diagnosis, assessment, and treatment* (pp. 41–66). New York: Guilford Press.

Rapee, R. M. (2014). Preschool environment and temperament as predictors of social and nonsocial anxiety disorders in middle adolescence. *Journal of the American Academy of Child and Adolescent Psychiatry, 53,* 320–328.

Rapee, R. M., Gaston, J. E., & Abbott, M. J. (2009). Testing the efficacy of theoretically derived improvements in the treatment of social phobia. *Journal of Consulting and Clinical Psychology, 77,* 317–327.

Rapee, R. M., & Heimberg, R. G. (1997). A cognitive-behavioral model of anxiety in social phobia. *Behaviour Research and Therapy, 35,* 741–756.

Rapee, R. M., & Lim, L. (1992). Discrepancy between self- and observer ratings of performance in social phobics. *Journal of Abnormal Psychology, 101,* 728–731.

Rapee, R. M., & Spence, S. H. (2004). The etiology of social phobia: Empirical evidence and an initial model. *Clinical Psychology Review, 24,* 737–767.

Reimer, S. G., & Moscovitch, D. A. (2015). The impact of imagery rescripting on memory appraisals and core beliefs in social anxiety disorder. *Behaviour Research and Therapy, 75,* 48–59.

Reisberg, D., Pearson, D. G., & Kosslyn, S. M. (2003). Intuitions and introspections about imagery: The role of imagery experience in shaping an investigator's theoretical views. *Applied Cognitive Psychology, 17,* 147–160.

Rodebaugh, T. L. (2009). Hiding the self and social anxiety: The Core Extrusion Schema measure. *Cognitive Therapy and Research, 33,* 90.

Rodebaugh, T. L., Woods, C. M., Thissen, D. M., Heimberg, R. G., Chambless, D. L., & Rapee, R. M. (2004). More information from fewer questions: The factor structure and item properties of the original and brief Fear of Negative Evaluation Scale. *Psychological Assessment, 16,* 169–181.

Salkovskis, P. M. (1991). The importance of behaviour in the maintenance of anxiety and panic: A cognitive account. *Behavioural and Cognitive Psychotherapy, 19,* 6–19.

Salkovskis, P. M. (Ed.). (1996). *Frontiers of cognitive therapy.* New York: Guilford Press.

Saulsman, L. M., & Page, A. C. (2004). The five-factor model and personality disorder empirical literature: A meta-analytic review. *Clinical Psychology Review, 23,* 1055–1085.

Scaini, S., Belotti, R., & Ogliari, A. (2014). Genetic and environmental contributions to social anxiety across different ages: A meta-analytic approach to twin data. *Journal of Anxiety Disorders, 28,* 650–656.

Scheier, M. F., & Carver, C. S. (1985). The Self-Consciousness Scale: A revised version for use with general populations. *Journal of Applied Social Psychology, 15,* 687–699.

Seebauer, L., Froß, S., Dubaschny, L., Schönberger, M., & Jacob, G. A. (2014). Is it dangerous to fantasize revenge in imagery exercises?: An experimental study. *Journal of Behavior Therapy and Experimental Psychiatry, 45,* 20–25.

Shamir-Essakow, G., Ungerer, J. A., & Rapee, R. M. (2005). Attachment, behavioral inhibition, and anxiety in preschool children. *Journal of Abnormal Child Psychology, 33,* 131–143.

Sheehan, D. V., Lecrubier, Y., Sheehan, K. H., Amorim, P., Janavs, J., Weiller, E., et al. (1998). The Mini-International Neuropsychiatric Interview (M.I.N.I.): The development and validation of a structured diagnostic psychiatric interview for DSM-IV and ICD-10. *Journal of Clinical Psychiatry, 59,* 22–33.

Skocic, S., Jackson, H., & Hulbert, C. (2015). Beyond DSM-5: An alternative approach to assessing Social Anxiety Disorder. *Depression and Anxiety, 30,* 8–15.

Spence, S. H., & Rapee, R. M. (2016). The etiology of social anxiety disorder: An evidence-based model. *Behaviour Research and Therapy, 86,* 50–67.

Stangier, U., Heidenreich, T., Peitz, M., Lauterbach, W., & Clark, D. M. (2003). Cognitive therapy for social phobia: Individual versus group treatment. *Behaviour Research and Therapy, 41,* 991–1007.

Stapinski, L. A., Rapee, R. M., Sannibale, C., Teesson, M., Haber, P. S., & Baillie, A. J. (2015). The clinical and theoretical basis for integrated cognitive behavioral treatment of comorbid social anxiety and alcohol use disorders. *Cognitive and Behavioral Practice, 22,* 504–521.

Stein, M. B., & Deutsch, R. (2003). In search of social phobia subtypes: Similarity of feared social situations. *Depression and Anxiety, 17,* 94–97.

Stein, M. B., Torgrud, L. J., & Walker, J. R. (2000). Social phobia symptoms, subtypes, and severity: Findings from a community survey. *Archives of General Psychiatry, 57,* 1046–1052.

Stopa, L. (2011). Imagery rescripting across disorders: A practical guide. *Cognitive and Behavioral Practice, 18,* 421–423.

Stopa, L., Brown, M. A., & Hirsch, C. (2012). The effects of repeated imagery practice on self-concept, anxiety and performance in socially anxious participants. *Journal of Experimental Psychopathology, 3,* 223–242.

Stopa, L., & Jenkins, A. (2007). Images of the self in social anxiety: Effects on the retrieval of autobiographical memories. *Journal of Behavior Therapy and Experimental Psychiatry, 38,* 459–473.

Turner, S. M., Johnson, M. R., Beidel, D. C., Heiser, N. A., & Lydiard, R. B. (2003). The Social Thoughts and Beliefs Scale: A new inventory for assessing cognitions in social phobia. *Psychological Assessment, 15,* 384–391.

Vassilopoulos, S. (2005). Social anxiety and the effects of engaging in mental imagery. *Cognitive Therapy and Research, 29,* 261–277.

Vriends, N., Bolt, O. C., & Kunz, S. M. (2014). Social anxiety disorder, a lifelong disorder?: A review of the spontaneous remission and its predictors. *Acta Psychiatrica Scandinavica, 130,* 109–122.

Watson, D., & Friend, R. (1969). Measurement of social-evaluative anxiety. *Journal of Consulting and Clinical Psychology, 33,* 448–457.

Watson, D., Gamez, W., & Simms, L. J. (2005). Basic dimensions of temperament and their relation to anxiety and depression: A symptom-based perspective. *Journal of Research in Personality, 39,* 46–66.

Weeks, J. W. (2015). Replication and extension of a hierarchical model of social anxiety and depression: Fear of positive evaluation as a key unique factor in social anxiety. *Cognitive Behaviour Therapy, 44,* 103–116.

Weeks, J. W., & Heimberg, R. G. (2012). Positivity impairments: Pervasive and impairing (yet nonprominent?) features of social anxiety disorder. *Cognitive Behaviour Therapy, 41*, 79–82.

Weeks, J. W., Heimberg, R. G., Fresco, D. M., Hart, T. A., Turk, C. L., Schneier, F. R., et al. (2005). Empirical validation and psychometric evaluation of the Brief Fear of Negative Evaluation Scale in patients with social anxiety disorder. *Psychological Assessment, 17*, 179–190.

Weeks, J. W., Heimberg, R. G., Rodebaugh, T. L., Goldin, P. R., & Gross, J. J. (2012). Psychometric evaluation of the Fear of Positive Evaluation Scale in patients with social anxiety disorder. *Psychological Assessment, 24*, 301–312.

Weeks, J. W., Heimberg, R. G., Rodebaugh, T. L., & Norton, P. J. (2008). Exploring the relationship between fear of positive evaluation and social anxiety. *Journal of Anxiety Disorders, 22*, 386–400.

Weeks, J. W., & Howell, A. N. (2012). The bivalent fear of evaluation model of social anxiety: Further integrating findings on fears of positive and negative evaluation. *Cognitive Behaviour Therapy, 41*, 83–95

Wells, A. (1997). *Cognitive therapy of anxiety disorders: A practice manual and conceptual guide.* Chichester, UK: Wiley.

Wells, A., Clark, D. M., & Ahmad, S. (1998). How do I look with my mind's eye?: Perspective taking in social phobic imagery. *Behaviour Research and Therapy, 36*, 631–634.

Wild, J., & Clark, D. M. (2011). Imagery rescripting of early traumatic memories in social phobia. *Cognitive and Behavioral Practice, 18*, 433e443.

Wild, J., Hackmann, A., & Clark, D. M. (2007). When the present visits the past: Updating traumatic memories in social phobia. *Journal of Behavior Therapy and Experimental Psychiatry, 38*, 386–401.

Wild, J., Hackmann, A., & Clark, D. M. (2008). Rescripting early memories linked to negative images in social phobia: A pilot study. *Behavior Therapy, 39*, 47–56.

Wittchen, H. U., Stein, M. B., & Kessler, R. C. (1999). Social fears and social phobia in a community sample of adolescents and young adults: Prevalence, risk factors and co-morbidity. *Psychological Medicine, 29*, 309–323.

Wong, J., Gordon, E. A., & Heimberg, R. G. (2014). Cognitive-behavioral models of social anxiety disorder. In J. W. Weeks (Ed.), *The Wiley–Blackwell handbook of social anxiety disorder* (pp. 1–23). Chichester, UK: Wiley–Blackwell.

Wong, Q. J. J., Gregory, B., & McLellan, L. F. (2016). A review of scales to measure social anxiety disorder in clinical and epidemiological studies. *Current Psychiatry Reports, 18*, 1–15.

Wong, Q. J., & Moulds, M. L. (2009). Impact of rumination versus distraction on anxiety and maladaptive self-beliefs in socially anxious individuals. *Behaviour Research and Therapy, 47*, 861–867.

Wong, Q. J., Moulds, M. L., & Rapee, R. M. (2014). Validation of the self-beliefs related to social anxiety scale: A replication and extension. *Assessment, 21*, 300–311.

Wong, Q. J., & Rapee, R. M. (2016). The aetiology and maintenance of social anxiety disorder: A synthesis of complementary theoretical models and formulation of a new integrated model. *Journal of Affective Disorders, 203*, 84–100.

Woody, S. R., Chambless, D. L., & Glass, C. R. (1997). Self-focused attention in the treatment of social phobia. *Behaviour Research and Therapy, 35*, 117–129.

Yonkers, K. A., Dyck, I. R., & Keller, M. B. (2001). An eight-year longitudinal comparison of clinical course and characteristics of social phobia among men and women. *Psychiatric Services, 52*, 637–643.

Index